A
PLAGUE
ON ALL OUR **SPORTS**

Bill Ribbans and Mark Saggers

A PLAGUE
ON ALL OUR SPORTS

When Covid and Sport Collided

First published by Pitch Publishing, 2024

Pitch Publishing
9 Donnington Park,
85 Birdham Road,
Chichester,
West Sussex,
PO20 7AJ
www.pitchpublishing.co.uk
info@pitchpublishing.co.uk

A CIP catalogue record is available for this book
from the British Library.

ISBN 978 1 80150 668 7

Typesetting and origination by Pitch Publishing
Printed and bound in India by Replika Press Pvt. Ltd.

Contents

Introduction

'A plague on both your houses'

Romeo and Juliet. Act 3. Scene 1. William Shakespeare

In May 2023, the World Health Organization (WHO) declared the COVID-19 global health emergency over. It estimated 20 million people had died worldwide; 225,000 had perished in the UK alone. Numbers may have been dwarfed by the 1918–19 Spanish flu pandemic but the scale of the disaster was simply unimaginable in the modern world.

It was all so different on New Year's Day 2020. Pre-Christmas, the UK electorate had returned Boris Johnson and the Conservative party with a landslide majority of 80 seats and a mandate for delivering Brexit.

As 2019 became 2020, British sport sailed serenely on.

The busy Christmas English league football programme made way for the Football Association (FA) Cup third-round weekend thoughts. Traditionally, lucky minnows take on Premier League football giants during the first weekend of January. In 2020, AFC Fylde visited Sheffield United, Port Vale travelled to Manchester City and Gillingham entertained West Ham United. All games kicked off late as fans listened to a Prince William-narrated video on mental health before battle was joined. Sadly, there would be no major giant-killing feats during these clashes but, unforeseen by anybody, the nation's physical and psychological fortitude was about to be tested in a way not witnessed for 80 years.

At New Year, Liverpool were 13 points clear, chasing their first league title for 20 years – their first of the Premier

League era. Norwich City were adrift at the bottom of the table heading back to the Championship from whence they had emerged in 2019. In Scotland, Glasgow Celtic sat atop the Premiership table – which they had occupied for all but one week of the season en route to their record-equalling ninth successive title. The round of 16 draw in the Union of European Football Associations (UEFA) Champions League, which had produced mouthwatering ties, was awaited in February.

In cricket, England were touring South Africa. Barmy Army supporters had travelled in their thousands. In the first week of January, they had arrived in Western Province to enjoy the delights of a Cape Town Test match interspersed with visits to the neighbouring winelands. England squared the series 1-1 after beating their hosts by 189 runs. Joe Root's team would go on to a clinch a memorable 3-1 Test series win.

In rugby union, the European Rugby Champions Cup was proceeding through the final stages of the pool games in the early new year. Fans looked forward to the Six Nations Championship. It started at the beginning of February with home victories for Ireland, Wales and France.

For indoor sport enthusiasts, both the PDC World Darts Championship at Alexandra Palace and the BDO World Darts Championship at the O2 in London were completed at the beginning of the year. Alexandra Palace hosted the Masters snooker championship later in the month. Potters Leisure Resort in Great Yarmouth staged the World Indoor Bowls Championships for most of January.

Jamaica, New Zealand and South Africa joined their English hosts for the 2020 Netball Nations Cup in late January. The Manchester Velodrome accommodated the 2020 British National Track Championships on January's last weekend.

Winter would surely give way to spring and with it more events to savour. Those sporting occasions stored in our collective memories from previous instalments awaited. The Cheltenham and Aintree horse-racing festivals, the university Boat Race, and the denouement of the football and rugby union seasons.

For many sports fans, international sport starts in Melbourne each year. The tennis Australian Open commences in late January, Formula 1's Grand Prix season opener in March. In the USA, the February American Football Super Bowl precedes the April Augusta Masters golf tournament.

The year 2020 would be extra-special. Football's Euro 2020 championships would reach their climax with a Wembley final. Tokyo would host the Summer Olympics and Paralympics.

These examples, and many more, are indicative of the rich tapestry of sporting events that annually greet the beginning of the British and global sporting year. What could possibly interfere with its progress?

It was all to be brought to a shuddering halt by an invisible foe measuring 0.1 microns in diameter.

The pandemic's onset was terrifying. Via media outlets, we witnessed the human suffering in places such as China and Italy. We knew that it would wash up on our shores before long. Its arrival was associated with a paralysis of society, the economy … and sport.

This book analyses the way COVID-19 brought global sport to its knees, tranquillised it, and threatened its subsequent revival via a combined health and economic apocalypse affecting every type and echelon of sport.

It charts sport's response to lockdown, recovery planning, obstacles faced and modifications required to re-emerge. It reviews the agility needed to rebuild seasons and sporting events that usually take years in the planning. It examines the financial effects, and questions what the pandemic taught us about the robustness of sporting enterprises.

At the human level, athletes' responses to the crisis and imposed restrictions varied hugely. Like most of society.

Many, unselfishly, gave time and resources to support people less fortunate. Others tarnished the reputation of themselves and their sports by behaving in a selfish and, occasionally, dangerous manner – the 'covidiots'.

It reminded us of the importance of sport in our national life. The response of society to its triumphs, trials and transgressions informed us of the deep and delicate bonds that bind and position sport in our collective consciousness. Society's tolerance of institutional and individual sporting indiscretions appeared most stretched at times of maximal fear – April 2020, January 2021 and late 2021.

While the media concentrates upon the sporting gods, what was the effect upon mere mortals? The majority – who want to run, swim, cycle, Zumba, or any other form of exercise that keeps body and mind together? For some, it was a disastrous sporting shutdown. For others, it offered opportunities to pursue new recreational horizons – with mixed results.

What were the psychological effects of periods of padlocked gyms, domestic detention, and banishment from football terraces? What were the long-term effects on mental health for professional athletes confined to 'bubbles' to ensure the continuation of elite sport and financial streams?

COVID-19 resembled a mythical sea monster with huge humps representing the pandemic's waves. It possessed a long and powerful tail that could cause chronic disability to previously fit and healthy individuals afflicted by long COVID; create injury to overburdened athletes with challenging calendars; deprive many of sporting success through loss of opportunity.

Writing in the aftermath of this tumultuous period in our lives carries the risk of applying Boris Johnson's retrospectoscope too liberally. It is inevitable. To improve context and understanding, the authors have tried to place the decisions and events surrounding sport alongside the contemporaneous happenings in wider society.

The book's two authors have spent long careers in sport. One has spent 45 years as a radio and television sports journalist with the BBC, Sky, talkSPORT and TalkTV. The other has worked medically and surgically with athletes for 43 years. Like everybody, their professional lives were turned upside down from March 2020 onwards. Both were intimately involved and witnessed from the 'inside' the endeavours required to permit the sporting phoenix to rise from the ashes – from sitting in empty sports stadia during Project Restart to witnessing Euro 2020 final spectator chaos; from planning sporting authority risk assessments to showing professional sports people how to put lateral flow test (LFT) swabs up their noses. This has allowed the book to encompass a narrative of events from a wider perspective but also to include personal observations from the authors' own experiences and others that they interacted with along the way.

We hope that the result is both an informative and reflective contribution that chronicles one aspect of the most damaging and frightening periods of recent times.

Chapter 1

The New Beast from the East

The birds have flown the nest
The Bird's Nest stadium in Beijing, China hosted the 2008
Summer Olympics

While the United Kingdom enjoyed its 2019 seasonal festivities and traditional sporting winter fayre, a particular bug became no longer snug in a rug in mid-eastern China.

Wuhan has a rich 3,000-year-old history, with a busy industrial metropolis of 11 million inhabitants and a scientific institute of international repute in coronavirus research. The first Wuhan resident to develop COVID-19 officially became symptomatic on 1 December 2019. It is unlikely he was patient-zero. People were probably infected months earlier.

Cases were linked to the Huanan seafood market which was closed on New Year's Day. By that stage, the virus had flown the nest. Literally. Wuhan is a well-connected transport hub boasting non-stop flights to 117 destinations in 15 different countries. COVID-19 was identified in Italian sewage on 18 December. A Parisian, married to a Charles de Gaulle airport worker, required hospital treatment during Christmas week.

In January, people were travelling ahead of the Chinese New Year on the 25th; 450 million people crisscross China and the globe in the world's biggest annual human migration. Seven million Chinese were scheduled to travel abroad. Sixty thousand passengers flew from Wuhan to 382 foreign cities in the fortnight before lockdown. Some took the bug with them and created a 'perfect viral storm'.

The die was cast for a global pandemic even before the WHO knew of its existence. It would wreck lives and livelihoods, and wreak havoc with global sport. Starting in China.

In 2020, China had scheduled a wide range of important sporting events. Its reputation as both a global sporting superpower and country capable of hosting varieties of sporting occasions seemed ready to be cemented. The World Athletics Indoor Championships, Olympic qualifying tournaments in football, boxing, wrestling and basketball, Winter Olympic skiing test events, international golf, badminton, motor racing, field hockey, tennis and snooker events were all scheduled to land in China in the first quarter of 2020.

The sporting consequences of the pandemic would commence in China and move rapidly to engulf the world. Rather than ripples spreading from the middle of a pond, the damage resembled the after-effects of a fast-moving tsunami across the oceans.

While we were most aware of the damage to our local sporting scene, the carnage wrought by the pandemic globally reminded us that elite sport calendars are put together like giant jigsaw puzzles. Each piece represents a competition or fixture somewhere. The planning is complex. The repercussions when pieces are lost reverberate widely.

The beginning of the Year of the Rat

By 5 January, a Shanghai laboratory had genetically sequenced the new virus – a close cousin of SARS (severe acute respiratory syndrome virus) that had killed at least 774 people between 2002 and 2004. The Chinese government released the genetic sequencing information a week later and immediately closed the responsible laboratory for 'rectification'.

On 11 January, the first death in Wuhan was reported – but WHO denied that the virus was capable of human-to-human transmission. Within days the virus had spread to Thailand, Japan, South Korea and Singapore. Nine days later, China finally admitted that the disease might be capable of inter-human spread. It had been obvious in Wuhan for weeks.

It was ironic that the epicentre of the global outbreak, Wuhan, was due to host some of the first of the Chinese 2020 international sporting bonanzas. Olympic qualifiers in boxing and women's football were scheduled. On 22 January, the International Olympic Committee (IOC) announced that both would be removed from Wuhan. The Chinese government advised people not to travel in or out of the city. Concern was sufficiently high in the UK that SAGE (Scientific Advisory Group for Emergencies) met in London the same day.

Boxing was rescheduled for Amman, Jordan. The women's football shifted to Nanjing – 333 miles away. However, within days, that venue was also deemed unsafe. The tournament was switched to Australia.

The next day (23 January), Wuhan went into lockdown. It would not be lifted until April. The virus was reported to be three times more infectious than normal influenza. It was believed that 7 million residents fled the Wuhan area before lockdown was enforced. Southampton University research estimated that 10 per cent of people flying out of Wuhan and other infected Chinese cities carried COVID-19 with them. Many Chinese students were returning to British universities.

From late January, Chinese national and international sporting fixtures fell like dominoes. Important events in rallying, golf, football, basketball, tennis, field hockey and the Chinese National Winter Games were either suspended, cancelled, played behind closed doors, moved abroad or postponed.

On 24 January, COBRA (an abbreviation for Cabinet Office Briefing Rooms) met in London for the first time in the crisis. Matt Hancock, the health minister, announced that the UK risk was low. Prime Minister Boris Johnson met Chinese dancers outside 10 Downing Street to celebrate the forthcoming Year of the Rat.

Following hasty competition reorganisation and travel rearrangements, the Chinese women's football team landed in Australia and went into quarantine. Despite the chaos, China progressed to the next stage of this Olympic marathon tournament and were scheduled to play South Korea home and away. After numerous postponements, the tie was finally completed in April 2021 – 13 months late.

In the midst of these difficulties, the Australian Open tennis tournament took place from 20 January to 2 February. During the qualifying tournament, there was more concern with the pollution caused by bushfires than COVID-19. The Melbourne air quality was rated temporarily as the worst in the world. It would be the last 'normal' Aussie Open until 2023.

On 29 January, the first official cases in the UK were reported. A Chinese student and family had travelled from Wuhan to York. With reported cases in at least 17 countries, including several European nations, WHO declared a global Public Health Emergency of International Concern the next day. It would last over three years.

The escalating health crisis required more extensive action to be taken by the Chinese and international sporting authorities.

Nanjing's World Indoor Athletics Championships were postponed and rescheduled for 2021. It would be put off again until March 2023 and, for a third time, until 2025. The first alpine test events for the 2022 Beijing Winter Olympics were cancelled. The Beijing-hosted China Open snooker was the last ranking event before the World Championships in Sheffield with prize money of over £1m. It was cancelled and not rescheduled.

For the UK, 31 January represented Brexit day. Boris Johnson signed the withdrawal treaty from the European

Union. Three days later, the prime minister gave an upbeat speech at Greenwich warning that 'there is a risk that new diseases such as coronavirus will trigger a panic'. Privately, SAGE was warning the government that Chinese cases were likely to be 200,000 to 300,000 and doubling every four to five days. Hancock reassured parliament the next day that the UK had '50 specialist beds and a further 500 beds are available in order to isolate people'.

Spreading its tentacles

January 2020 had seen a significant proportion of Chinese sport brought to a halt. February would see more postponements and spread to engulf most of the Far East.

On the first weekend of February, Chinese cases jumped by 50 per cent. In the Philippines, a man became the first to die outside of China. On 11 February, WHO officially named the disease COVID-19 (coronavirus disease 2019) and the virus responsible as severe acute respiratory syndrome coronavirus 2 (SARS-CoV-2).

The Chinese Lingshui Masters Badminton tournament was cancelled. It was a prestigious tournament with Olympic qualification on offer. It would not reappear until 2023 because of the persistent virus.

Chinese motorsport events stalled. Most importantly, the Shanghai Chinese Grand Prix set for April was axed. It would have no new place in the shortened and revised 2020 schedule. It was omitted altogether from the 2021, 2022 and 2023 Formula 1 calendars.

Travel bans on Chinese athletes abroad affected their participation in Olympic qualifying tournaments. The Yangzhou-hosted April beach volleyball tournament was buried in the sand by mid-February.

By late February, and before most countries abroad had even contemplated severe restrictions of personal liberties, China had started to bring the pandemic officially 'under control' in most of its regions. On 25 February, the incidence of new cases from the rest of the world exceeded China's for the first time.

By early March, China was 'reporting' less than 100 new cases daily. It had witnessed thousands daily at the peak of the crisis. Pockets of infection would arise subsequently. These would be subjected to stringent containment policies as part of the country's 'zero-COVID' policy that would not be lifted until December 2022.

Postponements, rescheduling and cancellations were taking their toll. Finally, in early July, the Chinese General Administration of Sport announced that no further international sporting events would be held in China for the rest of 2020. The exception was trial events for the 2022 Winter Olympics. Later, table tennis would reappear with four international tournaments in November. All the events were dominated and won by Chinese players.

Coming to a country near you

By early February, sporting fixture chaos began to spread beyond China's borders.

The European golf men's tour only reaches its own continent in May. Prior to that, it meanders around the sunnier spots of the globe. Three Asian tournaments – Malaysia, India, and China – were cancelled. Only the Indian Open had reappeared by 2023. Women's golf tournaments scheduled for Thailand and Singapore for late February were cancelled.

The Asian Champions League football tournament was suspended in March and not restarted until mid-September. Remaining group matches and knockout stages were centralised in Qatar. It took two months to complete the tournament – one month later than originally planned. The Malaysian government denied their representatives, Johor Darul Ta'zim, permission to leave their country. Al-Wahda could not leave Abu Dhabi because of COVID-19 afflicting their squad. Even worse, the defending champions, Al-Hilal from Saudi Arabia, made it to Qatar but could not complete their fixtures when the virus swept through their team. They were unbeaten at the time. Eventually, Ulsan Hyundai from South Korea took the title.

Asian Football Confederation (AFC) international cup games were suspended in mid-March and cancelled completely in September. Qatar 2022 FIFA World Cup qualification began in June 2019 for the AFC. By early March 2020, the whole continent's qualifying tournament was halted and, eventually, postponed for 14 months until summer 2021. The final Qatar qualifiers, Australia, would not be known until June 2022 – three years after it started.

Rugby union suffered next. The world-famous Hong Kong and Singapore Sevens tournaments tried in vain to move from April to October. The World Rugby Sevens Series for 2019–20 was intended as a ten-tournament competition. The sixth leg was played in Vancouver in early March. In June, World Rugby cancelled the remaining four tournaments. New Zealand were awarded the overall title. The Sevens Series did not appear again until September 2021 and contained only two Canadian events.

The FIBA quadrennial men's basketball Asia Cup was due to be hosted by Indonesia in August 2021. Qualifying games had commenced three years earlier. The tournament finale would be delayed by a year. The Asian weightlifting championships were moved from Kazakhstan to Uzbekistan but postponed and rescheduled for 2021. The Asian Olympic wrestling qualifiers in Bishkek were postponed indefinitely on the insistence of the Kyrgyzstan government, who had postponed all sporting events. The event had already been moved from the Chinese city of Xi'an because of the epidemic.

Organisers tried to rescue events by moving to behind-closed-doors events. In Singapore, the One Championship 'King of the Jungle' in mixed martial arts survived by this manoeuvre in late February. It would be the last such hostilities until the aptly named Bangkok 'No Surrender' event in July.

South Korean national and international sport was next in line for the fast-spreading virus. Its football K-league season was delayed and eventually shortened. Busan was due to hold the World Team Table Tennis Championships in March. After serial rescheduling, it was finally offered the event in 2024. The World Short Track Speed Skating Championships in Seoul were abandoned by the International Skating Union.

Japan reported its first COVID-19 case on 15 January in a patient who had returned from Wuhan. The disease appeared to be relatively well controlled. By the end of February, only 230 cases and five deaths had been announced. Despite low numbers, Japanese schools were closed.

A second outbreak in mid-March was brought into the country by travellers from abroad and proved more deadly. A state of emergency was declared in Tokyo in early April and soon extended to the whole country. This state was not lifted from the whole country until late May.

The centre of sporting attention for the country was the hosting of the XXXII Summer Olympiad from 24 July to 9 August. The Paralympics were due to follow from 25 August to 6 September.

This great sporting event came hot on the heels of the successfully hosted autumn 2019 Rugby World Cup in Japan. The success of the national team in reaching the quarter-finals for the first time, losing to eventual champions South Africa, boosted the sport in the country. Sadly, the national team, the Cherry Blossoms, would not be able to play any games in 2020. Critical momentum to the development of the game would be lost.

The Japan Rugby Top League (JRTL) announced in late March that the 2020 season which had been halted mid-season would be cancelled completely for the year. The 2021 JRTL season was delayed from its planned mid-January start after 62 players and staff from six teams tested positive for

COVID-19. It started five weeks late, reformatted, and was completed within three months.

In late February 2020, the IOC stated that it was 'business as usual' for the Tokyo Olympics. On 24 March, the IOC announced that the Olympics and Paralympics would be delayed for one year. On the day of the announcement, from a Japanese population of 126 million, the country had recorded a total of 1,128 cases and 42 deaths. In comparison, the UK's population of 68 million had had 8,077 cases and 694 deaths identified up until then.

The Japanese football J1-league season lasted four days in late February. It did not restart until July behind closed doors. After two rounds of matches, a maximum of 5,000 spectators were admitted. This was increased to 50 per cent stadium capacity in August. Away fans were banned. The season was completed before Christmas with all 34 games played.

The Japan Racing Association made all horse racing behind-closed-doors events and stopped off-track betting except for phone and online wagers.

The baseball season was due to open in March. As the virus reached Japanese shores, the Nippon Professional Baseball League teams were in pre-season training and fans banned from these sessions. The season finally started in mid-June behind closed doors. Some fans were admitted in July, and this rose to 30,000 by the end of the season. The scheduled 143 games were reduced to 120 for each of the 12 sides. The season finished a month late in November. Yomiuri Giants beat Hanshin Tigers 4-0 in the Japan Series finale. It was the eventual winners who had caused concern earlier when two of their players tested positive in June, creating worries about the viability of the season. Fortunately, the fears were not realised.

The professional sport of sumo is organised in a series of six *honbasho* tournaments from January to November. In 2020, there was to be an additional Olympic exhibition in July. The first tournament, the Hatsu *basho*, took place without interference. The Haru *basho* in March took place without spectators. The May Natsu tournament became only the second *basho* to be cancelled since 1946 – because of the state of national emergency. The Olympic exhibition had already been stopped following the Games postponement. However, the remaining three events in July, September and November took place – but all in Tokyo. Nagoya and Kyushu were deemed unsafe. In July, limited numbers of spectators were admitted to the *basho* but all socially distanced and masked. The final November *basho* had 5,000 spectators admitted – half of the venue's capacity.

Sumo did not escape COVID-19. The first case was announced in April. The next month, a 28-year-old sumo wrestler died from complications of COVID-19. He was the first Japanese person in their 20s to die. Apart from his weight, he was also diabetic. Five days later, the Sumo Association announced regular testing programmes. In September, the whole of the Tamanoi stable of wrestlers were withdrawn three days before the *basho*. Out of 19 cases, 11 needed hospital admission. Two more stables would report outbreaks in December.

The lands of the sporting setting sun

By the end of February, the sporting landscape in the Far East had been devastated. It would not be long before Australasia would suffer. Competitions which had been years in the planning were swept away. Some countries' pandemic policies were infinitely tougher than the UK and Europe. Consequently, many sporting seasons and events were delayed, shortened or cancelled. Some international events remained un-resurrected for years.

Organisers and athletes had had to learn to become adaptable and reactive. They had to contend with rescheduling, quarantining, altered travel arrangements and missed competitive opportunities. Elite sports people are used to working to carefully developed training programmes geared to peak performance on a certain planned future date. All that was thrown into confusion and doubt. Most importantly, it became apparent that even elite athletes were not immune from the serious health effects of COVID-19.

Soon the whole sporting world would follow suit and experience similar setbacks, misfortunes and, in time, tragedies.

Chapter 2

March to Lockdown – UK style

VERY EARLY in 2020 it was apparent to members of the UK health community that COVID-19 had the capacity to cause both national and global harm. On 24 January, Graham Medley, Professor of Infectious Disease Modelling at the London School of Hygiene and Tropical Medicine, said this virus 'was going to kill an awful lot of people very quickly in the UK'. The same day, Professor Neil Ferguson, from London's Imperial College, warned that the UK needed to lock down to cut transmission rates by 60 per cent.

By mid-February, SAGE concluded that the pandemic was uncontainable. Public Health England (PHE) only had the capability to cope with 50 cases and trace 800 contacts weekly. Despite media coverage of shortages of personal protective equipment (PPE), the government donated 279,000 items to China. Later, we would buy PPE back from China. On 25 February, SAGE modelling calculated that, without controls, the UK needed 220,000 intensive care beds – England had 3,766 – and could sustain deaths of up to 370,000 by the end of 2021.

The scale of the problem was witnessed in our own lounges.

Television carried speeded-up footage of the 1,000-bedded Huoshensan hospital's construction in Wuhan. 'Foundations to functioning' in nine days at the end of January. In late

February and early March, we viewed the harrowing sight of the near collapse of parts of the Italian health system as cases rocketed. Italy recorded its first official case on the same day as the UK. The UK was only weeks behind.

Sport could not be immune from this natural disaster for much longer.

Amazingly, Premier League football, the English Football League (EFL), the FA Cup and their Scottish equivalents continued through until early March. The Carabao Cup was completed on 1 March when Manchester City defeated Aston Villa at Wembley. Six Nations rugby union started on 1 February and completed three of its five rounds by 23 February. The new rugby league season – Super League XXV – would start in late January. Joe Root's England, having completed their South African Test series, started six one-day cricket internationals against the Springboks in the first half of February.

However, problems were beginning to occur on mainland Europe. On 23 February, Italy suspended all sport in Lombardy and Veneto. The next day, it was announced that all Serie A games in Italy would be played behind closed doors.

The viral presence in Europe would create considerable problems for the UK. Much of it was related to sporting pursuits including 1.5 million Brits going skiing annually.

The first person in the UK not to have caught COVID-19 from direct Chinese connections was identified on 6 February. He had been to Singapore before flying on to the Alps to go skiing and then home to Brighton. The virus followed. Four days later, television showed people in hazmat suits deep-cleaning a Brighton GP practice. During the February half-term holidays, thousands of British families went to the Alps. Many returned with more than the usual bumps and bruises from the piste and piano bars.

The virus was coming at the UK from all directions – at least 1,000 separate sources in early 2020. In fact, direct spread from Chinese sources was very much in the minority. Sixty per cent of microbial imports arrived from France, Italy and Spain.

Having completed the Six Nations third round, the organisers revealed that they were monitoring the 'situation' closely. On 26 February, it was confirmed that the crisis in Italy was so desperate that the 7 March Ireland–Italy game would be postponed, preventing visiting supporters bringing COVID-19 to the Emerald Isle. The same day, Matt Hancock announced plans to 'contain, delay, research and mitigate' the pandemic. By the end of the week the global stock markets had their worst week for a decade. In the UK, some schools closed voluntarily.

The virus had reached the Middle East, forcing the cancellation of the United Arab Emirates (UAE) cycle tour after positive cases.

On Friday, 28 February, Boris Johnson asked the nation to 'wash their hands for 20 seconds' as 'the issue of coronavirus is something that is now the government's top priority'. The same day, Switzerland became the first European nation to halt senior football. Over the weekend, Serie A postponed seven games in Italy.

On 1 March, Hancock appeared on radio and asked the nation to either sing 'Happy Birthday' or 'God Save the Queen' while undertaking their ablutions. The next day, Boris Johnson attended his first COBRA meeting – he had missed the first five – but still encouraged people to 'go about business as usual'. SAGE minutes stated that there was 'no evidence that banning very large gatherings would reduce transmission'. Spectator sport was given the green light to 'carry on regardless' – for the moment. Meanwhile, in the Far East, Middle East and Africa numerous international events were cancelled.

Some sports teams were beginning to get concerned about travel. Ireland pulled out of a women's cricket tour to Thailand. Professional cycling teams Mitchelton-Scott and

Team Ineos withdrew from events in early March. Other cycling teams would quickly follow suit.

Britain's first official death from COVID-19 was announced on 5 March. In fact, later analysis suggested that the first death had occurred five weeks earlier – a day before the first official notified case in York. The deceased had never travelled abroad in his lifetime. Viral containment was no longer possible. Still Boris Johnson appeared on morning TV and said, 'What the experts say is that … things like closing schools and stopping big gatherings don't work as well, perhaps, as people think. One of the theories is perhaps you could take it on the chin.' It was 'herd immunity' in anything but name. Similarly optimistic soundbites came from Thomas Bach, IOC president, in relationship to the Tokyo Summer Olympics and Paralympics.

Johnson confirmed that he would continue to shake hands in hospitals. The same day, Premier League football announced that pre-match handshakes would be banned. UEFA would follow suit within days.

Despite the evidence and actions of others from around the world, our country's internal messaging was that sport in the presence of spectators should continue.

However, the Rugby Football Union (RFU) announced that it was not safe for either the men's or women's teams to play Six Nations games in Rome in mid-March. On 6 March, the Scotland–France women's game was postponed with a positive case and seven in isolation in the home camp – only 24 hours before kick-off. The Scottish team had been in Italy two weeks beforehand when their game was called off similarly only hours before.

Mass participation events like the Rome and Paris marathons in the spring were postponed. Major European-based events in cycling, motor racing, football, athletics and skiing were delayed.

The Six Nations fourth round was scheduled for the weekend of 7–8 March – Ireland–Italy had already been an early casualty. Boris Johnson was one of 81,000 fans at Twickenham for England v Wales. He posted a video of himself on Twitter shaking hands with five women in the crowd. The next day at Murrayfield, 67,000 Scots and French enjoyed the game. One French fan required admission to hospital and died four days later – the first COVID-19-related death in Scotland. It was the same day that France banned any public gatherings greater than 1,000 in its own country.

The same weekend, England's men's cricketers started their short tour of Sri Lanka. It had been announced in advance that fist bumps would replace handshakes. On Saturday, 7 March they began a warm-up game in Katunayake ahead of two Test matches later in the month. Neither would happen.

The wheels were beginning to fall off the government's advice towards sport and their policy towards the pandemic in general. The next week would witness the strategy collapse like a pack of cards.

Chapter 3

'That Was the Week That Was'

A satirical BBC television show hosted by David Frost. 1962–63

A week like no other … in politics and sport

9–15 March 2020

The news from Europe was bleak on Monday, 9 March. Italy was reporting that ten per cent of COVID-19 cases required intensive therapy unit (ITU) support. Italian premier, Giuseppe Conte, placed the whole country into a rigid lockdown. All Italian sport ceased. Other countries toyed with holding sporting events behind closed doors. Paris Saint-Germain played Borussia Dortmund in an empty stadium in the Champions League two days later.

The official UK stance on sport was still encouraging. The government believed there was no rationale for cancelling sports events. Sir Patrick Vallance (Chief Scientific Adviser to the government) stated that gatherings 'actually don't make much difference' and that 'what you can't do is suppress the thing completely … because all that happens is that things pop up later in the year'. The global stock markets didn't agree. The Financial Times Stock Exchange (FTSE) fell by eight per cent, its worst day in 12 years.

That evening Leicester City beat Aston Villa 4-0. It would be exactly 100 days before another Premier League football game would be played.

Traditionally, in March, first-class cricket counties fly to warmer climes – the Caribbean, South Africa and Middle or Far East. Several counties called off their tours at short notice. Others curtailed their plans and headed back home. However, Northamptonshire left for Singapore on 9 March. This was after much internal discussion and liaison with the Singapore authorities, who had taken a more rapid and strict approach to viral containment. When they returned to England on 17 March (virus-free), they found the sporting landscape had shifted.

The USA had confirmed COVID-19 cases before the UK – 20 January. President Trump declared a public health emergency 11 days later and placed restrictions on Chinese flights. The great American sporting calendar continued with the New England Patriots beating the Los Angeles Rams in the Super Bowl in Atlanta on 3 February.

'And I can feel it coming in the air tonight, oh Lord'
Lyrics from 'In the Air Tonight' by Phil Collins. 1981

By the beginning of March, with cases rising, sport began to close down. The California Indian Wells tennis tournament is called the 'fifth slam'. It became the first major North America sporting casualty when it was cancelled two days before starting on 9 March. The next day, the National Basketball Association (NBA) and National Collegiate Athletic Association (NCAA) announced that games would be played behind closed doors. Spain, France and Germany agreed similar measures for football in the hope that games could be saved.

The same day, the last EFL fixtures were played, and the first UK COVID-19 football-related patient was announced – Nottingham Forest owner Evangelos Marinakis. Italian football was already considering that the Serie A season may not finish and weighing up their options.

On Wednesday, 11 March, the government and its medical advisers were still upbeat for UK sport. Jenny

Harries, the Deputy Chief Medical Officer, told the prime minister on TV that face masks are 'really not a good idea and doesn't help'. On sporting events, she said, 'These sort of events and big gatherings are not seen to be something which has a big effect. So, we don't want to disrupt people's lives unduly.' Boris Johnson referred to the problem as a 'mild to moderate illness' and told viewers of breakfast television that one possible strategy was 'take it all in one go ... and allow the disease ... to move through the population'.

WHO was not so sure. It declared the crisis a global pandemic with 4,300 deaths worldwide already reported.

COVID-19 cases had infected German and Italian footballers. The French football League Cup Final and Spanish Cup Final (both scheduled for April) were postponed. A raft of other major events in North America and Europe scheduled for March, April and May were deferred. Meanwhile, football fixtures were completed in Scotland.

In England, Manchester City versus Arsenal on 11 March was postponed as a precaution. Several Gunners players were self-isolating as contacts, after the owner of Greek club Olympiacos contracted COVID-19. He had been at Highbury two weeks before. The Premier League announced that they had no plans to cancel the weekend's fixtures and 'all necessary measures are being taken'. Brighton announced that their Saturday game with Arsenal would go ahead. 'The risk is considered extremely low,' they claimed.

By the next day, Thursday, 12 March, the mood music was beginning to alter in UK government circles. Slightly. The prime minister admitted that 'this is the worst public health crisis for a generation ... families ... are going to lose loved ones'. He admitted to considering stopping sporting fixtures – but not yet. However, the term 'herd immunity' was first used openly by a government insider, Dr David Halpern. Vallance reiterated that 'it's not possible to stop everybody getting it and it's also not desirable because you want some immunity in the population'. The FTSE outdid its dismal performance on 9 March and plunged another ten per cent.

In Italy, Juventus reported that 121 players and staff were self-isolating. Spain, Holland, Denmark and the USA joined Italy and Switzerland in suspending senior football. UEFA announced that it was calling an emergency meeting on 17 March to consider postponing the Euro 2020 tournament for one year.

Abroad, athletes and sporting authorities were taking decisions into their own hands. Australia's female cricketers refused to travel to South Africa and the men's series between Australia and New Zealand was cancelled. In the USA, both the NBA and National Hockey League (NHL) suspended their seasons. Major League Basketball (MLB) announced that the start of its season on 26 March would be delayed. Teams were sent home from their Florida pre-season training bases.

The English Premier League remained hopeful. However, the health crisis was beginning to control the footballing agenda. Arsenal's manager, Mikel Arteta, tested positive, their training ground closed, and the entire squad and staff of over 100 were put into self-isolation. Leicester City and Manchester City announced that they had players at home.

That evening on BBC television's *Question Time*, Professor John Ashton, one of the country's leading public health doctors, said, 'I'm embarrassed by the situation in the country.' Later analysis suggested that the UK had 130,000 cases at the time but only one in 200 was being detected by contact tracing.

Friday the 13th

Friday the 13th would live up to its reputation. The global media news had difficulty keeping up with the speed of events. The National COVID Inquiry heard that one of the country's senior civil servants told the prime minister that day,

'We are in huge trouble … I think we are absolutely f***ed … This country is heading for disaster.' Vallance defended the government's decision not to ban large sporting events that morning. By the evening Downing Street contradicted him, stating a ban would soon be implemented.

The Premier League was one of the last global football competitions standing – albeit with fans awaiting the outcome of an emergency meeting. France and Germany had suspended their leagues. At about 11.00 GMT, the Premier League, EFL and Women's Super League (WSL) and Championship announced that no football would take place until April. Scottish football took the same decision simultaneously. Southampton and Manchester City elected to take each other on at 'noughts and crosses' remotely instead.

BBC Sport's Dan Roan reported that a Premier League and EFL restart on 3–4 April was privately deemed 'almost impossible'. Chelsea confirmed that Callum Hudson-Odoi had tested positive a few days before and the Chelsea squad were in self-isolation with the training ground being 'deep cleansed'. Everton and Bournemouth had players with COVID-19 or identified as close contacts and were at home. Watford's Troy Deeney revealed much later that he had spent four days in hospital on a ventilator after his club's last pre-lockdown game. Leicester's boss, Brendan Rodgers, became the second Premier League manager to contract the virus and was ill for three weeks.

In Galle, the England cricket team were playing a four-day game against the Sri Lanka Board XI. Before tea, the players left the field and returned to their hotels to pack for the flight home. Elsewhere in world cricket, the Indian Premier League (IPL) delayed its start from 29 March. India cancelled its one-day series with South Africa. In Pakistan, the Super League play-offs were condensed and some of the overseas stars headed for the airport.

On Saturday, 14 March, the only Six Nations fixture that remained was at the Millennium Stadium, Cardiff, for Wales–Scotland. Like its Premier League football counterparts, the Welsh Rugby Union (WRU) performed a volte-face in rapid time. On the Friday morning (and before the Premier League football suspension announcement), the WRU confirmed that the game would go ahead. Less than five hours later, they announced its cancellation with both sides in the middle of their final training sessions.

In the afternoon, the April Augusta Masters was postponed. The prestigious PGA Players Championship was being played in Sawgrass, Florida. The organisers decided that the tournament would go ahead with spectators before doing an about turn during the first day's play by announcing that the final three days would take place behind closed doors. At the end of the first day's play, the organisers went further. The entire event was cancelled. Half the prize money was shared amongst the players – $52,000 per competitor. The golfers departed early. Slightly richer.

Cycling events were punctured. The indoor Manchester event for the weekend was cancelled. The Paris–Nice classic was in full throttle that week and operating 'behind closed doors' on 'open roads'. However, the final stage on Sunday, 15 March was scrapped. One of the three blue riband events of road cycling, the Giro d'Italia, scheduled for May, was postponed.

Weekend in a new England

'Weekend in New England' by Barry Manilow. 1976

By Saturday, 14 March, Britain was beginning to take fright. In response to empty shelves of pasta, hand gel and toilet paper, the UK retailers' association asked people not to panic buy.

FA chairman Greg Clarke told the Premier League that he did not think the season would finish. He found an ally in Karren Brady, vice chairperson of West Ham United, who called for the season to be declared 'null and void'. Her club were in a relegation battle at the time. Remarkably, half of the fixtures in English football's tier five and six (the National Leagues) took place that weekend.

The problem of testing symptomatic players was already apparent. With pitiful testing capacity available through public health, private companies stepped into the gap. Peterborough United had two players in isolation. Their chairman, Darragh MacAnthony, complained, 'The testing kits are £150 each which is mad.'

In the Far East, the optimistic Japanese prime minister, Shinzo Abe, said, 'We will overcome the spread of the infection and host the Olympics without problem, as planned.'

On Sunday, 15 March, there was reported to be turmoil inside Downing Street. Politicians and health advisers met to discuss 'Plan B'. It was decided that next day, Boris Johnson, flanked by Chris Whitty (Chief Medical Officer for England) and Vallance, would begin daily televised Downing Street media briefings. It was hoped that such occasions would provide clear and unambiguous messaging. They would become a staple teatime diet for British families for 92 consecutive days until 23 June.

Across the UK, some sport took place. An international swimming meeting in Edinburgh and the final day of the All England Open Badminton Championships in Birmingham were held.

In Britain, horse racing took place with crowds. Five fixtures on Saturday and two on Sunday; 8,400 fans watched the Midlands Grand National at Uttoxeter. Irish meetings were already behind closed doors. Race organisers knew the same fate was imminent in Britain. Martin Cruddace of Arena Racing and owner of 16 tracks believed that the restrictions could last until the end of June.

Other events had to justify their decisions. Six thousand, two hundred runners participated in the Bath half marathon despite an outcry over it taking place. Andrew Taylor, the event's director, said he had not received any advice from public health officials to abandon. The Rugby Football

League (RFL) defended their decision to play games over the weekend, saying, 'Government guidance was that there was no medical rationale to call off games this weekend.'

Individual athletes were not impressed. Wayne Rooney believed the government and football authorities had treated footballers as 'guinea pigs'. 'The rest of sport – tennis, Formula 1, rugby, golf, football in other countries – was closing down and we were being told to carry on. I think a lot of footballers were wondering is it something to do with money being involved in this? Why did we wait until Friday? Why did it take Mikel Arteta to get ill for the game in England to do the right thing?'

A trio of sporting misadventures

There were three major sporting events during this week that caught the concern of medics and public alike. One took place in the lee of the Cotswolds hills, another on Merseyside, and the last across the other side of the world in Melbourne.

The annual Cheltenham Festival is the pinnacle of jump racing in the British Isles. Every March, around 150,000 horse-racing fans descend on the Cotswolds course. In 2020, the four-day equestrian extravaganza was scheduled from 10–13 March. Despite warning notices and hand-sanitiser facilities, the stands were packed and the bars overflowing. Twenty thousand Irish spectators attended – not to the approval of everybody in their own country. 'If Cheltenham was being held in Ireland, I don't think it would be on, quite frankly,' Simon Coveney, the Irish deputy prime minister said.

By mid-April, Gloucestershire Hospitals Trust had recorded more than double the number of deaths compared to adjacent hospitals in Bristol, Bath and Swindon.

The government defended its decision to allow the festival to proceed. The culture secretary, Oliver Dowden, said the risk at mass gatherings was no greater than it would have been in pubs or restaurants. One local resident later described the race meeting as a 'petri dish' and 'breeding ground for COVID-19'. Comedian Lee Mack, footballer Charlie Austin and Queen Camilla's ex-husband, Andrew Parker Bowles, were all struck down.

The exact contribution of the event to pandemic spread will probably never be known due to the absence of contemporary effective testing, tracking and tracing. Therefore, the source of the infection that led to the deaths of such people as a local publican near the course and the chairman of Lancashire County Cricket Club, David Hodgkiss, who attended the meeting, remains unclear. At the end of the meeting, course director Ian Renton stated that, 'The team here has done a highly competent job in putting on the extra precautions and measures in line with the advice of the medical authorities, and the crowd has responded really responsibly … For the large numbers who came here it has remained a wonderful four days of racing.'

On Wednesday, 11 March, Liverpool entertained Atlético Madrid in the second leg of the Champions League round of 16. Over 40,000 home supporters were joined by 3,000 fans from the Spanish capital – despite Madrid being the epicentre of the escalating crisis in that country with its schools having closed the day before. La Liga had decided to hold all games behind closed doors on the day of the match and Spain went into national lockdown three days later.

The Anfield game took place on the day that the WHO declared COVID-19 a pandemic. A WHO statement declared that 'we are deeply concerned both by the alarming levels of spread and severity, and by the alarming levels of inaction'. The *Liverpool Echo* reported on 3 June that Merseyside had experienced a spike in deaths one month after the football match. More than one expert was scornful of the decision-making. Ex-north-west regional director of public health and Liverpool season ticket holder, Professor John Ashton, declined to attend Anfield, claiming 'I think it was clinical and policy negligence' when viewing the government's strategy at the time. His namesake, Matthew

Ashton, Liverpool's public health director, commented three weeks later, 'It was not the right decision to stage the match.' He tried to calm the situation by adding, 'People don't make bad decisions on purpose – perhaps the seriousness of the situation wasn't being understood across government at that time.'

King's College London's Professor of Genetic Epidemiology Tim Spector stated that the Liverpool and Cheltenham events had 'caused increased suffering and death that wouldn't otherwise have occurred'. A 2021 parliamentary inquiry agreed. 'Subsequent analysis suggested that there were an additional 37 and 41 deaths respectively [Liverpool and Cheltenham] at local hospitals after these events. However, it is not clear whether those deaths were as a result of attendance at the events themselves or associated activities such as travel or congregation in pubs.'

The Formula 1 global caravan assembles traditionally in Australia for the opening Grand Prix of the season. The country is an epicentre of world sport in the first quarter of every year. Test cricket series, the January tennis Australian Open and the March Australian Grand Prix keep us wedded to our television screens in the cold of the northern hemisphere winter.

It is a massive feat of logistics to get cars, parts, staff and drivers – let alone the accompanying media – around the world. It has been part of the World Championship since 1985 and held initially in Adelaide before switching to Melbourne in 1996. It had been the championship's opening race in 12 of the previous 14 years. In 2019, 324,000 people had attended the weekend celebration. The dates of 12–15 March would witness the 2020 edition. Twenty-one further races were planned to complete that year's World Championship.

The first COVID-19 case in Australia occurred on 25 January 2020. Although patient numbers were low in the country, in comparison to China and Europe, there was still disquiet amongst some teams regarding travel to the Victorian state capital. The two Italian-based teams, Ferrari and Alpha Tauri, expressed reservations about their teams' ability to leave the quarantine zones in northern Italy. They had witnessed first-hand the distressing scenes of an overwhelmed health service within their own country. Italy at the time was the most infected nation in Europe. The Chinese race on 19 April had already been postponed.

Victorian state leader Daniel Andrews was criticised for allowing the race to go ahead. He felt that cancelling would be a disproportionate reaction to the advice his state government had been given. However, prior to race weekend, and with fans arriving from all over the world, Health Minister Jenny Mikakos warned that positive tests at Albert Park could stop the race.

On Thursday, 12 March world champion Lewis Hamilton expressed surprise that the race was proceeding: 'It seems like the rest of the world is reacting ... you see the NBA has been suspended, yet Formula 1 continues to go on.' Media pictures taken inside the track on the Friday morning showed team staff not socially distancing and an absence of face masks.

One of the British-based teams, McLaren, announced that eight of their staff were being quarantined. When one of their mechanics tested positive after developing 'flu-like symptoms', the team withdrew from the race on the Thursday evening. At a meeting that night, only three teams were willing to compete (Red Bull, Alpha Tauri and Racing Point).

The race weekend was cancelled on Friday as fans queued outside the venue. It provoked angry reactions. It was rumoured that drivers Sebastian Vettel and Kimi Raikkonen had flown out of the country by the time the race was called off. Fourteen more McLaren staff were quarantined. The same day the Bahrain and Vietnam Grands Prix were cancelled. It was an ignominious early end to the weekend as the Formula 1 circus jetted off back to their factories and domiciles.

There is a worrying footnote to this saga as the respective teams nestled back in their home countries. On 30 March, the 76-year-old Red Bull head of driver development, Helmut Marko, gave an interview to Austrian TV. He wanted to set up a camp for his ten drivers to get the virus before the season restarted. This included Max Verstappen, Daniil Kvyat, Pierre Gasly and Alex Albon. A week earlier, the Dutchman, Verstappen, had admitted he was terrified of contracting the disease. The media claimed Marko was well known for his outlandish comments and he admitted, 'Let's put it this way, it has not been well received.'

In the space of one week, national and global sport had ground to a halt. It could be argued that the public and, for once, sporting authorities were ahead of government policy and announcements. The reaction of many in emptying supermarket shelves confirmed that the populace had made up its own mind. Lockdown was inevitable.

The week's delay in the UK, in terms of human suffering, will be reviewed in the next chapter. Meanwhile, major sports, used to holding great authority in the self-governance of their activities, found themselves powerless. Major media outlets, used to filling their pages and screens, wondered what to schedule in their place.

All of us just watched, listened and waited.

Chapter 4

Reaction and No Action

16–23 March 2020

BY MONDAY, 16 March most British sport had been suspended. That evening on television, Boris Johnson advised the population to work from home if possible, increase social distancing and avoid pubs and restaurants. Although the official number of UK cases that day was 602, back-modelling suggested that actual infections had reached 320,000.

Imperial College London's scientists had calculated that the UK death toll would exceed half a million if no measures were instituted – more than the total military UK deaths in the Second World War. SAGE advised the government to lock down the population. France had announced similar measures that day. The advisory board warned of the danger of NHS facilities being overwhelmed with demand for ITU beds outstripping provision thirty-fold in early April.

The next day, new chancellor Rishi Sunak announced a £350 billion support package to an unmasked House of Commons chamber. The Bank of England went on to cut interest rates to the lowest in its 325-year-old history.

To raise the nation's mood, the Queen tried to 'rally troops' with a speech from Windsor on the Thursday.

'In the middle of a chain reaction'

Lyrics from 'Chain Reaction' by Diana Ross. 1985

Further major sporting events were cancelled, including the university Boat Race, Grand National horse race, Isle of Man TT motorbike racing, national hockey leagues, English Premiership rugby union, gymnastics and netball leagues. French players and teams refused to travel to the UK for rugby league fixtures for the upcoming weekend and the Super League was suspended. Triathlon, boxing, basketball and athletics would follow the next day. London was hosting Olympic-qualifying boxing bouts, which were due to finish on 24 March but were cancelled mid-tournament.

Abroad, the German Bundesliga was suspended, and the Italian Football Federation called for Euro 2020 to be postponed. In Brazil, the previous day, players from the Grêmio club had taken to the field wearing face masks in protest at being made to play.

In America, the MLB announced an indefinite delay to the start of the season, and the National Football League (NFL) decided that its normally glitzy April draft extravaganza would proceed without the planned hoopla in Las Vegas. The Kentucky Derby horse race was moved back to September.

The NHS intended to discharge thousands of patients to free up beds. Many would end up in care homes and spread COVID-19. In January 2020, an estimated 3,450 acute hospital beds were occupied daily by 'medically fit' patients ripe for discharge as the disease swept through the country. The move was ruled unlawful by the High Court in April 2022.

British horse racing ran its last cards for 76 days at Wetherby and Taunton without spectators before closing the stable doors. UEFA took the early decision to move Euro 2020 to 2021 while recognising that such a decision would have knock-on effects on many other scheduled football tournaments – including the women's Euros, men's under-21 Euros, the Nations League and new FIFA Club World Cup. Major cycling events like the Tour de Yorkshire, Paris-Roubaix and Liège-Bastogne-Liège were parked in the long grass. The 24-hour Le Mans motor race was postponed from June until September.

In cricket, the first high-profile player, Alex Hales, tested positive after returning from the Pakistan Super League. The same day, the English Cricket Board (ECB) started its weekly online medical meetings with all 18 first-class counties' doctors to plot their way through the crisis. Such meetings continued for two years. They proved pivotal in disseminating information and receiving reports from around the country. It allowed planning for a safe return of professional cricket later in the summer. Other professional sports followed suit.

By Wednesday, the prime minister announced that all schools would close two days later. Traffic had reduced by one third nationally and the pound fell to its lowest level against the US dollar since 1985. It was not only people's cars that would remain idle but their occupants as well. The nation's 675 Saturday morning parkruns were stopped. The ECB advised that all recreational cricket activity should cease with immediate effect.

Formula 1 'boxed and coxed' by announcing that its 'mid-season' three-week break would move forward from August to April – even though it had not managed to hold any events yet. Three further Grands Prix would be postponed the next day – including the iconic Monaco race in May.

Bundesliga club Borussia Monchengladbach revealed that players and staff would be taking pay cuts. The American soccer league (MLS) was suspended until at least 10 May and English football announced that the 2019/20 season would be extended indefinitely. No thoughts of abandonment.

As school gates closed on Friday, 20 March, the grim statistic of 50 UK COVID-19 deaths was reached. It has been estimated that 790,000 people were infected – even though official figures were around 700. Boris Johnson announced that from that night all cafes, pubs, bars, clubs, restaurants, gyms, leisure clubs, nightclubs, theatres and cinemas would close. People swarmed into pubs as though it would be their last-ever drink. A clearly distraught ICU nurse, Dawn Bilbrough, having completed a 48-hour shift, addressed the public from her vehicle in a supermarket car park after finding no essential foods. 'Just stop it,' she pleaded.

The World Snooker Championship at the Crucible in Sheffield was postponed. The rugby union season in England and Wales below the elite levels was stopped – with no relegation or promotion enacted. The English cricket season would be delayed by at least seven weeks.

The weekend of 21–22 March was chaotic. It was Mothering Sunday and the good spring weather caused thousands to surge into parks and other spaces. The term covidiots was first used to describe their behaviour. The prime minister warned the nation of tougher measures if people did not respect social distancing, and Environment Secretary George Eustice pleaded with people to stop acting like plagues of locusts emptying shopping aisles.

WHO announced that the virus was spread via droplets and not airborne-mediated. This shaped policy and educational messages across the world – an error not corrected for another 13 months. It was announced that 5,500 nurses had offered to return to the medical front line to join retired doctors who had been encouraged to dust down their stethoscopes. John Lewis closed its stores – something that neither World War had accomplished.

Germany joined Italy (11 March), Spain (14 March), France (16 March) and most other countries in a full national lockdown. In frustration at a lack of national decision-making, London Mayor Sadiq Khan took unilateral action and instructed the capital to lock down. One and a half million vulnerable people received letters instructing them to stay isolated.

Formula 1 world champion Lewis Hamilton tested positive (for the first time) – believed to be due to contact with actor Idris Elba. Ex-Manchester United player Marouane Fellaini caught COVID-19 while playing in China and spent three weeks in hospital recovering. In Spain, ex-Real Madrid president Lorenzo Sanz died from the disease. Later in the month, Marseille's Senegalese former president Pape Diouf died, aged 68, after contracting the virus. Meanwhile, in Southampton, chief executive Martin Semmens expressed the view that Premier League football could return before population restrictions were lifted.

In response to requests to consider the wisdom of proceeding with the 2020 Tokyo Olympics – from countries such as USA and Brazil – the IOC gave itself a four-week deadline to come to a decision.

Within 24 hours, the Japanese government and IOC announced jointly that the Games would be delayed by one year. The 25th Dubai World Cup horse race scheduled for 28 March was postponed and its $12m prize money moved to 2021.

Even for a prime minister with libertarian views, the pressure to 'close the country' had become overwhelming. Most others had made up their minds in the previous week. The general population had confined themselves to barracks, and sporting institutions had locked the stadia. Any lingering view that 'herd immunity' might be the way forward was doomed as the majority had decided they would prefer to 'pass' on that option.

So, at 8.30pm on Monday, 23 March, Boris Johnson informed the British population that coronavirus was 'the biggest threat this country has faced for decades'. Stay at home was the message. Only go to work if absolutely necessary and to the shop for essential items. As regards exercise, we would only be allowed out once per day – either alone or accompanied by a household member. All golf courses shut. The next day, the Irish Taoiseach Leo Varadkar put the republic into lockdown and Clonmel witnessed the last horse racing in the Emerald Isle.

Down under, Aussie Rules football had tried to continue behind closed doors but stopped when the country joined the UK in lockdown. UEFA postponed the end of May club finals in the Champions League, Women's Champions League and Europa League. The eighth Formula 1 (F1) Grand Prix, in Azerbaijan, on 7 June was postponed.

For whom the delays tolled

The former UK Chief Scientific Adviser Sir David King described the delayed lockdown as 'grossly negligent'. Imperial and Oxford universities estimated that the decision not to lock down nine days earlier had increased cases from 200,000 to 1,500,000. Imperial College's Professor Neil Ferguson estimated that the ten-day delay in locking down the country doubled the death toll in the initial stages.

In a few short weeks, the impossible had happened. Throughout the world, sport (from the recreational gym user to the elite performer) had been mothballed. Professional sport scheduling and finances were in chaos and individual athletic dreams at all levels of attainment lay in tatters.

Chapter 5

The Good, the Bad and the Downright Ugly

IT IS a truism of modern life that personal misdemeanours receive more media column inches than virtuous deeds. Never was this truer than during COVID-19 restrictions. The more prominent the miscreant the more coverage their acts would receive – especially if they were famous sports people.

Public tolerance of rule-breaking often reflected anxiety levels experienced during different pandemic phases. Concerns included not only worries of death or severe illness from the virus, but lack of access to other vital medical services, and social isolation. At times, British people were being asked to restrict their liberties to a degree not seen since 1945.

The transgressions of sports people, suggesting a mindset of privilege and allowance of being 'above the law' or flying in the face of popular opinion (and risking public health in the process), were frowned upon. When many people's financial survival was at risk, the huge wealth of many sports people and organisations was poorly tolerated – especially when the latter attempted to hijack government monies to furlough staff.

Adverse public opinion seemed to reach a crescendo at three specific times. Initially, during the first spring 2020 lockdown, when the world was coming to terms with a new and terrifying risk to life without clear effective treatments, vaccination programmes and, even, sufficient testing capacity. The second period was in the early months of 2021 when a wearied and battered population was faced with a new viral variant resulting in further lockdown – having believed its 2020 sacrifices would lead to better days. The final period of resentment and hostility occurred during the latter part of 2021 when the anti-vax stance of many athletes created poor messaging of the importance of the protective programme.

Inevitably, some athletes' behaviour reflected the society from which they had emerged. Between 27 March and 11 May 2020, the English and Welsh police issued 14,000 fines for lockdown breaches. Nearly 120,000 people had received fixed penalty notices by the end of the pandemic. Overall compliance during early 2020 reached 97 per cent – but was inevitably lowest in 18- to 29-year-olds, who received nearly two-thirds of all fines. Numerous football managers pleaded that their young charges be viewed similarly to others within society. However, rule adherence overall would diminish in response to poor examples set by individuals in the public eye – including politicians and sports people.

From mid-March to the end of April, there was scant sport to follow and much to ponder. With little to fill normally busy sports schedules, a new game appeared: 'spot the offending athlete'.

Going out, out

On 17 March, Chelsea player Mason Mount played five-a-side football with his childhood friend, West Ham's Declan Rice. At the time, the whole Stamford Bridge club were isolating after Callum Hudson-Odoi had tested positive. Mount's club were suitably unimpressed.

Following the 23 March lockdown announcement, it did not take long for a trickle of sacrificial sporting lambs to offer themselves up to the altar of media and public opinion. Repeatedly, rule-breaking would be compounded by hypocrisy.

Step, or stagger, forward Aston Villa star player Jack Grealish. The Brummie midfield maestro's misdemeanour on 29 March was compounded by his decision the day before to take to Twitter. He pleaded with followers to 'only leave your home to buy food, buy medicine or for exercise …' It had been viewed 250,000 times. He ignored his own advice and went to a friend's home for a party, which neighbours described as 'going on all night. It was unbearable.' Then 'there were a series of almighty collisions which reverberated through the flats'. The footballer's £80,000 Land Rover had struck several parked cars and railings. At 08.00 hours, the player was pictured on the street wearing shorts and odd shoes. He was fined by his 'deeply disappointed' club. Grealish admitted that 'I am old enough now and mature enough to know I'd done wrong'. Later, he would be banned from driving. Sadly, his reflections did not extend to vowing not to err again. The episode did not stop Manchester City spending a £100m British transfer record fee for him in August 2021. Indeed, at his new home he would have found sympathetic souls.

In a sad repetition of his future team-mate's decision-making, Kyle Walker had urged 1.7 million people on Instagram to follow government guidelines. Then, on 31 March, he hired two escorts at a cost of £2,200 to spend several hours in his Cheshire apartment. After discovery, he said, 'I want to apologise to my family, friends, football club, supporters and the public for letting them down.' The player was fined £240,000 by his club. A month later, he issued another apology after visiting family at two separate Sheffield addresses and was spotted the next day cycling with a friend in Manchester. Walker claimed to have been 'harassed' by the media. His manager, Pep Guardiola, said, 'I judge my players with what happens on the pitch.'

Not to be outdone by players, the 'Special One' appeared next on the media's list of COVID-19 sinners. On 7 April,

Jose Mourinho was filmed in north London parkland dressed in Tottenham Hotspur kit and holding a stopwatch. He was apparently supervising a training session for three players. Three other Spurs players had been caught training in breach of regulations. London Mayor, Sadiq Khan, took aim at Mourinho, saying, 'My concern is people, particularly children who may support Spurs or follow football, will watch these images and say, "If it's OK for them, why isn't it OK for me?" The Portuguese manager did not apologise but encouraged others to follow regulations. Following a well-worn path, Mourinho had appeared in March in a FIFA video with Arsene Wenger and Mauricio Pochettino asking people to socially distance.

Later in the summer, another Manchester City ace, Benjamin Mendy, would 'run a horse and cart' through COVID-19 restrictions with a 22-year-old Greek woman called Claudia. By 29 June, all UK arrivals had to undergo a 14-day self-isolation period. Mendy had invited his guest after an online exchange. *The Sun* reported that Mendy informed her, 'U stay in my house. It's ok they don't gonna check.' The four-day 'romp' included an unexpected bonus. Claudia reported, 'One day he took me to Leeds where he saw his dentist.' Like Grealish and Walker, he would break regulations again.

These were not the only footballing covidiots. Later, Everton would fine forward Moise Kean £100,000 for hosting a 'raunchy party' and Wolverhampton Wanderers would discipline midfielder Morgan Gibbs-White for partying in London.

In September, Phil Foden and Mason Greenwood made their England debuts in Iceland in a Nations League match. They celebrated by inviting two females to their hotel. They had contacted them on social media before arriving. The girls posted pictures of their nocturnal adventure online. The players were fined by the Reykjavik police and dropped by England.

Furlough furore and salary savings

When sport closed in March 2020, Premier League clubs were not short of 'a bob or two'.

It was not surprising that there would be a backlash after some clubs applied for government funding to 'furlough' staff. The scheme had been announced by Chancellor Rishi Sunak on 20 March. Eighty per cent of salaries of non-working employees would be paid up to a maximum of £2,500 per month. It was unprecedented in UK economic history and provided a lifeline for many families and businesses; likewise, parts of professional sport. Some sports and organisations further down the food chain had no choice. But did Premier League football clubs?

The rocky road started at the new Tottenham Hotspur stadium. On 1 April, Spurs announced a 20 per cent wage cut for all 550 non-playing staff. Chairman Daniel Levy announced that Tottenham would be 'utilising, where appropriate, the government's furlough scheme' – potentially claiming £1m monthly from the Treasury. Simultaneously, Spurs announced an operating profit of £178m. Levy received £7m and their star striker, Harry Kane, £10m annually. Spurs' owner Joe Lewis had a reported fortune of £4.36bn and the club had paid out £11m to players' agents in 2018–19. Henry Winter wrote in *The Times* that 'the public will surely feel disgust at the thought of clubs going cap in hand to the government'.

Undeterred, Newcastle United, Norwich City and Bournemouth announced plans to follow suit.

Abroad, Juventus players agreed to forsake their salaries for four months to save the club £80.7m. Bayern Munich negotiated a 20 per cent reduction, and Atlético Madrid and Barcelona a 70 per cent pay cut. In cricket, it was reported on 29 March that the ECB's centrally contracted players like Joe Root, Ben Stokes and Jos Buttler would take £200,000 pay cuts. The ECB would go on to cut 62 jobs centrally during the pandemic.

Opprobrium rained down on elite football from all quarters. Players supporting low-paid workers in their clubs by voluntary pay cuts was mooted in the press.

London Mayor Sadiq Khan said, 'Highly paid football players ... should be the first one to ... sacrifice their salary rather than the person selling the programme or the person who does catering.' Conservative MP Julian Knight, chairperson of the Digital, Culture, Media and Sport (DCMS) House of Commons Select Committee, stated that 'this isn't what [the scheme] is designed for ... this exposes the crazy economics in English football and the moral vacuum at its centre'. He believed that clubs furloughing staff should be subjected to a windfall tax. Labour MP David Lammy felt that 'it's criminal that Premier League footballers haven't moved more quickly to take pay cuts and deferrals. And completely wrong that taxpayers are now being asked to subsidise cleaners, caterers, and security guards at these clubs instead.' Gary Lineker joined in the criticism of his ex-club Spurs. Meanwhile, a relatively small club, Huddersfield Town, announced that its senior management had volunteered to take salary deferrals for two months to ensure that all members of staff, both full- and part-time, would receive full pay – even though some would be furloughed.

On 2 April, the minister of health, not so fresh from recovering from the disease himself, waded into the debate. During the daily government briefing, Matt Hancock trained his guns on footballers: 'Given the sacrifices that many people are making ... I think the first thing the Premier League footballers can do is make a contribution, take a pay cut.' Former Premier League manager Harry Redknapp agreed with him, to safeguard non-playing staff.

The fightback started immediately. Reference to footballers being easy targets, the large tax bills paid, and the good works and monies already pledged were raised.

On 3 April, it was reported that the Premier League had 'woken up and smelt the coffee'. It wanted players to accept a

30 per cent pay cut to protect jobs. Additionally, they would give £125m to the EFL and National Leagues and £20m to the NHS.

The Professional Footballers' Association (PFA) calculated a £500m saving if such reductions were agreed and which could 'harm' the NHS by removing £200m in tax revenues. The PFA preferred a wages deferment for the Premier League and EFL rather than pay cuts. Stijn Francis, Spurs defender Toby Alderweireld's agent, claimed that footballers should be allowed to terminate their contracts and leave a club for free if wages were cut. A YouGov poll revealed that 92 per cent of the population supported lower incomes for leading footballers. The FA tried to set an example by announcing that England's manager, Gareth Southgate, would take a 30 per cent pay reduction and senior management 15 per cent. Eddie Howe, David Moyes and Graham Potter – Bournemouth, West Ham and Brighton managers respectively – announced that they would do similar. Later, in April, Sheffield United manager Chris Wilder and club senior executives would take salary reductions for six months to try and safeguard salaries of other employees.

Collective talks broke down over the 4–5 April weekend and clubs began individual negotiations with their players. Matters were further complicated by the players' own wishes to channel their donations in areas that they supported. Before the Premier League announcement, Jordan Henderson, Liverpool's skipper, had led discussions with fellow captains on pay cuts, deferrals, and establishing a collective charitable funds to support the NHS and other causes.

Football was smarting at politicians' interference. Wayne Rooney vented his spleen. 'How the past few days have played out is a disgrace. First the health secretary, Matt Hancock, in his daily update on coronavirus, said that Premier League players should take a pay cut. He was supposed to be giving the nation the latest on the biggest crisis we've faced in our lifetimes. Why was the pay of footballers even in his head?

Was he desperate to divert attention from his government's handling of this pandemic?' Sean Dyche, the Burnley manager, had equally strong feelings. He told talkSPORT, 'I have seen footballers do so many good things, so many things financially, so many things with time, care, effort and attention.'

Despite the mounting criticism, Liverpool FC announced, on 4 April, that they would be following the furlough path. Facing a severe backlash from fans and ex-players alike, they quickly reversed their decision. The chief executive of the world's seventh-biggest club, Peter Moore, announced two days later, 'We came to the wrong decision last week and are truly sorry for that.'

Like Liverpool, Tottenham (13 April) and Bournemouth (14 April) reversed their decisions to take government aid. However, Newcastle and Norwich were joined by Sheffield United in furloughing some of their non-playing staff.

The controversy rolled on despite Liverpool's decision. The next day, Oliver Dowden, the culture secretary, wrote in the *Daily Telegraph* that the Premier League should be 'thinking very carefully' about their next move. 'Leaving the public purse to pick up the cost of furloughing low-paid workers, while players earn millions and billionaire owners go untouched, is something I know the public will rightly take a very dim view of ... at a time of national crisis, our national sport must play its part. I expect to see the football authorities judge the mood of the country and come together with an agreement urgently.'

Rob Green, ex-England goalie, did not support the furloughing clubs: 'Clubs have become such big businesses now, worldwide figures rather than just the heartbeat of the community, and I think they forget that sometimes ... The numbers that are going around in football, it does seem disproportionate to furlough those people.'

Premier League CEO Richard Masters defended the right of clubs to use the furlough scheme, stating, 'We face a

£1 billion loss, at least, if we fail to complete season 2019/20.' In contrast, Spanish football announced that it would not be seeking any government financial support despite La Liga already losing £133m in sponsorship and ticket revenue by 7 April.

Towards the end of April, the decision on Premier League footballers' wages became clearer. Some clubs paid salaries in full (like Chelsea, Crystal Palace and the two Manchester teams), some negotiated wage reductions for a limited period (like Arsenal and Tottenham), and others agreed a percentage of wage deferrals (like West Ham, Southampton and Watford). The row had escalated into one of the most serious disagreements in history between the league, the PFA and the players.

It had taken a month to reach these decisions during which time the wealth of elite footballers had become an unwelcome distraction from the real fight against the deadly virus and relegated the time, energy and money many had spent helping others less fortunate than themselves. The truth is that most sporting organisations and athletes followed the rules and, where possible, sought to provide support wherever they could.

#Players Together

Out of the meetings of Premier League captains, orchestrated by Henderson, the #Players Together movement was established. Henderson's unstinting work in supporting various charities throughout the pandemic was recognised with an MBE in June 2021.

The initiative was formally announced on 9 April. Their decision to partner with NHS Charities was 'warmly welcomed' by Matt Hancock, who called it a 'big-hearted decision'. However, the minister's support did not appease everybody.

Ex-Premier League striker Jonathan Walters told BBC Radio 5 Live, 'Players would have done their own things anyway, donated in their own way, and a lot of players have helped the local hospitals or the local food bank but to get 500 Premier League players to come together as one force is a difficult thing so it's taken a couple of weeks and I think it was happening long before Matt Hancock was having his say and sort of called the players out. It's a fantastic initiative and one that will help a lot of people.'

On the same radio station, Rob Green continued the criticism of Matt Hancock. 'I think it's lazy, it's deflecting from the inefficiencies of his own job and something that he was desperate to do in that press conference. It deflected away from the questions he was getting at the time about ventilators, the testing, coming out with 100,000 [daily tests] by the end of the month. The lads are sat there in their own houses, doing what they're told, working hard on trying to keep fit and through no fault of their own get called out and all of a sudden it becomes a political debate against footballers when there were already wheels in motion.' Burnley captain, Ben Mee, explained, 'Initially, Jordan Henderson contacted us and since then we've come together, we wanted to do something really positive. And we think it's a great time to show togetherness; I think that's what the country needs right now, a lot of togetherness. I think the idea came about to try and really do something positive and something really good to help out and support those in need.' Ten days after its launch, #Players Together were able to announce that £4m had already been raised. An online auction of 500 signed football shirts raised £1m alone in June 2020.

Continuous pressure

In the week before lockdown, furious calculations were undertaken by government and its advisers about the likely resources required by the NHS and its ability to fight the virus. A little late in the day.

On 16 March, government asked businesses to support the supply of ventilators. The NHS had access to 8,175 ventilators. Information from abroad, especially Italy, estimated that up to 30,000 might be needed. Blue-chip companies like Rolls-Royce and Dyson, with no experience of manufacturing such equipment, were asked for help. Much of what followed was chaotic, with changing specifications, plans shelved and orders (like those with Dyson) cancelled.

The day after the call to arms, three professors supped a pint in a Bloomsbury pub and discussed the looming ventilator crisis. They included experts in intensive care medicine, a Formula 1 designer and healthcare engineer. They phoned a Mercedes engineer for advice. The latter produced 'engines that power Lewis Hamilton'. Rapidly a team was formed – split between University College Hospital (UCH), London and the Mercedes base in Brixworth, Northamptonshire. They decided to manufacture an alternative to a 'full-blown' ventilator, which would be expensive to make and labour-intensive to supervise. Early Italian evidence suggested that CPAP (continuous positive airway pressure) machines were suitable in half the patients requiring breathing support – but easier to use. One of the principal collaborators, Professor Mervyn Singer, described it as halfway between an oxygen mask and a ventilator.

The Brixworth factory was repurposed. Mercedes threw the 'full might' of their team behind the project. Other companies such as Oxford Optonix opted in. Such a project would normally take two years to design, build, test and pass regulatory standards. Working to plans designed in London, a prototype was built in less than 100 hours from first meeting. At ten days and, after rapid approvals were obtained, it was being trialled on the wards at UCH. By 4 April, following success with seven patients, the government placed an order for 10,000 CPAP machines to be delivered within two weeks. Mercedes made design details freely available online for others to follow.

Other UK-based Formula 1 companies joined the battle with Mercedes to boost the country's ventilator capacity.

McLaren, Red Bull, Williams, Renault, Racing Point and Haas were all involved in three separate projects under the banner 'Project Pitlane'. Together they contributed a further 10,000 ventilators for use by the NHS. Abroad, it was reported that controversial football super-agent Mino Raiola was trying to organise footballers to purchase ventilators for Italy. Formula E team Envision Virgin Racing's owners, a China-based green energy technology company, produced over one million masks by early April 2020.

This incredible story of ingenuity and determination was only made possible by the collaborative efforts of these experts in different fields. To turn a dream into such reality was achieved by a sport used to rapid problem-solving and the ability to work 24/7 to meet tight deadlines.

The sporting world in unison

Within weeks of lockdown, examples of charitable works instigated via sport worldwide could be found. Some were acts of major organisations, others from wealthy owners and many more from individual athletes trying to support communities close to their hearts. On 19 March, an Australian gin distillery, owned by Shane Warne, turned its hand to sanitiser production.

Before the end of March, the American NFL had donated £28m ($35m) to various agencies, gifted from owners and players. New England Patriots owner Robert Kraft used the team's plane to deliver 1.2 million protective masks from China to the USA. In April, the NFL announced that its annual player draft would become a three-day virtual fundraiser for six COVID-related American charities.

The Spanish La Liga organised a virtual festival featuring players and musicians performing from their homes, raising more than 1m euros. Dutch players and main football sponsor ING made an 11m euros contribution towards amateur football. Germany midfielder Marco Reus donated 500,000 euros to small businesses in Dortmund. Through their foundation, Paris Saint-Germain helped support 100,000 healthcare workers in the French capital. The UEFA Foundation for Children announced plans to help the world's poorest communities cope with the pandemic.

In tennis, Novak Djokovic donated 1m euros to buy medical equipment in Serbia. Controversial Australian Nick Kyrgios offered to personally deliver to anyone short of food in his locality. The impressive Springbok rugby captain, Siya Kolisi, used his foundation to supply protective equipment to hospitals across South Africa.

British-based sports people raised funds to help overseas. Manchester City manager Pep Guardiola donated 1m euros to help fight coronavirus in Spain. Chelsea player Antonio Rudiger raised money for face masks for his mother's country, Sierra Leone. Paul Pogba of Manchester United pledged to set up a fundraising page to help UNICEF support children affected by the coronavirus.

England wicketkeeper Jos Buttler auctioned his 2019 World Cup Final winning shirt to support heart and lung centres dealing with the coronavirus response. It sold for £65,100. Olympic gold medallist Adam Peaty auctioned the swimming trunks he wore in the Rio Games for £13,000.

McLaren Formula 1 driver Lando Norris shaved off his hair and raised $12,000. Gary Lineker donated his BBC salary for two months to the Red Cross. Ex-McLaren Formula 1 boss Ron Dennis used his foundation to develop a scheme for providing a million free meals to NHS workers during the crisis using a £1.5m budget.

Premier League clubs reached out to their local communities and contributed meals and other essential items to the vulnerable and NHS staff. Arsenal, Chelsea, Crystal Palace, Leicester City, Manchester United, Norwich City, Tottenham Hotspur, Watford and West Ham were particularly prominent and generous – some even turned over their own stadium kitchens for the purpose.

Others provided accommodation for fatigued NHS workers trying not to take the virus home to their families. Chelsea allowed use of the Millennium hotel at Stamford Bridge; Watford converted executive boxes into bedrooms and counselling suites for health staff. Gary Neville allowed key workers to stay free in his Manchester Hotel Football.

Other clubs like Manchester City, Manchester United, Tottenham and Burnley made their stadia available for NHS use. Later, Brighton & Hove Albion converted the Amex Stadium into a drive-in coronavirus testing centre.

In other sports, Durham cricket offered the Riverside ground to NHS staff and Warwickshire turned its Edgbaston car park into a drive-in testing centre. Rugby union side, Llanelli Scarlets, announced plans to convert their training facilities into a temporary hospital ward. The Cardiff Millennium Stadium was turned into a field hospital.

Prominent managers like Tottenham's Jose Mourinho and West Ham's David Moyes could be seen personally delivering food to the needy. There were countless examples of similar acts of kindness throughout the British football pyramid. Many vulnerable and self-isolating fans received phone calls from their footballing heroes.

Taking on the government

Manchester United's Marcus Rashford's activism for charitable causes began before the pandemic. The youngest of five children, brought up by single parent Melanie, in Manchester, Rashford knew first-hand the sacrifices his mother had made to raise her children and put meals on the table. Building on ambitions he harboured as a youth player at Old Trafford, he partnered with Selfridges to deliver essential items to the homeless at Christmas 2019. With his mother, he personally hand-delivered the gift boxes.

The March lockdown provoked a crisis in nutrition for children from poor families. School closures threatened a loss of adequate food for many. In 2019, 16 per cent of nursery and primary school children qualified for free school meals. Rashford collaborated with the charity FareShare to distribute meals across the Greater Manchester area. The campaign gained momentum and spread nationwide using £20m in donations raised. The initial target of helping 400,000 children expanded to four million meals by July 2020. Southampton FC had similarly joined forces with FareShare to deliver 1,000 weekly meals for those in need on the south coast in the first week of lockdown.

Based on his own experiences, on 15 June Rashford wrote an open letter to the UK government encouraging greater efforts to eradicate childhood poverty. Next day, a policy U-turn was announced and £15 weekly food vouchers for 1.3 million children would be delivered across the looming summer school holidays. Rashford's action was described by *The Guardian* as 'a political masterclass'.

As schools prepared to return for the new school year, Rashford announced on 1 September that he had formed a Child Food Poverty Task Force with several major food brands. After setbacks in the Houses of Parliament, the government announced finally on 8 November that £400m of funding would be provided over the next year to support poor families' food and household bills. Rashford received an MBE in October 2020. Rashford's tireless campaigning across many issues linked to eradicating poverty would continue.

What did we learn from April 2020 about our relationship with sport?

The first month of lockdown had proven bruising for professional sport in many respects. In normal times, its exponents are idolised by many for their skill and commitment. Their endeavours are celebrated and briefly take us out of our own less glamorous world. However, that bond proved to be not without limits. Faced with physical, psychological and economic hardship, society re-evaluated that relationship and its tolerance of the antics and financial clout of elite sport. Particularly football.

Footballers' private lives are not that anymore. Social media has accelerated that process. The added fame and influence that brings has been courted by many sports people. When that same exposure uncovers immature, hedonistic behaviour, a lack of respect for the law and hypocrisy, the perpetrators are duly castigated.

However, April 2020 demonstrated that the overwhelming majority of professional athletes used their wealth and privileged position to engender positive results to benefit the most vulnerable in our society.

In early April, FIFA president Gianni Infantino stated that 'football that will come after the virus will be totally different ... more inclusive, more social, and more supportive, connected to the individual countries and at the same time more global, less arrogant, and more welcoming. We will be better, more human and more attentive to true values.'

David Moyes reflected on the experience. He hoped the pandemic might mean a 'reset' of football: 'I hope we will all look back and think: "Maybe we were indulging too much."'

The next two years would demonstrate whether football had learnt any lessons.

Chapter 6

I'm a Sports Celebrity ...
Get Me Out of Here!

ON 13 May 2020, the UK government published its guidelines for elite sport's return. It was 51 days since lockdown started. During those seven weeks, many opinions were given on the desirability and timing of sport's return, and what changes needed to be made to maximise participants' safety.

Evidence given to the National COVID Inquiry suggested that the government machinery was in chaos in the early pandemic weeks and struggling to develop coherent policies. The enormity of the impact on sport was apparent. Suddenly, it seemed sadly irrelevant compared to the struggles experienced by every family and hospital in the country. It was an uncomfortable position. Initially, the government and its public health advisers simply did not have the time or energy to elevate elite sport above its new position on an extremely low rung of the priorities ladder.

The period from early April to mid-May witnessed many with a stake in sport's return taking to the media. Involved 'parties' appeared to be jockeying for position, ensuring their views were centre stage ahead of the critical decisions. What were the principal areas of debate?

Decisions had to be played out against a background of the national situation. Views on the morality of prioritising and playing sport were expressed. It was necessary to consider the financial implications of returning as against 'shutting up shop' for the summer. Legal connotations. Furloughed employees. Expiring contracts. Medics and players had their own concerns. What were the risks to athletes and staff? Athletes' mental state had been affected by lockdown and could be damaged further when conscripted back into action. How would consent be gained? How were personnel going to be assessed clinically? Where was PPE going to be sourced at a time of national shortage? What would the protocols look like, and would alterations to sport be needed for safety? How would athletes access healthcare? What were the increased injury risks from inadequate preparation and condensed fixture lists? Where would games be played? What pressures were coming from government and major sporting bodies to get sport restarted?

A nation in crisis

Nearly 34,000 UK citizens died from COVID-19 in April 2020. It would be the worst month for the disease during the entire pandemic.

In the same month, the country's prime minister nearly succumbed to the virus. The NHS was close to being overrun. Less than ten per cent of hospital deaths from COVID-19 had access to ITU. Clinicians were told to reuse PPE if stocks were running low. On 22 April, Chris Whitty said that it was 'wholly unrealistic' to expect life to return to normal in the short term. Captain Thomas Moore walked 100 laps of his garden, raising £32m for NHS charities.

On 30 April, a recovered Boris Johnson said the UK was 'past the peak' and that he would set out a 'comprehensive plan' for easing lockdown shortly.

'If I were a rich man'
Song from the musical Fiddler on the Roof. 1964

Professional sport needed financial stability.

On 7 April, FA chairman Greg Clarke said football faces 'the danger of losing clubs and leagues' amid economic challenges 'beyond the wildest imagination'.

The Premier League employed 12,000 people and supported a further 94,000 UK jobs. It would contribute £3.6 billion in taxes during the COVID-19-hit 2019/20 season. Its contribution to the UK's gross domestic product (GDP) was £7.6 billion. If it were a country, the league would be the world's 155th-richest – sitting above Bermuda and Monaco. Yet, in the 2017/18 season, over one third of Premier League clubs posted losses.

Many clubs had speculated that the gravy train would keep on arriving and allocated future revenues – mostly on players' salaries; £1.6bn in outstanding transfer fees were due to be paid that summer. Finance expert Rob Wilson warned 'football clubs don't tend to plan long-term financially, and that's why they are being found out a bit now'. He predicted redundancies and ripped-up contracts. Football business analysts Vysyble stated that 'for some time now, wages and transfer fees have been beyond any kind of economic sense'. The clubs' main sources of income – television, matchday revenue, merchandising and sponsorship – were all affected.

On 11 May, Premier League clubs were told they would have to repay a combined £762m to broadcast partners if the season was not restarted. The sting in the tail was that they were still liable to repay £350m – even if games were completed with schedule changes and fans' absence. Normally season ticket renewals provide pre-season income but deadlines had to be lifted. Expiring and starting sponsorship deals, for instance on shirt suppliers, needed consideration.

Further down the football food chain matters were worse. All football below the National Leagues – tier 7 and below – was ended, with results expunged on 26 March. On 22 April, tiers 5 and 6 – the three National Leagues – abandoned their regular season. A points-per-game formula was used to determine placings but end-of-season play-offs were contested and finished in early August.

In early April, the EFL remained optimistic that it could complete its three divisions' seasons in 56 days behind closed doors. However, the potential financial apocalypse concentrated minds. Luton CEO Gary Sweet warned that clubs 'at every level' were at risk and needed 'a swift and material aid package'. Ex-FA chairman David Bernstein said, 'I don't think football is going to handle this and settle this without some outside help. The trouble is football does not like outside interference, but frankly I think that we're past that point now.'

Championship clubs had been spending £1.06p for every £1 earned. It was 'Mr Micawber' financial planning. Ex-FA CEO Mark Palios believed a 'double figure' number of EFL clubs could become insolvent. The EFL and PFA proposed clubs defer up to 25 per cent of Leagues One and Two players' wages for April. Championship clubs were expected to make individual decisions.

EFL clubs rely on gate money with figures rising to 40 per cent of income. In comparison, only 17 per cent of Manchester United's income came from ticket sales and matchday revenue. Even 'smaller' Premier League clubs' revenues dwarfed those in lower divisions. Watford's 2018/19 income at £148m was larger than all 24 League One clubs put together.

Women's senior football was taking hard decisions. Semi-professional AFC Fylde disbanded. Reading became the first WSL team to furlough players.

On 30 March, Aberdeen urged Scottish authorities to 'put a stake in the ground' regarding league resumption. The club predicted a £5m shortfall if the season did not restart.

The divide between the 'haves and have nots' was stark and would prevent most of professional football restarting. Other sports would come to similar decisions.

Ploughing your own furlough

In many sports, large swathes of employees had to be furloughed. Coronavirus Job Retention Scheme (CJRS) regulations had to be complied with. It did not differ if the furloughed person was a widget assembly line worker or a professional athlete.

Furloughed staff could study or 'train' to improve effectiveness. They could not provide services, engage in business activities or generate revenue. The employer could contact the employee to relay business progress, maintain social contact or address welfare issues. The employee need not check emails or reply to messages. An employee who undertook work without the employer's knowledge might breach their own furloughed status.

This left difficult conundrums within sport. Early legal advice was that players could not train together in organised sessions, attend virtual meetings with coaches or undertake media work. Individual self-generated exercise (allowed for everybody) could not be restricted. On 24 March, the ECB offered home training packages for its national cricket squads – including, ironically, 'medicine balls'.

Later, whether and when to un-furlough staff had to be carefully considered. For competitions, without significant television contracts or crowds to generate income, bringing back employed players would deepen the financial crisis. Premier League football and Test cricket could reappear first alongside some community sports. County cricket was caught in the middle and delayed. The latter had not the means to generate income to cover the extra costs of restarting.

'I Want to Break Free'

Song from *The Works* album. Queen. 1984

Most professional athletes have time-limited contracts with termination dates usually coinciding with a season's end. With the season in abeyance and no fixed plans for completion, chaos beckoned.

Eighty-six Premier League and 1,400 EFL players would become free agents on 1 July. Contract extensions for 28 days in emergencies could be granted if club and player agreed. There was a real threat that absent players might affect a restarted competition's integrity. Players planning to switch clubs during summer 2020 might not want to risk injury in a concertinaed fixture scramble.

On 6 April, it was agreed by FIFA and the Premier League that contracts ending an 30 June could be extended, and the summer transfer window delayed. However, on 16 April, half of all Premier League clubs wanted the season finished by 1 July because of contract concerns – even if some games were cancelled.

A similar issue was anticipated in cricket and rugby union.

Close to one quarter of professional cricketers were out of contract at the end of the summer. In modern cricket, different players have different contracts – some for red ball (four-day matches) and others for white ball (one-day and T20 games) only. Delays would inevitably bring changes to the different formats and, possibly, reduced opportunities to play and impress. The inaugural 100-ball competition promised excitement, increased media exposure and a substantial boost to selected players' incomes. Its cancellation removed their hopes. Fifty-five players across English rugby union's Premiership's 12 teams faced no job at the end of the current contract cycle. All faced the prospect of not being able to 'prove their worth' before collecting their P45s.

The long arm of the law(yer)

Elite sport would not feel the same without the omnipresence of lawyers. On 1 May, Nick De Marco, speaking about football's Project Restart, stated, 'It's inevitable there will be litigation arising from it.' There were 'four big legal issues' – broadcasters, sponsors, clubs and players; disagreement over finances if the season is cancelled, who would win the title, and who gets relegated and promoted. 'What if players don't feel that it's safe to return?' De Marco felt there was a 'very big problem' regarding player contracts. Clubs needed to understand their liabilities if players or staff members became seriously ill, having agreed to return.

In early May, the Premier League explored abandoning relegation and pulling up the drawbridge. The FA responded angrily and would block any attempts by invoking the 1991 Founder Members' Agreement. The EFL chairman, Rick Parry, warned it could lead to a 'very messy' legal action.

Ethics and morality

'A people that values its privileges above its principles soon loses both.'

Dwight D. Eisenhower. President of the USA 1953–61

Athletes were anxious to get back to work but many had concerns as to whether it was 'right and proper'. Apprehension reached its acme in early May.

Brazilian international and Nice captain Dante described Project Restart as 'indecent'. Gary Neville felt that 'we're hearing different things every day, but I think if this was a non-economic decision, there would be no football for months'. Bournemouth's Simon Francis, out of contract on 30 June, said, 'I'm not sure why the return of a contact sport is being considered.' Manchester City's Sergio Aguero, Chelsea's Antonio Rudiger and Brighton's Glenn Murray felt similarly. Andy Murray said tennis 'is not the most important thing at the moment'.

Crystal Palace chairman Steve Parish commented football 'cannot occupy any paramedic or ambulance that the NHS needs'. Wycombe Wanderers manager Gareth Ainsworth said, 'If on the same street, you've got one house celebrating a football result, and next door there's an ambulance outside … that just can't happen.'

On 12 May, as plans advanced, London mayor and Liverpool fan Sadiq Khan felt 'with the country still in the grips of this crisis, and hundreds of people dying every day …

it is too early to be discussing the resumption of the Premier League and top-flight sport in the capital'.

By that time Project Restart had gained unstoppable momentum and government plans for elite sport to resume were about to be published. In fact, preliminary discussions had taken place weeks earlier between government, health officials and sport with many principles for Restart already agreed.

Time out

Players, parents and managers expressed concerns about resumption. The Aston Villa manager, Dean Smith, revealed that he would be unable to field an asthmatic player and another who lived with a family member undergoing chemotherapy.

The BAME (Black, Asian and Minority Ethnic) community had apparent increased risks. Watford's Troy Deeney and Chelsea's N'Golo Kante delayed their return to football training while initial testing results were revealed, and early training protocols gauged. They had reasons to be worried and Deeney had first-hand knowledge of the dangers of the disease. In June, the government confirmed that the BAME community were more likely to die from COVID-19.

Danny Rose, Newcastle United and England defender, was critical and joined by Crystal Palace winger Andros Townsend's father. Troy Townsend said, 'I am a parent, and I am worried.' Parish confirmed that Palace would not force any player to play.

Education and consent would be crucial. The League and clubs needed to get players onside while respecting those who declined to return. Legal ramifications and risk-balancing were debated in the media. Some expected the players to wilt when confronted with pressures from clubs and peers. On 9 May, it was reported that up to 50 players might refuse to return. However, the authors are not aware of any ultimately refusing to play.

'Where's a doctor when I need one?'

Elite athletes are used to instant medical access. For most of 2020, many private hospitals were taken over by the NHS and subsumed into the national health effort. Some units became cancer centres to shield immunosuppressed patients from the virus rampaging through NHS hospitals. A footballer with a sprained ankle requiring imaging would not be welcome. Equally, injured athletes did not want to attend casualty departments and add to the burden of overstretched staff.

One of the authors of this book, Bill, was stopped from operating for four months. His first surgery in July 2020 was on a double Olympic gold medallist whose surgery had been deferred since March. Further guillotines would be imposed on his scalpel in early 2021. Many surgeons were 'repurposed'. Prevented from operating, some worked as porters turning ventilated ITU patients. Players and management had to be advised and avoid unnecessary risks.

If advice, scans and surgery were hard to access, what about other treatments? From experiences with previous viruses, it was acknowledged that steroid injections might suppress the immune system temporarily. Many hospitals would not sanction such treatments without wide consultation and in dire circumstances. Restrictions on use, delay and collegiality are not terms often applied to elite sports medicine.

Sport had to consider emergency services' availability for games. Normally ambulances are on-site for crowd and participants' safety. With such national services close to being overwhelmed, was it ethical to divert paramedics to an 'empty Anfield' even if they were paid for privately?

What would be the medical arrangements at training grounds and stadia? Sports medical departments are not governed by the same strict Care Quality Commission (CQC) regulations laid down elsewhere. Cleanliness was not always top of the agenda. Discarded tape and sweaty socks festooned many medical rooms. It had to change.

Sports needed to purchase PPE, thermometers, cleaning equipment, and dispose of potentially biohazardous contaminated materials at a time when the NHS was struggling to properly protect its key clinical workers. Enhanced contracts needed to be signed with cleaning companies. Isolation areas would have to be designated for staff developing symptoms at work.

West Ham's Karren Brady summed up the concerns on 11 April: 'What happens if games recommence, and players get injured when playing? ... One thing I know is that if you try managing an apocalypse, you can't.'

Physiotherapists were told not to treat trivial concerns. Bill brought physio staff to his clinic to observe safety procedures and PPE-donning routines. Physio rooms ceased to be players' social space. It was strictly 'one in and one out' followed by a thorough clean. Pitch-side emergency drills had to be modified. Aerosol generating procedures (AGPs), like heavy nosebleeds or maintaining the airway of an unconscious player, were potentially risky procedures for medics with high-level PPE needed.

Mind games

Athlete support emerged as a priority for sporting organisations who normally function as well-oiled performance machines. They had to metamorphose overnight into welfare establishments. Many had paid only lip service to the area before and were ill-prepared.

Mental toughness in the heat of battle does not always transfer to resilience in dealing with social isolation, job uncertainty, financial loss, health concerns and the postponement, or even cancellation, of sporting opportunities trained and competed for during their careers. For the 'chosen few', it was welcome to the 'normal world'. Requests from footballers for mental health support from the PFA doubled.

Many footballers and staff came from abroad – some accompanied by families, others separated from loved ones.

All needed contact from clubs to ensure they were coping. Some lost those closest to them. Pep Guardiola's mother had died in Barcelona.

The loss of the pinnacle of careers following the cancellation of the Olympics must have been devastating for many. The 2021 rescheduled date did not come with guarantees of selection, form and freedom from injury. Dina Asher-Smith, Britain's fastest-ever woman sprinter, was the 2019 world champion over 200m and one of the favourites for 2020 glory. A hamstring injury in the British trials meant that she did not feature in either 2021 sprint final – but managed a bronze in the relay.

There can be golden linings to these dire situations. A few athletes whose Tokyo dreams had been dashed by injury could rekindle dreams for 2021. Footballers, like Marcus Rashford and Harry Kane, with injuries that threatened participation in the denouement of the 2019/20 football season, experienced a reprieve because of lockdown. They were freed of concerns over missing Euro 2020.

At Northants cricket (NCCC), Zoom meetings of the welfare group were organised. Non-furloughed clinical staff, club chaplain, sports psychologists, and the Professional Cricketers' Association (PCA) representative participated. Overseas players, isolated individuals and contract issues were reviewed. Contact was maintained with players.

Bill sent out 18 weekly newsletters to inform NCCC players and staff of developments. Information from various sources – government, PHE, sporting bodies and medical journals – were distilled to make it relevant for the players. Advice was offered on health matters, explaining the local medical situation, and what a return to training might look like.

NCCC organised remote social events, like quiz nights, for players and staff to maintain morale and monitor those fully engaged – and those who were not. A well-established backroom staff paid dividends. Knowing the players (and families) well over years and understanding different personalities helped to interpret their 'messages'.

The NCCC board invited Bill to their Zoom meetings for health updates. Chairman Gavin Warren remarked that five years previously he had an insolvency expert advising the board but now needed a doctor. Different times, different priorities. Supporters were not forgotten, and online forums answered questions and disseminated information.

The doctor would like to see you now

At the end of March, the *British Journal of Sports Medicine* published an impassioned article from Italian doctors imploring football not to restart until the crisis was controlled. Italian law conferred team doctors with ultimate control over players' health. All Serie A doctors warned football administrators via letter about planning too early a return. Not a level of control commonly ceded to the UK's touchline medics.

A month later, the FIFA Medical Committee's chairman, Dr Michel D'Hooghe, thought it unwise to consider playing competitive football until 1 September. Simultaneously, Dr Brian McCloskey, London 2012 Olympics public health director, advised a 'bottom-up not top-down' approach with community sport first to return based on the logistical difficulties of staging elite sport. Scotland's national clinical director, Jason Leitch, believed recreational tennis and golf would reappear first while football would be a 'difficult challenge'. The Premier League had never pictured itself lower in the pecking order than the local tennis club's mixed doubles.

The week beginning 27 April was pivotal in the genesis of Project Restart. The government and their advisers prepared to sit down with the major sports' medical advisers via video link. PHE representatives, including Deputy Chief Medical Officer and Boston United fan Jonathan Van-Tam, Culture Secretary Oliver Dowden, and medics from UK

Sport, football, rugby, cricket and racing met on Friday, 1 May. Premier League clubs convened remotely afterwards to digest the implications and inform their forward planning. One immediate decision was that all academy football would be stopped.

Eamonn Salmon, chief executive of the Football Medicine and Performance Association (FMPA), commented about the opinions over resumption amongst English football club clinicians, 'There are those who think it can be done, there are those that are doubtful, and there are those that probably suggest it is an impossible task.'

In all major UK sports, the CMOs met regularly during the early weeks of the crisis. Premier League club doctors wanted assurances including their own liability and insurance cover if players contracted the virus. They asked the Premier League for clarity over medical protocols, testing and player welfare. Four club doctors went further and posed 100 concerns and questions to the League in a letter.

Cause for concern?

The challenges presented by coronavirus elevated ever-present injury concerns to a new level. What were the main concerns over and above the scarcity of health access and specific BAME concerns?

The long-term effects from the virus remained unclear at that stage. Elite sports people are more prone to suffer from asthma. One fifth of endurance athletes have chronic respiratory conditions. Professional sport 'trades' in small differences in fitness between its participants. Even minor lung damage from the disease could affect long-term aerobic capacity and performance.

Additionally, elite athletes in high-intensity training may be at increased risk of altered inflammation and immunity, potentially affecting their response to viral exposure, particularly if their training load was increased quickly. This included the potential for cardiac inflammation. Strenuous physical activity requires deep inhalations. Researchers believed that this could increase the risk of athletes depositing viral particles deep within their lungs and increasing risks of disease complications.

Young athletes were not the only people involved in getting the show back on the road. Staff were likely to be older and more at risk. One Premiership manager was 72 years old. Players and staff may have had vulnerable family at home who needed shielding. News that Leeds United and England legend Norman Hunter had died from the virus on 17 April and the previous week Kenny Dalglish had contracted COVID-19 while in hospital focused people's minds.

Data suggested that dangers to young athletes from COVID-19 were minimal. The virus was clearly more lethal for the elderly but, nevertheless, over 240 people under 35 died from the disease in 2020.

There was every reason for the sports world to be concerned. Carefully planned protocols needed developing for the assessment and gradual return to exercise of anybody post-COVID-19.

Location, location, location

As early as mid-April, the Premier League was discussing the use of limited venues. It was accepted early that games would be played 'behind closed doors'. *The Mirror* reported that players might spend six weeks in nominated hotels.

Cricket and rugby union were exploring similar strategies. In America, plans were afoot to isolate professional athletes from the outside world. Possibilities included all ice hockey games in North Dakota, a cruise ship for basketball and a biodome for baseball.

For the first half of May, the issue of neutral grounds became a trial of strength between clubs, the Premier League, police and government. Limited venues was the police's preferred option as they feared large crowds gathering outside shuttered local grounds in densely populated areas. 'Some people in football need to recognise there's a bigger picture here,' said the UK's head of football policing, Mark Roberts.

Limited venues would make more efficient use of emergency services and better organisation for injured or ill players or staff. The reduced travel and ability to remain at local hotels would improve player recovery in a frantic fixture period – experienced subsequently by the American NBA. On 1 May, the Premier League told clubs that it was either neutral grounds or the season would be over.

The FA offered Wembley and St George's Park and the Premier League were considering using rugby's Twickenham. A football agent proposed moving the 20 clubs to Western Australia to complete the season – the same country that had 'padlocked' its borders to non-residents on 20 March and was not letting many of its own overseas citizens to return. Predictably, the idea was not picked up.

Within days, clubs at the wrong end of the Premier League table were opposing neutral venues. They felt their teams would be disadvantaged if perceived easier home games against weaker opposition were moved to neutral venues and the integrity of the competition compromised. Other clubs agreed. Votes on such decisions within the Premier League required a 14-6 majority. It would not be forthcoming.

By 13 May, it was reported that the clubs were winning the argument with government, police and the Sports Grounds Safety Association. Only two days before, Mark Roberts had told the clubs to 'get a grip'. Further discussions had placated the authorities if certain safeguards and messaging were in place. However, as late as 24 May, the possibility of a hybrid model (some games played on neutral turf) was back on the agenda to assuage police concerns.

The clubs would get their way – although negotiations continued even after the players had come back into training. Eventually, all games were played at the intended home grounds. Commentators speculated that such open opposition to the government and police would backfire long term on the Premier League and cement their reputation as a self-serving and rapacious outfit.

Logistics and undercooked bodies

After 11 March, 440 games in the Premier League, EFL and FA Cup remained in England to be completed. Four clubs were left in Europe with additional fixtures to be played. As the days ticked by the logistics of rescheduling became increasingly problematic. Producing a fixture list was one thing but a pre-season had to be scheduled and reasonable rest allowed before the 2020/21 season started.

No matter how diligent players were with home and individualised training, there would be an element of deconditioning increasing injury risk. As early as 3 April, Manchester City's Kevin De Bruyne expressed such concerns from being rushed back quickly. Returning players ideally needed their usual programme of carefully planned incremental workloads. Would there be enough pre-season games to regain match 'hardness'? Many sports injuries occur further down the track due to cumulative fatigue – both physical and mental. The spectre of the clash between player long-term welfare and short-term performance was ever-present.

Testing times … or not?

Sport's return required minimising athletes' risk of being infected or infecting others. The ability to identify a person with COVID-19 was critical. The question was how? Methods and means.

Ex-England team doctor Ian Beasley said, 'From a medical standpoint, I can support the prospect of games returning but with one key caveat. This can only be done by testing, testing, testing. But how do you test, when do you test, and how often do you test?'

The UK's capacity to test for such an eventuality was pitiful. Matt Hancock admitted the UK was starting from a 'lower base' in biotech capacity compared to Germany. Four days before lockdown, Boris Johnson promised an antibody test would be available soon in industrial quantities. 'A total game changer' that was fast 'coming down the track'. It veered off into a side turning and was all 'hot air'.

The UK was relying on the COVID-19 PCR (polymerase chain reaction) antigen test. The problem was that not many tests could or were being performed. On 28 March 2020, the government reported that only 177 tests were processed – utilising under two per cent of the nation's available laboratory capacity. The country had no ability to mass test potentially infected patients, health and social services staff, and thousands of elderly and infirm decanted from hospital beds into the community. This produced a moral debate over prioritising sports people for testing. Even if undertaken privately.

On 30 April, Chelsea's manager Frank Lampard said, 'It's important for football to take its place – I don't think it would sit well with me or anyone if we didn't make sure people were being tested on that front line.' Football feared a public relations disaster if it were seen to be receiving preferential treatment. This was recognised by the League Managers' Association's (LMA) chief executive, Richard Bevan, stating that tests must be made available first to NHS workers and patients: 'Once that's happened, by all means let's access it in sport.'

Even if capacity and ethics could be solved, testing was not without further problems. Pooled global studies reported an average of 40 per cent of patients with positive COVID-19 tests were asymptomatic. A positive test had a lot to do with timing during the disease process. Some continued to test positive long after they had ceased to be contagious. How would that be interpreted for a footballer champing at the bit to begin rehabilitation?

What would be the cost of testing athletes twice weekly? A single PCR test was expensive – £100 or more. The EFL calculated its 71 clubs' testing regime required 66,000 tests at a total cost of £6.6m or £93,000 per club. Without gate money, where would the funds come from unless the government stepped in? They wouldn't.

The Premier League was on a different financial planet and contracted with Hong Kong-based company Prenetics. Forty thousand home-testing kits would be ordered to cover ten weeks of training and playing to finish the season. A £4m bill. The decision did not meet with the approval of all in football. Watford's goalkeeper Ben Foster told BBC's *Newsbeat*, 'Footballers are not essential key workers; we shouldn't have access to tests before front-line workers.'

Beyond the specific COVID-19 tests, players and staff would require layers of health testing. Well-being questionnaires and apps needed to be completed before leaving home. Temperature testing was required prior to entry for training and games. Attending media and security staff would need including.

Each sport needed to consider the specific risks of their own activities. Where were likely points of cross-contamination? What changes were required to the training and stadia environment? Did any changes need to be made to the conduct of the game itself?

The development of risk assessments and protocols was going to occupy sports administrators and medical personnel for weeks.

Under pressure and keeping up with 'the Schmidts'

'Pressure, pushing down on me'
'Under Pressure'. David Bowie and Queen. 1981

As well as the logistical, financial, ethical and personal reservations about Project Restart, many felt that external forces were pressuring elite sport to return and override multiple misgivings.

Football had emerged from its bruising early-April battle with politicians on pay cuts and furlough decisions. Less than a month later, the sport found itself being courted by the ruling classes.

The prime minister said football would 'provide a much-needed boost to national morale'. A desire by the government to provide entertainment for a population growing weary of lockdown restrictions? The Norwich striker Todd Cantwell responded that 'we are people too' in a social media post.

UEFA was pressing for decisions and action. On 2 April, the Belgian Pro League had announced the season's abandonment. The next day, UEFA threatened leagues and teams with expulsion from the following season's European competitions for not trying to fulfil fixtures. The organisation was concerned that larger leagues faced massive financial problems if broadcast income was lost. There was the real danger of the Champions League and Europa League not being completed if clubs ceased playing domestically. On 28 April, UEFA gave European leagues a 25 May deadline to provide restart details. As Sir Alex Ferguson might have said it was squeaky bum time.

During April, the French and Dutch joined Belgium in abandoning all football – contributed to by their governments' stances on pandemic restrictions. However, Italy and Spain remained confident of getting the 'soccer show' back on the road despite the devastation the pandemic had wrought on their societies. Even Denmark's SuperLiga would restart before the end of May.

It was the sight of the German Bundesliga cranking up to play that could be seen as both a blessing and a curse to English domestic football. By virtue of its superior testing capacity and provision of ITU beds, Germany had fared better than most in the early months of the pandemic and, thus, better equipped to restart football. Additionally, it had been first to put in the hard yards on testing and protocols from which the rest of the sports world could learn. However, jeopardy lay close to the surface. A significant viral outbreak, despite sensible measures, could prove curtains for all other endeavours.

The Premier League has a view of its own position within the pantheon of global sport. It did not want to be left behind by its German, Italian and Spanish cousins.

The darling buds of May

There were so many factors to weigh up and so little time to achieve it as English football moved through the first weeks of May. We had all become conversant with terms like bio-secure bubbles, Project Restart and PCR testing.

Some Premier League clubs had allowed players to return to individual training from 27 April. At the beginning of May, managers and players located abroad were asked to return to England.

The government was onside and doctors and major sports were working hard to exchange ideas. It appeared that some parts of football would be able to re-emerge. The Premier League had won its battles with the police and sections of the media. As Dr Ian Beasley commented, 'When it comes to deciding whether Project Restart should go ahead, it is more of an economic question than a medical one.'

The timing and extent of that return would hinge on negotiations that occupied the middle of May.

Chapter 7

On Your Marks …
for Project Restart

13 May–17 June

Domestic planning regulations

On 13 May 2020, the government published its long-awaited roadmap for elite sport's return. All sport would follow its principles in their quest to return to training and, ultimately, competition.

'Step One' defined who qualified as an elite athlete. It permitted a return of organised individual training in a prescribed performance facility while adhering to social distancing. Guidance was clear on areas such as facility cleaning and staff and athlete testing. It mandated organisations to identify 'COVID officers' and 'COVID medical officers' for developing risk assessments and ensuring adherence to protocols.

Sports like running and cycling were easier to reintroduce. Other activities could be undertaken with social distancing. It meant angling and singles tennis could restart from 13 May in England. Golf could commence as a solitary pastime or with household members.

While Brits chewed over solutions, Germany had taken the plunge. The Bundesliga was already back in training and looking forward to an imminent return of football matches. How were they coping?

The Germans show a clean pair of heels

March was not out before the Bundesliga confirmed its determination to complete the nine outstanding rounds of matches of their season. Before the end of June.

Like in the UK, football faced opposition. Virologists called for the season to be declared null and void. They questioned the ethics of tens of thousands of COVID-19 tests being required while there remained a shortage for the general population. Some believed no football would be possible for a year. Players were clearly conflicted. Fears of contracting the virus through team-mate contact was tempered by the financial necessity of completing the season.

In early April, the potential apocalypse of not finishing the season was clear. It was estimated that, if no more games were played, 13 of the 36 clubs in the Bundesliga and Bundesliga 2 would declare bankruptcy by June. Some had already spent 'forward' revenues servicing debt, assuming monies would continue rolling in. The authorities decreed that clubs entering insolvency proceedings would not suffer the usual points deduction – losing only three points instead of nine.

On 6 April, some clubs came back into training. Players had to socially distance, train in small groups, arrive at the ground changed and avoid contact. Germany had experienced a seventh of the deaths of the UK overall. That day, the country reported 92 daily deaths from COVID-19 compared to the UK's toll of 1,038. By mid-April, Germany was conducting 100,000 daily tests. It was several weeks ahead of the UK in their ramping-up ability. Deaths, hospitals at breaking point and relative lack of testing was why English football resumption lagged behind the German restart.

On 23 April, the Bundesliga released its 41-page handbook outlining the protocols required for football restarting. A maximum of 322 people would be allowed inside a ground for matches. Each would be subject to stringent security and medical controls. COVID-19 tests and temperatures would be scrutinised. Procedures for transportation, arrival, changing rooms, post-match showering and team benches were mapped out. This involved segregation, social distancing, mask wearing and sanitisation. Post-match media conferences would be virtual. Among those who failed to make the cut were club mascots. This included Cologne's Hennes the goat, who had led out the side for every home game since 1950. There had been nine caprine reincarnations to date. Even players' wives and partners had to agree to either regularly test, live separately or compile contact tracing lists.

With no fans in the ground, some clubs became inventive. Borussia Monchengladbach announced that fans could pay for cardboard cut-outs of themselves to put in the empty stadium. At a cost of 19 euros each. On 23 May, thousands of stiff spectators were silenced as their side slid to a 1-3 home defeat by Bayer Leverkusen. Monies raised were donated to charities. Other clubs and countries would follow suit. FC Seoul in South Korea's K-league had to apologise to fans for filling the stands with blow-up sex dolls advertising pornographic websites.

The Premier League's chances of a return depended upon the Bundesliga successfully negotiating this 'viral minefield'. UK clubs, doctors and government officials assiduously took notes. The Premier League's medical adviser, Dr Mark Gillett, reported that discussions would take place in the coming weeks over whether clubs would follow the German protocols and isolate teams in hotels pre-resumption.

Angela Merkel, German Chancellor, gave the green light on 6 May. Games would start ten days later. The Bundesliga moved from starting non-contact training to matches in 40 days following a 24-day complete shutdown. Tackling in training only began in early May. Before that, FIFA had announced the five substitutes rule to ease player injury concerns during a compressed season. Individual competitions, such as the Bundesliga and Premier League, would have the discretion to implement it or not.

Football would not be the first sport to return in Germany. Exhibition professional tennis matches started behind closed doors on 1 May. Even cricket training was allowed to start mid-May with friendly warm-up matches pencilled in to follow.

Regular testing of players, staff and officials had already commenced. On 1 May, FC Cologne announced that three people had tested positive. One Cologne player called the Bundesliga 'irresponsible' for planning to resume the season. Three days later, ten cases were reported across the two leagues. On 4 May, ex-Chelsea striker Salomon Kalou was suspended from training by Hertha Berlin. The Ivorian had posted a social media video of him fist-bumping, clapping hands with team-mates and barging in on another player's coronavirus test.

The teams were due to spend one week from 9 May in hotel isolation ahead of the first game. Players would even have their own condiments sachets at mealtimes. It would be the beginning of 'bubble life' that would become so familiar to elite athletes across the world for the next two years. Presciently, Tim Meyer, the Bundesliga's head of coronavirus task force, warned about requiring teams to stay in quarantine for long periods: 'We do not know … what the consequences of it are … not just on a medical but also a psychological level.'

The cat was put amongst the pigeons that day when Bundesliga 2 side Dynamo Dresden placed their entire squad and coaching staff into a fortnight's isolation after two players tested positive. The club, who were bottom of their league, had to postpone their first two games. The decision by Dresden local health authority was at variance with the ruling made by the Cologne authorities a week earlier, who deemed that there had been no close contacts with the 'infected ones' – an observation challenged by a Cologne player. The Dynamos never regained their spark and were relegated at the end of June.

Isolation proved too much for some. On the eve of his team's first game, the Augsburg head coach, Heiko Herrlich, breached quarantine by leaving the team hotel to buy toothpaste. He had to sit out his club's opener against Wolfsburg but at least he had clean teeth. As later in the UK, regulations were hard to follow in the heat of the moment. Players had to be reminded of guidelines after Hertha Berlin's players celebrated during their 3-0 win at Hoffenheim. Later, six Borussia Dortmund players, including England international Jadon Sancho, were warned after taking selfies while having their hair cut without face masks.

For avid watchers in England, several trends were noticeable in the early German matches. There were increased injuries. The pressing intensity of teams, which is such a feature of the Bundesliga, was reduced. Increased goals from set pieces was noted. Hot weather, reduced fitness and tactical sharpness were all potential contributory factors. Additionally, the lack of crowds was reducing home advantage.

Despite all the regulations and concerns, the Bundesliga was completed on 27 June. To demonstrate that even in those unprecedented times some things never change, Bayern Munich won their eighth successive title.

And so, the blueprint was set for other football leagues and sports around the world to follow. Game on.

'But soon you will find that there comes a time for making your mind up'

Lyrics from 'Making Your Mind Up' by Bucks Fizz. Eurovision winner. 1981

For elite British sport, the middle of May was make your mind up time. Who would be capable of returning? Who could not financially contemplate abandoning their season? In which parts of sport did the maths not add up? In the 12 days between Steps One and Two government publications, a lot of difficult decisions had to be made.

Every sport and club laid the Step One blueprint on to its own activity and assessed whether it could comply safely to minimise employee risk. The same week, Boris Johnson and his team attended a wine and cheese gathering in the Downing Street garden, and COVID-19 protests were held at venues around the UK.

It was appreciated that not all sports would restart at the same time. Some would deem it unsafe to return for the immediate future. Analysis was undertaken of training and game situations. Various sports began to scrutinise pinch points within their activities. Rugby union's scrums and mauls came under scrutiny. Football games had to be examined. A Danish study found that footballers spent 98 seconds on average within the 'exposure zone' of an infected fellow player. Strikers and centre-backs were most at risk because of their 'duelling frequency'. One virologist, Copenhagen's Professor Thomsen, believed football would not be a problem in fanning contagion but that rugby codes and American football were of concern.

Following the 13 May Step One publication, frenetic activity involving meetings of government and health officials, the Premier League, PFA and League Managers' Association took place over safety and medical protocols.

'You say goodbye and I say hello'

Lyrics from 'Hello Goodbye' by The Beatles. 1967

While the elite end of football was busy planning their restart, stark realities hit the lower tiers. With players furloughed, no spectators, and ruinously expensive testing and safety regimens, League One and Two clubs faced significant losses in trying to complete the season.

Two days later, on 15 May, League Two clubs unanimously announced their wish to end the season with final positions determined on a points-per-game basis. However, they would have to wait for EFL ratification.

League One clubs had reached a stalemate. Six clubs were determined to carry on. The Peterborough chairman took to Twitter: 'We have no desire for voiding the season, points-per-game scenarios or letting a computer decide our footballing fate.' It would not be until 9 June that the EFL decided to abandon League One's season and for League Two's earlier decision to be confirmed. Inevitably, there would be disgruntled clubs. Peterborough's (again) director of football Barry Fry told the BBC, 'I feel my club has been cheated out of promotion.'

The top two clubs in League One and top three clubs in League Two would be promoted automatically. The next four teams in each division were allowed to enter the play-offs behind closed doors in June and July. Similar numbers of clubs were relegated.

Stevenage should have joined Macclesfield in being relegated out of the Football League but were reprieved following Bury's demise. Their owner, Phil Wallace, explained the issues faced by all clubs at that level, 'It would cost us £140,000 for the tests, we would have to bring players out of furlough and comply with a 47-page health and safety document regarding sterilisation of stadiums, etc.' Until 11 August, Stevenage were bottom and relegated after the points-per-game calculations were undertaken. However, two months after the season was abandoned, and only one month before the new season started, it was all change at League Two base camp. After twists and turns that would have done justice to Harry Houdini, Macclesfield's accumulated misdemeanours and consequent penalty points caught up with them. They were dumped out of the League and replaced by Barrow from the Vanarama National League. Barrow's return ended a 48-year exile. In the autumn of 2020, Macclesfield were wound up and expelled from tier 5.

Meanwhile, north of the border, it was all too much for the Scots, who announced that their season would end. Celtic were named Premiership champions for the ninth successive season and Hearts were relegated. Welsh domestic leagues came to a similar decision.

'All together now … all together now'
Lyrics from 'All Together Now'. *Yellow Submarine* album.
The Beatles. 1969

On 18 May, London recorded no new COVID-19 cases for the first time. Premier League clubs agreed for Stage One training involving socially distanced small group sessions to start the next day. The Italian Serie A and Spanish La Liga would follow suit. Players had to submit a pre-arrival health questionnaire and have their temperatures taken on arrival. Methods of monitoring protocol adherence were mooted, including 'surprise inspections', GPS player tracking and video analysis. A maximum of five players could be included in a group. Training was guillotined at 75 minutes. All equipment was disinfected after every session.

The Premier League reassured the world that 'strict medical protocols of the highest standard will ensure everyone returns to training in the safest environment possible'. However, a survey revealed that half of Premier League and EFL doctors and physiotherapists did 'not fully understand their roles, responsibilities and potential liabilities' regarding return to training. Dr Eva Carneiro, the sports physician unceremoniously dumped by Chelsea in 2015, stated that football should not be rushed back until the long-term risks of COVID-19 on players' physiology was understood.

Even after the players were back on the training paddock, there was still no consensus on how and when competition would resume. On 20 May, the Secretary of State for Digital, Culture, Media and Sport, Oliver Dowden, announced the establishment of a task force that would look at how sporting and arts events could resume safely. It would be supported by eight working sub-groups, including sports' representatives.

On 25 May, Stage Two of elite sport's return to training was published. It allowed athletes to return to contact training – initially in clusters of two or three and expanding finally to full team training. It was incumbent upon clubs and sports to determine risks and ensure all protocols were in place. As for Stage One, the Premier League discussed the details with all and sundry and announced that contact training would begin the next week. The low infection rates and player GPS tracking to monitor close contact time helped assuage players' fears. GPS data demonstrated that players in squad training were halving their 'close encounters'. The same day, Dominic Cummings appeared in the Downing Street Rose Garden to explain his 'flight' to Durham. Three days afterwards, the UK's Track and Trace system finally became operational.

The appearance of the training grounds was different. At Liverpool's Melwood, physiotherapists and doctors in full PPE sought shelter under gazebos. Temporary gyms were erected pitch-side and makeshift outdoor urinals appeared.

Less than three weeks before kick-off, the possibility of a hybrid model of home grounds and neutral venues was still on the table. Two weeks before restart, the police were still insisting on having the final say on whether games deemed high risk for civil disorder, such as Liverpool and London derbies, could be moved to safer sites.

However, football could see light at the end of the tunnel. Three days after Stage Two's publication, the Premier League announced its season would recommence on 17 June – 100 days after the stoppage. Government needed to placate an increasingly weary population. It was announced that BBC would televise live league games for the first time since 1988. Sky TV and Amazon Prime would make certain games free to watch. Viewers could turn on artificial crowd noise via their red buttons.

However, all was dependent upon government approval. On 30 May, Dowden published Stage Three. It set out the conditions for the return of competitive sport behind closed doors from 1 June. The speed of events was becoming dizzyingly fast. Three weighty documents in 17 days from the government had landed on elite sports' doormats. Administrators, medical staff, coaches, and health and safety officers were having to digest the information and formulate plans for their organisations.

Football would not be the first to return. That honour would be held by greyhound racing, horse racing and snooker. The Premier League would have to wait for over another fortnight.

The English Championship elected to bring players back into training on 25 May. Although nearly a week behind the Premier League, they planned to restart only three days later. Not all clubs agreed. Especially those at the league's wrong end. Hull City opposed a restart. At the time, they were one place above the relegation spots and would eventually be relegated. Bottom-placed club Barnsley were even more vociferous in their criticism. They were eight points adrift of safety. 'If the 2019/20 season is completed, it will be completed with a lack of sporting integrity,' the club said. 'Some clubs will have unbalanced squads compared to competitors due to ending player contracts. Some clubs will lose home-field advantage for matches behind closed doors in respect to the reverse fixture earlier this season. This is especially true with big rivalries and the loss of the respective revenue. Those clubs unfairly and unlawfully relegated to a lower division would face further uncertainty and potential failure of their enterprise.' Ironically, in the end, they escaped the drop by one point.

Some high-profile footballers were still having trouble understanding lockdown restrictions. Spurs' Serge Aurier posted a picture on social media with his hairdresser – six weeks before the rest of the nation was allowed to stop resembling desert-island castaways. It was the right-back's third documented COVID indiscretion. Manchester City had to warn Phil Foden for playing an impromptu football match on a beach. Foden would continue to have problems social distancing in Iceland three months later.

What about the players who had expressed reservations about returning to training? Watford's Troy Deeney delayed his return until early June, having expressed concerns for the health of family members and the BAME community in general. Chelsea's N'Golo Kante returned initially with colleagues but then changed his mind. He trained alone at home – a move which his club supported. He rejoined team-mates only 12 days before the resumption's opening fixtures. With a family history of cardiac problems, Chelsea said they would be content if he elected to miss the rest of the season. He would go on to contract COVID-19 in the autumn of 2021 and miss important matches but without any long-term health implications. At the time, a government review confirmed that members of the BAME community were twice as likely to die from COVID-19. In the summer of 2022, Kante would be one of several Premier League players unable to travel for pre-season games in America because they were not vaccinated.

'Every positive value has its price in negative terms'
Spanish painter Pablo Picasso. (1881–1973)

The twice-weekly COVID-19 PCR testing started before clubs came back into training. It involved all players and staff. In the Premier League, over 10,000 tests were taken in four weeks before the first competitive ball was kicked in anger. Some clubs feared that rivals would lie about positive tests or deliberately bodge tests. Medical confidentiality precluded infected individuals being identified. Only 17 positive cases were returned. Championship testing involved over 11,600 tests for the 24 clubs with 43 positive cases. The testing of the eight clubs involved in the League One and League Two play-offs resulted in 17 positive cases from over 3,000 tests.

The frequency of COVID-19 cases deteriorated with league status. Premier League rates were 1:600 tests, the Championship at 1:270, and Leagues One and Two combined at 1:179. Whether that was due to better controls, resources and/or compliance in the Premier League is difficult to judge. There were no reports than any players or staff became seriously ill. No clubs witnessed major outbreaks delaying their season's start – as occurred at Dresden in the Bundesliga. The low number of Premier League positives encouraged clubs not to follow the Bundesliga with hotel quarantine before restart – not to mention that most hotels remained closed. Similarly, wives and girlfriends were not requested to move house or be regularly tested as in Germany.

In early June, clubs were given permission to play friendlies behind closed doors. There was some disruption. Stoke visited Manchester United's Carrington training ground. The players had arrived at the ground when news came through that the visitors' manager, Michael O'Neill, had tested positive. A hasty exit stage right for the Potters. Meanwhile, all visitors to the UK had to quarantine for 14 days.

Italian regulations were tighter. Players back in training were informed that the entire squad would be quarantined for two weeks if any player or staff member tested positive. Two days before kick-off, the sanctions were softened requiring only positive tests to isolate but everybody else would be subjected to extra testing including pre-game.

'Everybody Hurts'

Song by R.E.M. 1992

The publication of the rescheduled fixture list for the Premier League and FA Cup was accompanied by warnings of an impending potential injury crisis. Forecasters Zone 7 reported that playing eight games in 30 days increased a player's injury risk by 25 per cent compared to the more normal four to five matches over the same time span. Manchester City faced a potential 13 fixtures across three competitions in 49 days. The problem was compounded by the shortened pre-season. Managers including Watford's Nigel Pearson and Newcastle's Steve Bruce voiced concerns. Players would normally expect a number of pre-season warm-up games to regain fitness and sharpness. Now the sides would be using early competitive matches to ramp up.

From previously shortened pre-seasons (due to summer international competitions), Zone 7 had identified three quarters of clubs experiencing increased injuries in the first half of seasons. Thighs, groins, knees and ankles were specific areas of concern. One sports scientist predicted that players had lost up to 15 per cent of their fitness – which had to be regained in less than three weeks of squad training. Dutch conditioning coach Raymond Verheijen, who had worked at Barcelona, Chelsea and Manchester City, believed that football was playing 'Russian roulette with the health of players'. The early reports from the Bundesliga were not encouraging. The Germans experienced a 225 per cent increase in injuries after four rounds of matches.

Ex-England manager Fabio Capello said, 'I fear injuries more than the virus. The risk of muscle injuries is already high in training. If they play three matches in a week, the physical recovery time between one game and another will be difficult.'

Further afield concerns were raised about rushing athletes back into action. In America's NBA, coaches wanted a minimum of one month's physical preparation otherwise they predicted 'a mess'. Strength and conditioning coaches emphasised that managers needed to understand training-load principles and the importance of assessing individual players' physical status. In Australia, Aussie Rules players had similar concerns about the risks of a four-week build-up to a season reset.

Alarm bells were ringing for Championship players' welfare. Ex-Aston Villa and England international Tony Daley, who spent ten years as fitness and conditioning coach at Molineux, told the PA news agency: 'It's definitely a week, minimum, too early to come back [to playing]. Players will have been doing something to tick over but you can't substitute football fitness, contact, accelerating, decelerating and in two-and-a-half weeks. They will have been mentally switched off and to come back in two-and-a-half weeks, it's a big ask. It can be done but I won't be surprised if there's a large increase in muscle injuries.'

Replacement, rehydration and redesignation

As in the Bundesliga, English football announced that five substitutes could be used in the Premier League – an increase from three. However, changes could only be made at three opportunities to minimise game disruption. A drinks break in each half was announced to counter dehydration and fatigue from playing games un-seasonally in the height of summer. Game Day Protocols were agreed only six days before kick-off. Elaborate flow charts and designated colour zones of stadia were mapped out.

Finally, on the evening of 17 June 2020, Aston Villa and Sheffield United played out a 0-0 draw in front of an eerily silent Villa Park. La Liga had kicked off six days earlier and Serie A three days later.

Football was back – but, in so many ways, not as we remembered it.

Chapter 8

Football. A Game of Two Halves

The 39 steps

Games came thick and fast.

The Premier League's 'second half' involved 92 matches over 39 days. Its 20 clubs finished on 26 July. Most clubs had nine fixtures to complete – a few had ten. Additionally, European competitions and the final three FA Cup rounds needed completing. The 24 Championship clubs would play 108 games over 33 days – followed by the play-offs.

There was no doubting the public's appetite to watch football. Liverpool and Everton's first game back would be a Merseyside derby. It attracted five million viewers on 'free to watch' Sky – a record for a live Premier League match. It finished 0-0. Previously, the police had flagged the match as a potential powder keg worthy of consideration for a neutral venue. In the event, it was played as scheduled at Goodison Park.

'Let there be light(s), and there was light(s)'

Genesis 1:3. The Bible

Stadia were organised into three traffic light zones – red, amber and green. The red zone included the pitch, technical areas, tunnel and dressing rooms. Only 110 personnel could enter this zone and had to provide negative tests in the five days prior to kick-off. The amber zone covered the rest of the stadia interior not included in the red zones – including stands, concourses and pitch-side interview areas. The green zone represented the space outside the stadium including access control points and parking.

Every player, coach and clinician destined for the red zone completed a medical questionnaire and had temperature checks on arrival. Each would hold a 'clinical passport' either on mobiles or paper confirming negative COVID-19 status. Amber zone attendees, like the media, displayed the results of a self-administered test taken within 24 hours of kick-off on a smartphone. They were checked for a fever. It was not the tightest of bio-security protocols. Health security at Wembley was stricter with additional heart rate and oxygen saturation tests administered by clinical staff.

Only 300 people could be present inside grounds for games – less than in the Bundesliga. Each club's matchday squad would be capped at 20 to include seven potential substitutes and two 'spares' in case of sudden illness. Combined coaching and medical staff could not exceed 12 personnel – a problem for clubs like Manchester City, who frequently exceeded that number. Like German mascots, ball boys and girls failed to make the cut. Players would have to field their own balls with clean ones placed on cones around the sidelines. Broadcasters had a maximum team of 98 inside the ground and another 75 in the car park. Only 25 journalists and four doping control officers were permitted entry.

'Cause I'm leaving on a jet plane'

Lyrics from 'Leaving on a Jet Plane' by Peter, Paul and Mary. 1967

German protocols for prolonged hotel quarantine were not enacted. Indeed, clubs were asked to avoid them, if possible, while accepting that government guidelines allowed an athletes' exemption to use hotels if required. For clubs like Norwich, travel-distance issues might require overnight stays.

Clubs were encouraged to charter private planes for long-haul away travel. Some teams chartered larger-than-normal planes. Eco-friendly travel would have to be suspended for 'the duration'. On the ground, clubs might use two coaches – some of which were reconfigured by placing seats back-to-back. Coach drivers were expected to COVID-19 test. Home players were encouraged to use personal transport if possible.

Red routes and readying rooms

A 'sterile route' conveyed red-zoners to changing rooms, which were adapted to provide a two-metre socially distanced and stripped-back environment. If space was too small, other areas, like hospitality suites and dining areas, could be repurposed. Any person feeling ill at the stadium would be led to a designated isolation room pending further medical checks prior to being dispatched home if safe.

Sidelined

On the touchline, technical areas for managers and players were enlarged as substitute numbers were increased. A total of seven substitutes could be named but only five utilised. A further variance from the Bundesliga was that players and coaches could choose whether to wear masks on arrival at the stadia and on the bench. The Premier League's GPS data of 300 games concluded that 98 per cent of players spend less than five minutes in close contact during matches.

Substitutes could be observed strung out and draped over spectating seating in the empty stands. Fourth officials, despite being subjected to similar testing regimes, were required to mask up. Was their ability to contract and/or spread the virus different from players and managers? Physios and doctors donned PPE on the sidelines ready to attend stricken players.

Standard-bearers

Pre-kick-off, entry on to the pitch was restricted. Players were encouraged to socially distance in the warm-up. The two teams were not allowed to enter the arena side-by-side.

Players were expected to hand sanitise on entering and leaving the field. On the pitch, certain standards were expected. No handshaking, spitting or nasal clearouts were permitted. At the drinks intervals, players would have to swig from their own labelled bottles. Goal congratulations were expected to be socially distanced, and scorers directed to specific 'celebration cameras' to interact with supporters at home. Players were told not to surround or manhandle referees.

However, there did not appear to be any sanctions for players breaching guidelines. It was one reason why so many of the rules didn't survive first engagement with the enemy. Requests for retaining one's own bodily fluids, not approaching referees and polite socially distanced acknowledgements of goals went unheeded. Images on TV screens appeared of opposition managers 'elbow greeting' and then hugging each other.

'It's over, it's over, it's over'
Lyrics from 'It's Over' by Roy Orbison. 1964

At 90 minutes, players would disappear for their post-game socially distanced showers. No sharing of shampoo bottles would be the order of the day. Post-game treatments were limited to 15 minutes. Player recovery regimes were completed at home.

Anything touched by players or backroom staff was disinfected – balls, goalposts, substitution boards and corner flags. Dugouts and changing rooms were scrubbed.

Television would be able to get their 'pound of flesh' interviews around the pitch perimeter at a distance. However, the 25 media scribes would conduct post-match press conferences remotely via Zoom.

'All in all, you're just another brick in the wall'
Lyrics from 'Another Brick in the Wall'. Pink Floyd. 1979

Lack of spectator interaction was an irritant. Perhaps wisely the Premier League decided not to use cardboard cut-outs or 'questionable' inflatable dolls as replacements. In the stadia, instructions from the touchline and player interactions were clearly audible. As mentioned earlier, domiciled fans could add canned spectator noise to enhance their experience. Some clubs utilised the 'virtual fan wall'. Sixteen fans from each side could be selected. Their reactions to key moments were beamed on to huge screens at the ground while sitting on the sofa at home bedecked in their club's livery. In addition, each home side had the opportunity to decorate their empty lower stands with 'wrap arounds' and play music at key moments.

It was all very surreal and sterile – in more ways than one.

Scene setting

The completion of the English football season cannot be viewed in glorious isolation from the events nationally where the virus waned and then waxed during those 39 days.

Two days before the season restarted, compulsory face masks were introduced on public transport. However, cases were falling and reached their lowest point in early July. The public were becoming restless. In hot weather at the end of June, half a million flocked to the beaches around Bournemouth, earning a rebuke from the prime minister – who himself had enjoyed a less than socially distanced birthday party in Downing Street as the first games began.

Super Saturday was celebrated on 4 July as pubs and restaurants began to open. However, Leicester were playing their first home games in a city where cases were three times higher than any other UK metropolis and were put back into lockdown.

Mimicking football, the UK government announced a traffic light system of its own. It applied to safe 'travel corridors'. Travellers returning from 59 countries would not have to quarantine on arrival from 10 July. Holiday bookings had exploded amongst Brits suffering from cabin fever. However, cases rose across Europe. Spain was severely affected. Numbers surged in popular destinations like Majorca. On the last day of the Premier League season, a 14-day quarantine was reimposed from the next day for travellers returning from that country. Cue queues of angry Brits rushing to Iberian airports to escape re-incarceration.

By a country mile

At the time of the national lockdown in March, Liverpool was leading the Premier League by a massive 25 points. Two more wins from their remaining nine fixtures would clinch their 19th league title. Their triumph would be their first for 20 years and their first in the Premier League era. Their scintillating form led to the best-ever season's start in the history of the top five European leagues.

Their supporters were ready to celebrate this unforgettable achievement. If the season did not restart, Liverpool risked the same fate as Ajax in Holland. Despite leading the Eredivisie at the time of its March suspension, the Dutch club were not awarded the title when the Royal Dutch Football Association (KNVB) annulled the season. It would have been too much for the patient Koppites.

The red mist descends

Liverpool secured their title eight days after the restart when Manchester City lost at Chelsea. The Reds never managed to recapture the heights from the earlier part of their campaign. They lost two and drew two of their final nine games. Their final winning margin was cut to 18 points, and they fell one point shy of Manchester City's record total of 100 points. However, they achieved a double of sorts. They won the title earlier than anybody (with seven games to play) and won the title latest of anybody (in late June).

There would be no open-top bus parade, but their supporters came out in celebration. Within hours of confirmation of the title, thousands of supporters let off red fireworks and celebrated in the streets. Especially outside Anfield. Three hundred fans fought with police. The city council sent out a mixed message telling fans to 'have a great party' but continue social distancing. Fat chance. Liverpool's assistant chief constable more soberly reminded fans of their social responsibility as Merseyside had been 'disproportionately affected' by the pandemic. An MP from parliament's DCMS committee took aim at Jürgen Klopp and the players for putting videos on social media of wild celebrations at their own party. Afterwards a contrite Klopp asked fans to revel privately at home. Liverpool's case rate rose in early July before falling again over the next two weeks to their lowest levels of the pandemic.

Hamstrung

The remaining eight clubs in the FA Cup were all from the Premier League. The quarter- and semi-finals would be slotted in between league fixtures. The final would be held at Wembley on 1 August – six days after the Premier League concluded. In that game, Chelsea lost 1-2 to their London rivals Arsenal. Both clubs were playing their 12th game in 45 days. Chelsea sustained two serious hamstring tears to Azpilicueta and Pulisic and their substitute forward Pedro dislocated his shoulder. All could have occurred during a 'normal' season game but the hamstring injuries particularly raised concerns over the degree of muscle fatigue despite enhanced sports science conditioning.

The view from abroad

While the Bundesliga finished on 27 June, other major leagues abroad more closely mirrored the Premier League programme. Major leagues and sports were sharing intelligence across the globe. Consequently, most strategies were remarkably aligned. La Liga concluded on 19 July and Serie A on 2 August.

The completed Spanish season reduced potential financial losses from a predicted one billion euros to 300 million euros. Guidelines included details on how groceries would be delivered to players' homes during match weeks. La Liga installed one 'enforcer', or inspector, to each club to ensure compliance. Even players' social media posts were scrutinised. In Portugal's Primeira Liga, CD Santa Clara had to move their home games 892 miles to near Lisbon. They were based in the Azores that maintained a 14-day quarantine period during the restarted season.

The Euro(isolation) zone

The 17 June restart for English football was also a pivotal day in decision-making for the two main European competitions' completion. August 2020 would be devoted, football-wise, to the denouement of these enterprises.

The Champions League had reached the quarter-finals at the time of lockdown. Two neutral venues in Lisbon were chosen to host the finale. The original host, Istanbul, lost out. Two-legged quarter- and semi-finals were scrapped. The seven games were played over 11 days in mid-August – behind closed doors. England's sole remaining representatives, Manchester City, departed at the quarter-final stage. The four semi-finalists came equally from France and Germany. City had 'enjoyed' a four-week break after bowing out of the FA Cup in the semi-finals. However, the French teams had not played since March and the German domestic season was wrapped up by early July. It could be argued that no team had the optimal build-up to the continent's premier competition – that difficult balance between sufficient rest and match sharpness.

In the UEFA Europa League, the first legs had not been completed in the round of 16 when the pandemic struck. Eight return legs and two first legs remained. Glasgow Rangers and Wolverhampton Wanderers had begun their campaigns in July 2019. Over 13 months later, they were still soldiering on. The final 15 games would be completed in 16 days with the last nine games held as one-legged occasions at various locations in Germany. Venue decisions were made on the day

English football re-emerged and reflected the Bundesliga's successful early return. The original venue for the final was Gdańsk in Poland. The decision to move to Germany was taken even though Poland's Ekstraklasa league had restarted at the end of May and by 21 June was playing before one-quarter-full stadia. Sevilla took their seventh title in Cologne when they beat Inter Milan 3-2 on 21 August. Rangers fell in the round of 16 having not played a competitive game for five months. Wolves bowed out in their quarter-final, and Manchester United in the semi-finals.

Home bankers and cautionary tales

What effect did empty stadiums have on results? In the Premier League, many of the clubs at the wrong end of the table campaigned energetically against neutral venues. In the event, no English games were switched by the police from their designated grounds.

Reading University researchers examined the effect of behind-closed-doors football across 17 countries. They compared 1,498 games after the restart compared to 4,983 before the pandemic. The results were revealing. Despite early restart rounds in the Bundesliga showing a reduced home advantage, the final analysis demonstrated only a 1.6 per cent fall overall. In English Premier League and Championship games, home wins fell only from 43.4 per cent to 42.0 per cent. However, the influence of fans in grounds was revealed in refereeing decisions. The production of yellow cards overall fell – but more for the away sides.

'Didn't they do well?'

Catchphrase of Bruce Forsyth. *The Generation Game* on TV. 1971

Testing of players and staff continued twice weekly once matches started again. The impressively low rates of positive results in the Premier League during training continued and even improved during the 39 days. Only three positive tests were returned over five weeks. The overall rate of positive tests throughout the entire Project Restart was 1:1,165 (or 0.09 per cent) for the Premier League. Similar notable falls in positive cases were witnessed in the Championship and League One and Two play-offs once competition was rejoined.

The elite of English football had successfully negotiated its remaining fixtures. Not a game had been lost because of large-scale outbreaks in clubs. Positive cases amongst the teams had been gratifyingly low and a protocol blueprint had been established. It would have to be dusted off again later in the pandemic. Financial losses had been reduced and none of the Premier League's or EFL's 92 clubs had declared bankruptcy.

It was onwards and upwards to the 2020/21 season – which was just around the corner flag.

Chapter 9

Restrictions and Recreation. The Regulations Roller Coaster

'Spinnin', and spinnin', and spinnin' around'
Lyrics from 'Spinnin and Spinnin" by Syreeta. 1974

Although people knew it was coming, the speed and totality was still a shock. No one younger than 75 years old had lived through such constraints.

On Friday, 20 March, Boris Johnson announced that all gyms and leisure centres would close. Three days later, total lockdown followed. People could take only one form of outside exercise daily, either alone or with a household member.

For 16 months, revised restrictions and regulations played havoc with accessing grassroots sports. It was bewildering and, at times, illogical. In sports terms, there would be isolated winners. However, most pursuits lost big time. In general, individual sports fared better than team sports; outdoor activities more than indoor endeavours. There would be nuances. The more socially distanced a team sport could be the more rapid its return. At times, permitted activities varied across the Union. Even when team sports returned, where and who you could play might be limited.

How this short-term convulsion translated into long-term change for sport and health will be explored later. This account gives an overview on the recreational roller coaster experienced by all.

'Please release me, let me go'
Lyrics from 'Release Me' by Engelbert Humperdinck. 1967

Exercise limitations, other than walking, cycling, or running, remained for 51 long days.

Major recreational winter sports such as football, rugby union and hockey had their seasons abandoned. On 20 March, the RFU cancelled all rugby below the Premiership. One week later, the FA declared all non-league football seasons null and void. With all results expunged, some clubs felt aggrieved. Jersey Bulls, in football's Combined Counties League Division One, had won all 27 matches that season. They were 20 points clear and guaranteed promotion. No more. The new cricket season was only weeks away. Players would have had a long wait in the pavilion – if it had not been locked and bolted.

On 13 May, people were allowed to meet and take exercise with one person from another household. The day brought other gifts. Anglers perched by the riverbank and tempted tench. Singles tennis could take place across a net acting optimistically as a microbial barrier between combatants. Golfers could wander the fairways alone or with a household member. Other members of the Union would be slower opening up – a theme repeated throughout the pandemic. Wales were behind England by five days and Scotland a further 11.

Recreational sport continued to tread this careful path as outdoor opportunities gradually increased. From 1 June, the 'rule of six' people meeting outside was introduced.

On 4 July, pubs and restaurants reopened with strict restrictions on 'Freedom Day'. On this 'Super Saturday', national cases reached a 2020 daily low of less than 600 official infections. Afterwards, cases steadily mounted again. One week later, outdoor swimming facilities reopened and sports involving a single ball touched by multiple players could restart – with stringent safety regulations. Recreational cricket opened the batting followed by football a couple of weeks later. On 19 July, Boris Johnson confidently predicted there would be no need for further nationwide lockdowns – describing the option as a 'nuclear deterrent'.

In late July, gyms, indoor swimming pools and leisure centres reopened after four months. Now, Johnson warned that the UK was 'not out of the woods' with cases bubbling up across Europe. As a result, bowling alleys could not reopen until mid-August. However, during that month, the nation dined out cheaply as the government subsidised 160 million meals in the 'eat out to help out' scheme. The initiative cost the taxpayer £849 million and linked later to between eight and 17 per cent of new COVID-19 infection clusters.

By early September, with academic establishments reopening, rising infections were causing concern. NHS Test and Trace apologised for laboratories struggling to keep up with demand. Some people travelled several hundred miles for virus testing. In mid-September, social gatherings in England were limited again to six people indoors and outdoors.

It was all going 'pear-shaped'. Health advisers requested a two-week circuit breaker to avoid deaths climbing. Johnson felt that it would have 'disastrous' financial consequences for the country. On 21 September, Vallance and Whitty held their own press conference warning of 200-plus daily deaths by mid-November. Labelled as 'Messrs Witless and Unbalanced' by Tory MPs, it was later appreciated that they had under- rather than over-estimated the developing situation. The government imposed 10pm curfews on pubs and restaurants and 1,700 Manchester students had to isolate in university halls for a fortnight after an outbreak.

Thirty outdoor pursuits had been exempted from the rule of six – including football, rugby, cricket and hockey – so long as they were 'organised'. Park 11-a-side football matches with erected goalposts passed muster. Impromptu games with 'jumpers for goalposts' were limited to three-a-side. Grouse shooting had been in full flow since the 'glorious 12th' of August. Rumours of rows within the corridors of power circulated. Should blood sports be exempt? In the end, the 'happy hunting season' continued. Meanwhile, indoor sports suffered. Netball and basketball could only be played outdoors.

'You can check out any time you like, but you can never leave'

Lyrics from 'Hotel California' by The Eagles. 1976
Quoted by residents of Leicester during their long local lockdown.

By the end of September, one quarter of the population – 16.8 million – was under local restrictions. The good burghers of Leicester never experienced Super Saturday. Instead, they had over 100 days of additional restrictions imposed because of local case numbers. There were illogical national directives. The prime minister urged people to sit in cinemas but banned them from watching their local football club outside.

The measures were not working. Cases had risen in 19 out of the 20 local areas under restrictions for over two months. Something needed changing. By mid-October, there were more COVID-19 patients in hospitals than when the first lockdown started. A three-tier national system was implemented in England. Liverpool was alone in Tier 3 with pubs, cafes and leisure centres closed. Northern Ireland and Wales introduced four-week firebreaks. The latter banned people from COVID-19 hotspots elsewhere travelling to Wales. Germany and France went into second lockdowns.

There was a risk that the NHS would be overrun. Johnson announced a second lockdown from 5 November to 2 December. Gyms closed. Outdoor recreation was encouraged but only with one other person from outside of your household. It was *The Darling Buds of May* revisited.

People canvassed for grassroots sport to continue, extolling the positive physical and mental benefits of exercise. Many local football leagues had only restarted in October and managed a handful of games. Indoor sports facilities' closure was not met with the same universal obedience as in

March. Some gyms refused to shut. One owner was fined £67,000. A Liverpool gym was reported to have closed only after armed police arrived.

'*Tears for souvenirs are all you've left me*'

Lyrics from 'Tears' by Ken Dodd. 1965

On Wednesday, 2 December, the country re-emerged blinking. Pandemic indicators remained worryingly high. Grassroots sport could restart. Gyms, pools, golf courses and leisure facilities were permitted to reopen after their four weeks' closure.

Post-second lockdown arrangements were announced. A 'beefed-up' three Tiers approach would be reimposed. Only the Isle of Wight, Isles of Scilly and Cornwall would be in Tier 1. Tier 3 included large swathes of the Midlands, North East and North West, including Greater Manchester and Birmingham. The good news was that five days later the COVID-19 vaccination programme started. The first nation in the world to put 'jabs in arms'. Good times surely would follow?

Restrictions on recreational sport depended upon which Tier people lived in. Some local authorities chose more restraint based on public health grounds. Lancashire FA banned all football-related activity in high case areas. It rescinded the restrictions before Christmas only to find the deteriorating national situation putting the sport into reverse again at the end of the month.

'On the fifth day of Christmas, my true love sent to me …'

In late November, a five-day Christmas amnesty had been announced. Three households could meet. Sleepovers were allowed. However, as Christmas approached, the population were warned to be cautious. SAGE advised people to avoid board games and put female family members at the centre of decision-making: 'Women carry the burden of creating and maintaining family traditions and activities at Christmas.'

On 14 December, the Christmas mood music dampened further with the announcement by Matt Hancock that a new COVID-19 variant (later called Alpha) had been identified in Kent and elsewhere. Large parts of the south-east were elevated to Tier 3. Thirty-four million people were banned from the pub at Christmas.

Having claimed on 16 December that it would be inhuman to cancel Christmas, the prime minister torpedoed the festive plans three days later. A new Tier 4 was announced. Into it was placed London and the south-east – with restrictions like November. The message was simple – no mixing at all. Gyms would be amongst those ordered to close in these high case areas. Non-elite sport would have to stop again. There would be no Christmas family bubbles for those in Tier 4. The new regulations came into effect that midnight, creating crowds at London railway stations as people sought to disappear to all ends of the country – taking their viruses with them.

The rest of the country could only meet family on Christmas Day. The next day, mainland Scotland, Wales and Northern Ireland announced Tier 4 restrictions. Two-fifths of England would face similar limitations. Many countries halted flights and ferries to and from Britain.

The respite for the rest would not last. On 4 January, Boris Johnson announced England's third lockdown. Hospital admissions were now 40 per cent higher than the April 2020 peak. There would be similar restrictions to the first lockdown in March 2020, including school closures except for children of key workers and vulnerable pupils.

'Here I go again, far beyond control'
Lyrics from 'Here I Go Again' by Archie Bell and the Drells. 1969

The public would be barred again from the gyms and other exercise parlours that they relied upon traditionally to shed the festive mince pies and Christmas puddings. There was criticism as to why naturally socially distanced sports like golf and tennis should be banned – while elite sport, and walking, running and cycling continued.

On 22 February, a new national roadmap to exit lockdown was published. It was all very déjà vu. People's patience was wearing thin. Unseasonably mild weather had brought large crowds on to parks and beaches; £66,000 worth of fines were issued in London for illegal parties on one weekend. Health experts warned, 'We could blow it by breaking the rules now.' Not heeding the warnings, the public did the same at the end of March.

On 29 March, the rule of six was reapplied for a third time. Outdoor sports like golf, tennis, basketball and outdoor pools could reopen. Organised outdoor team sports, like football and cricket, could tentatively begin – but in the absence of spectators. On 12 April, indoor leisure facilities, such as gyms and swimming pools, could reopen – but only used individually or in household groups. Five weeks later, indoor group sports and gym classes began. Finally, 2021's version of Freedom Day arrived on 19 July. It was the date for all legal limitations to be lifted.

'I'm in pieces, bits and pieces'

Lyrics from 'Bits and Pieces' by The Dave Clark Five. 1964

Sport could begin to see the light at the end of the tunnel. However, it was only the beginning of the end. Over 20,000 people would die from COVID-19 in the UK in the second half of 2021. Delta and Omicron viral variants would emerge and claim more lives. For the individual, trying to keep body and soul together and maintain their sporting pursuits, it had been disconcerting. Trying to keep up with all the activity restriction changes, while fretting about other areas of their lives, was an achievement by itself.

The effect of the 'stop–go policy' of varying restrictions on the nation's general physical and mental fitness had been laid bare before the parliamentary DCMS committee at the end of 2020. Pre-March 2020, two-thirds of the population engaged in at least the recommended 150 minutes of weekly exercise. By 1 December, that number had dropped to one quarter. There was a real concern that the combination of working from home, lack of sporting opportunities and people's reluctance to mix in crowded spaces would compromise long-term fitness and accelerate the ever-growing rise in obesity levels.

How individual community sports fared and the long-term effect on the nation's fitness and health will be explored later.

Chapter 10

Community Spirit

THE UMBRELLA effect of restrictions throughout 2020–21 on grassroots recreation and personal health has been explored. But how did individual sports and activities cope? It is instructive to begin with the more solitary activities that flourished under lockdown and follow with those that had to hang on to lifebuoys – with apologies to any sports that have been overlooked.

'But I would walk 500 miles, and I would walk 500 more'
Lyrics from 'I'm Gonna Be (500 Miles)' by the Proclaimers. 1988

Our Fitbits encourage us all to achieve 10,000 daily steps. That number was a marketing ruse by promoters of a Japanese pedometer in 1964. However, there is an association between steps and health. Pre-pandemic global-wide data suggested that the world strutted on average only half that number. Increasingly, walking had become a 'utility function' for commuting, business and shopping over recent decades.

A 2020 study reported that during a ten-year period, over-40 Americans averaging 8,000 steps daily had half the mortality compared to those walking half the distance; 12,000 steps would reduce the risk further to one third.

During the first month of the 2020 lockdown, WHO reported that the world reduced its step count by one quarter.

Others showed people were 30 per cent less active and spent 30 per cent more time sitting during home confinement.

Humans were in danger of becoming 'sitting ducks' for the virus. Literally. Many struck back.

The simple pleasure of walking for recreation was rediscovered by people during the first lockdown. Quiet highways and byways, more proximity to the Hobnobs (occasioned by home working) and lack of alternative exercise opportunities meant Shanks's pony became Hobson's choice.

Incarcerated at home and needing escape from endless Zoom meetings, people took to the lanes and footpaths for leisure. Previously, walking patterns had varied little since 2005. While 'utility walks' dropped by two fifths in 2020, total miles walked per person increased by the largest amount since 2002. We rambled longer. Walks greater than one mile increased by a quarter. One third of all trips involved walking compared to a quarter in 2019. The trend was maintained in 2021. People continued to stroll further, with two-thirds of all walks undertaken for leisure. Sore bunions, anyone?

The Loneliness of the Long Distance Runner
A book (1959) by Alan Sillitoe and film (1962)

Running was one of the few recreations permitted for long phases of 2020–21. It became a form of physical and mental release from the cabin fever many were developing from enforced domiciliation.

Many people with little previous, or recent, running experience donned their trainers and took to country lanes. Weekend warriors were freed to become daily lockdown lopers. Regular runners increased by seven per cent in 2020. However, it was very different for organised events that had become firm fixtures for many runners.

Pre-lockdown, 350,000 Brits turned up at weekends to run 5km across hundreds of open spaces. The parkrun phenomenon started in 2004. From meagre beginnings in London's Bushey Park, the Saturday morning spectacle spread to 22 countries. With lockdown, runners were left to their own devices and timetables. Some embarked upon improbable schedules, hoping to revisit the triumphs of their youth. As 2020 wore on, Bill's clinics became increasingly populated with post-gambolling shin splints, aggravated arthritic ankles, stress fractures and bulbous Achilles tendons. Joggers were missing both the social element and sensible restraint that communal running delivers. It would be fully 16 months, in July 2021, before it came again under starter's orders; 100,000 runners appeared at 500 different venues.

For more dedicated runners, half and full marathons are the order of the day. London and the Great North Run figure prominently in their diaries. The 2020 London Marathon became an early pandemic casualty – jettisoned on that fateful Friday, 13 March. A rescheduled October event was announced, but it would be an elite-only race with a parallel 'remote' event organised. People could run their own marathon close to home. The virtual race required an entry fee donated to charity. 'Finishers' received a medal. Times recorded on the event app could be used in applications for the 2021 edition. A Guinness World Record for a remote marathon was recorded. Thirty-eight thousand athletes did laps of their locality – many robed in fancy dress. They were refuelled from the back of relatives' cars and trestle tables erected in front gardens. The event's remote nature meant runners from 109 countries participated.

Hopes of the London Marathon returning to its April slot in 2021 evaporated even before the 2020 event took place. However, the 2020 virtual event's success encouraged organisers to adopt a hybrid model for the delayed October 2021 running – 40,000 entrants ran remotely; 40,000 'in-person' competitors were organised into staggered starts to improve social distancing.

The organisers made an early call to maintain the 2022 event as an autumnal offering. On 2 October, over 42,000 runners completed the traditional course. There would be no 'remote' entrants. Finally, after four years, the 2023 London Marathon reverted to its April slot on St George's Day. All went well. England's patron saint must have been smiling down kindly on the event.

The world's biggest half marathon is held in early autumn in Newcastle. The 2020 Great North Run should have been the 40th anniversary edition of the event pioneered by Sir Brendan Foster. Sixty thousand people held much-coveted entry cards. With a start date of mid-September, the organisers hoped that easing restrictions would be enough for the race to proceed. However, by mid-June, with the rule of six and no 'sleepovers' allowed, the race was cancelled. Although it reappeared in 2021, the finish on the iconic South Shields promenade was binned for a finale on the Great North Road. Like London, spaced starting timeslots were the order of the day. Finally, on 11 September 2022, the event returned to its traditional route with a record number of runners.

It had been a long, lonely and winding road for the nation's joggers.

'Round, round, wheels go round and round,
down, up pedals, down, up, down'
Lyrics from 'The Pushbike Song' by The Mixtures. 1970

Cycling comprised less than two per cent of all journeys made in England and only one per cent of total mileage accumulated on our roads before the 2020 pandemic. This was despite cycle traffic increasing by two-fifths across the UK in the previous quarter of a century.

This increased appetite for cycling coincided with a sea change in British successes in major championships, including the Olympics, Tour de France, Giro d'Italia, and Vuelta d'Espagna. In 2018, 2.5 million bikes were bought in the UK.

However, compared to the post-Second World War years, cycling journeys were relatively uncommon– less than a quarter of 1949 total mileage. In recent years, it is the middle-aged men in lycra (MAMILS) who undertake most leisure-based rides. Youngsters got out of the habit long ago of cycling to school. In 2016, only two per cent of primary school children cycled to UK schools compared to 49 per cent in Holland. Another contributor to the obesity crisis afflicting the country.

March 2020 provided a chance to reconsider our transport and recreation choices. Encouraged by much emptier roads, good spring weather and a preference to avoid public transport, people took to their bikes in droves. In spring and early summer 2020, cycling numbers more than tripled at weekends and doubled during the week. Miles cycled on British roads were the highest for 50 years.

Transport Secretary Grant Shapps announced a £2bn package in early May 'to put cycling and walking at the heart of our transport policy'. Many local authorities and government agencies invested in infrastructure and schemes to encourage this trend. Pop-up bike lanes, cycle and bus-only corridors and safer junctions were planned 'within weeks' as part of a £250m emergency active travel fund. Greater Manchester announced its intention to create 150 miles of protected cycle routes. Transport for London (TfL) announced schemes for cycle-only roads and bridges and a 'bike Tube' network above Underground lines. This was often in opposition to local councils, residents and motorists. Kensington and Chelsea council spent £320,000 installing a bike lane in Kensington High Street in 2020. It was quickly used by 4,000 cyclists daily. It was ripped up seven weeks later because it was slowing up motor vehicle flow. Within weeks, analysis showed that the freed-up car lane was blocked 80 per cent of the time by parked vehicles.

The government announced a £50 'Fix your bike' repairs initiative to coax 7 million rusted cycles out of garages and sheds. From summer 2020 until late 2021, 400,000 vouchers were issued. Bicycle shops (which were allowed to stay open as essential stores) and online sites were inundated with bike enquiries. Many sold out, creating long waiting lists. In the first full month of lockdown, bike sales rose 60 per cent month-on-month. One retailer revealed that their wholesaler had cleared their entire annual stock that month; 2020 saw an extra £1bn spent on bicycle sales. MAMILS were being elbowed aside with noticeably increased sales to women and families. The cycling boom was seen across the world with similar initiatives by authorities abroad.

Even as the novelty was wearing off, TfL recorded an increase in cycling of seven per cent in inner London and 22 per cent in outer London in autumn 2020 compared to pre-pandemic numbers. Nationally, 2021 saw even more people cycling regularly than the year before and over a quarter more than five years previously.

Perhaps all those lockdown cyclists would agree with Sherlock Holmes's creator, Sir Arthur Conan Doyle:

'When the spirits are low, when the day appears dark, when work becomes monotonous, when hope hardly seems worth having, just mount a bicycle and go out for a spin down the road, without thought on anything but the ride you are taking.'

'Gone Fishin' Instead of Just A-wishin''
Song by Bing Crosby and Louis Armstrong. 1951

Angling was one of the first sports to reappear in May 2020. Its oft solitary nature lent itself to social distancing. Accordingly, the 750,000 UK fishing licence holders stocked up on maggots, dusted down their flies and headed down to the riverbank. The summer of 2020 saw a boom in the activity. An additional 100,000 people bought fishing licences.

In the early 2021 lockdown, angling was accorded a different status to the previous 2020 incarnations. It was reclassified as an exercise that could be undertaken either alone or with a household member. Regular angling numbers had been falling in the pre-pandemic years – nearly 20 per cent from 2015 to 2019. However, by 2021, the numbers had risen again and were close to 2017 levels. Pre-pandemic, it had supported 27,000 jobs and was worth £1.4bn to the UK economy.

Bunkered

In March 2020, 2,577 British golf courses summarily closed. 'Big Berthas' lay idle in golf bags. For seven weeks, not a ball was hit in anger out of the rough. Its restart in mid-May saw clubs besieged by players eager to tee off. Llanymynech Golf Club had an issue. Some of its course lay in England and the rest in Wales – where golf was banned for a further five days.

However, it would not be golf as members remembered. Changes had to be made.

Booking tee-off times was mandatory. Players could only play with housemates or one non-household member. Golf shops remained closed. Many clubs had staff still on furlough. Courses were not in their normal pristine condition. Flagsticks could not be removed, bunker rakes were unavailable and ball washers decommissioned. The 19th watering hole remained out of bounds and changing had to be done in the car park. On 4 July, golf clubhouses reopened if they were COVID-19 secure. Club treasurers breathed a sigh of relief. It would be a brief respite.

The mid-October Tiers introduction caused access issues for golfers in high case areas. Within weeks, all golf stopped as the country endured the November lockdown. A 250,000-signature petition was presented to the House of Commons contesting that golf was a safe outdoor pursuit. The government remained in its bunker.

Briefly in December, fairways reopened but facility access varied. Clubhouses in Cornwall (Tier 1) could serve drinks at tables without food. Those in Devon (Tier 2) could only serve drinks with substantial meals. A clubhouse in north Somerset (Tier 3) could not open its doors but was permitted to serve takeaway meals. The pre-Christmas introduction of Tier 4 areas heaped further misery. Tier 3 and Tier 4 residents could not travel outside of their area unless necessary. 'Necessary' did not include sport. Many golf clubs were in difficulties with members who lived the other side of a Tier boundary and were therefore unable to travel to their own course. A Lancashire golfer complained that he could walk his dog legitimately on his golf course during the November lockdown but could not cross the Tier boundary in December to play golf at the same venue.

All these concerns became academic when the government announced the third national lockdown for the new year. All golf courses closed again. The arguments resurfaced for keeping them open. The government replied that no sport would be exempted.

It would be the end of March before golfers could take to the tees. Despite losing five out of 12 months in 2020 to 2021, the sport amazingly boomed. Deprived of alternative sports, people flocked to the courses. The normal three million players mushroomed to over five million in 2020. It would be the highest number of participants this century. The average age of golfers dropped by five years and many women took up the sport. The game was urged to seize the opportunity. Time would tell if this would be a passing fad.

'Pump It Up'

Song by Elvis Costello and the Attractions. 1998

The modern British gym had 'taken wings' in the 1980s. Pre-pandemic, it had faced many challenges: the rise in popularity of cycling and parkruns, the utility of computer-based 24/7 accessible exercise programmes and smartwatches. They had all nibbled away at monthly gym membership direct debits. Nearly one quarter of UK adults were gym members but only half of them used the facilities regularly.

However, it remained a major player in the leisure industry. Pre-lockdown, there were over 7,000 UK gyms –

one third owned by local authorities. The industry generated £8bn annually and employed 180,000 personnel with a similar number of personal trainers utilising gym facilities. This access would be put into abeyance. Gyms acted quickly in March 2020 by freezing members' subscriptions – it stopped gym bunnies cancelling them never to restart.

Sitting at home didn't stop many becoming more curious about exercise. Being exiled from our gyms and other regular exercise venues was a shock to many. The phenomenon of keeping healthy through habit had been described pre-pandemic. For a lot of people, regular exercise times became as ingrained into our weekly timetables as the supermarket shop, going to work and watching the TV news. That Tuesday evening five-a-side football or 10am Wednesday spin class became regularised. The world was faced with the reality of habit discontinuity in all aspects of our lives – including exercise. Using Google trends, interest in online searches around the area of exercise peaked in the first two weeks of lockdown and remained above pre-pandemic levels for months afterwards.

The nation needed alternative ways to access their workouts. Step forward with a lunge, Joe Wicks. Starting hours before lockdown on 23 March 2020, the fitness coach took to YouTube to deliver daily exercise classes for children at home. By the second day, he had an audience of nearly one million drawn from all ages. He continued to broadcast until July and then reprised his sessions during subsequent lockdowns. From March to July 2020, home gym equipment purchases rose by 2,000 per cent. Sales of indoor recreational aides and virtual trainers, like Peloton and Zwift, soared.

After four months of initial closure, there was much debate over the second closure of gyms on Bonfire Night 2020. Inevitably, gym owners and staff detailed the extensive safety measures put into place and the mental well-being aspects of access to exercise. It would be to no avail. For all November 2020 and the first quarter of 2021, steppers, elliptical trainers and treadmills fell silent.

In September 2020, SAGE revealed that closing gyms and leisure centres might reduce the R number by only 0.1, but stressed how difficult it was to estimate. Test and Trace data placed gyms sixth on the list of places visited in the previous week by people contracting the virus – behind venues like supermarkets, pubs and senior schools.

Trying to run a business which is closed for over eight months out of 13 (and with restrictions during part of the 'open' months) was stressful. Despite using available economic survival packages, there was concern that the industry was teetering on a financial cliff edge by early 2021. However, people piled back into the gyms from the summer of 2021, encouraging owners and investors. In 2022, membership was back to 95 per cent of pre-pandemic levels and many of the early gym closures had been balanced by new venues opening.

'A natural vector of disease'

Just as the country was considering ending its first lockdown, recreational cricket was bowled a googly by the prime minister. Having claimed, in the House of Commons on 23 June, that a cricket ball was 'a natural vector of disease', he added nine days later that cricket had issues with 'teas and dressing rooms'. Later that day, it was announced that government guidelines on the game would be published shortly. Chris Whitty took a different view to the PM. He said that 'it was very safe' to resume playing.

The sport enjoyed regularly by nearly 300,000 adults every summer had been reprieved. The recreational game restarted on 11 July – 20 days before the professional County Championship and only three days after England's first Test match against the West Indies started in the 'hermetically sealed' bio-bubble at the Ageas Bowl in Southampton.

However, members of the village third XI were asked to refrain from hugging each other and putting sweat or saliva on the ball. Cucumber sandwiches would have to be prepared at home and eaten in isolation – in contrast to being able to sit in restaurants in August with team-mates to 'eat out to help out'. Players were only allowed to stand within one metre of each other when fielding around the bat. Players had to sanitise their hands every six overs. Umpires could no longer be used as human clothes hangers. Unworn players' jumpers and hats were placed over the boundary ropes. The ball could not follow a circuitous route back to the bowler after a delivery. Spectators could congregate in maximum groups of six. The dressing rooms were *hors de combat* and sweaty players had to return home for post-game showers.

The community game benefitted from being a summer sport. By the time the virus had returned with a vengeance in the 2020 autumn, bails, bats and boxes had been put away for the year. The winter restrictions meant no indoor nets for the amateur cricketer.

When the game returned in April 2021, similar restrictions applied on the pitch. However, the opening weekends of fixtures would feature no spectators. By mid-May, fans and cricket teas were back on the menu – subject to government guidance. Finally, on 19 July, all restrictions were removed – except for refraining from applying bodily fluids to the ball, a regulation which became permanent.

The sound of leather on willow might be echoing around the shires again – but not in the same numbers. Sport England revealed that playing numbers in 2021 had dropped by more than a fifth compared to pre-pandemic levels.

'It's touch and go'

Like all community-based team sports, junior rugby union clubs saw their season abruptly halted in mid-March 2020. Worries were aired that the game would be slow to return because of the close physical contact involved in elements of the game – like scrums, tackles and mauls.

On 4 June, the RFU published its six-stage plan (labelled A to F) for the graduated return of the community game: the Rugby Restart Road Map. Many amateur clubs began restricted outdoor training in early July. There was optimism that the 2020/21 competitive season might start in early autumn. However, as the COVID-19 situation deteriorated, such hopes would be dashed. In late September, the RFU announced no league matches below the men's top two Tiers and the women's Premier 15s would be played in 2020.

The community game was stuck at Level D of its Road Map. Clubs could play local rivals in non-contact fixtures based on the newly announced Ready4Rugby format. It was essentially ten-a-side touch rugby with kicking allowed. On 30 October 2020, the day before the PM announced the second national lockdown, all competitive leagues for the 2020/21 season were cancelled below elite levels.

After the second lockdown ended, the government approved the return of grassroots rugby union training from early December. However, it came with major strings attached – the adoption of 'law variations'. There would be no scrums or mauls. The grizzled old tight-head prop had no one to bind to. Friendly 15-a-side games could start just in time for Christmas. However, with the country in the grip of its new Tier arrangements, off-field social distancing and strict COVID-19 sanitary arrangements were the order of the day. The community game had reached Stage E of its Road Map. It was like a five-metre scrum close to the virus's try line. The early January third lockdown stopped that final shove. Penalty awarded to the coronavirus.

After the early 2021 lockdown, limited contact training was allowed from late March 2021. It would be another four weeks before games played under the law variations were allowed. Finally, on 19 July 2021, scrums and mauls could be reintroduced into community club training. Phase F – the Road Map's final phase – had been reached. Full contact friendly games started in early August and the new competitive season in September.

It remained to be seen how many superannuated hookers would be prepared to dubbin their boots and Vaseline their ears again. Pre-COVID-19, 224,400 adults turned out for their local teams. Participation numbers were already dropping in previous years. In 2021, this number dropped by 40 per cent – equivalent to 4,500 fewer teams playing on a Saturday afternoon compared to pre-pandemic. Many players had retired, and others had discovered new pastimes during 18 months of enforced exile. Previously thriving clubs were struggling to put out third and fourth XVs. Club finances had taken an almighty hit – dependent historically on bar takings and the rental of premises and grounds to external parties. RFU and government loans were welcome but would not compensate for the effect on the clubs and communities which they supported.

Unlucky 13

The 13-a-side rugby league game encountered similar difficulties to rugby union. It was a sport predicated on 'close encounters of an unwelcome kind' during a pandemic.

Furthermore, it had been a summer sport since 1996. Having finished the 2019 season in October, no more than a couple of games had been possible before lockdown. While other major summer sports, like cricket, rescued a shortened season with modifications, grassroots rugby league stayed closed. Some training was allowed in early autumn, but by late September it was announced that no normal fixtures would be possible.

Competitive grassroots rugby league restarted at the beginning of May 2021 – after a month of progressive easing of training restrictions. However, for aspiring young professionals, academies announced no formal competitive structure in 2021. Two full seasons would be lost for the tyro players. There were justifiable concerns about youngsters drifting away from the sport. Overall, the number of registered players, at all levels, dropped by a quarter in 2020.

As one of the most popular team sports, local rugby league clubs give identity and focus in many areas of social and economic deprivation, especially in its northern England heartland. A dividend survey calculated that the sport contributed £185m to the economy. Every £1 of money spent by clubs generated a social return of £4.08p.

It had been a bruising and dispiriting period both on and off the pitch for a sport which is often regarded as the beating heart of its local communities.

A tale of two courts

Netball is played all year round in the UK. In late 2019, the sport was on a 'high'. The national team's gold medal in the 2018 Commonwealth Games earnt the side the BBC's SPOTY (Sports Personality of the Year) Team of the Year award. In 2019, it hosted the World Cup. Interest had been more than piqued. Recreational participation increased by one fifth in 2019. It was easily outstripping other popular sports like rugby union. With 1.6 million participants, including children, the game was booming. Half of games were played indoors – in leisure centres and school gyms.

Like all sports, netball developed a roadmap for return. From mid-May, individuals could undertake netball training outdoors with one person from another household. On 1 June, up to six people could train socially distanced. From 18 August, up to 30 players could train outdoors and friendly matches were permitted.

The reopening of indoor facilities in late July 2020 did not allow sports like netball and basketball to return indoors. They would remain victims of the rule of six. England Netball emphasised that many young participants would not play in outdoor spaces because of body-image perceptions. Some Muslim women needed secure courts to avoid being seen by men. There were fears that participation numbers could be permanently damaged. Basketball and badminton faced similar dilemmas.

Netball had to adjust its recreational game to allow safe training and play with alterations to the game. Because of national restrictions, fellow players in Australasia were asked to trial the changes instead. These modifications included increasing social distancing between players, whenever possible, and introducing a form of walking netball. Twenty-six thousand volunteers were trained to administer the changes; 2,000 COVID-19 officers were appointed to provide support for every club. Training and games were restricted to outdoors in December 2020 and the former time limited in Tier 4 areas. The return was brief. Community netball was suspended again in early January.

The three lockdowns interspersed by repeated implementation of rules of six meant that indoor netball (and basketball) did not return until May 2021 – 14 months without access to an inside court.

Despite the difficulties of 2020, the number of participants playing the game recreationally held up remarkably well. In January 2021, England Netball were able to announce that 80 per cent of their members from pre-pandemic times had signed up again for the year. This was without knowing how much recreational netball would be possible that year. A fillip to the morale of the sport and its finances. The sport had proven its resilience and enduring attraction.

The collapsing pyramid

English football has an egalitarian pyramidal structure. It allows any club to rise and fall according to its playing performances. It contains at least 11 levels or tiers. Outside of this are numerous other clubs who turn out on Saturdays and Sundays to provide exercise and camaraderie for their participants. Collectively, this comprised 43,000 active clubs who provided games for over two million people to play regularly in pre-COVID-19 seasons.

Four days after the country was plunged into its first lockdown, all men's football below the National Leagues (level 5) was cancelled. The results of 2019/20 were expunged from the records. The same would apply to women's football below the Women's Super League and Championship level.

The 2020/21 season began tentatively to a background of rising national cases and varying limitations on social activities. Like other sports, organised grassroots football outside escaped the rule of six straitjacket. Football did not have the same issues as the two rugby codes and could more easily socially distance on the park. Thus, it escaped modifications to its conduct.

The plight of the all-conquering Jersey Bulls in Level 10 has been recounted earlier. They started their 2020/21 season in early September. By the time their league was suspended pre-Christmas, they remained unbeaten. However, they had managed only four fixtures. A fellow league side, Chessington and Hook United, had completed 15 games. The effects of COVID-19 infections on players, travel restrictions in certain regions and national lockdowns had created chaos across non-league structures.

The government revealed on 22 February 2021 that grassroots football could tentatively begin again in late March. The FA announced that community leagues had the option to continue their seasons until late June. Two days later, the FA published a survey of all teams involved in tiers 7 to 10 (non-league levels 3 to 6). Over three-quarters of fixtures remained outstanding. As a result, 76 per cent of clubs voted to stop the season. Many clubs regarded concerns over fixture congestion, player welfare, contracts and their own financial plight powerful reasons not to continue. The number of regular footballers at all levels had dropped 30 per cent by 2021.

The 2021/22 season would see the COVID-delayed restructuring of the pyramid. Clubs' new positioning would include factors such as their points per game accumulated over the previous two truncated seasons. Jersey Bulls would finally receive their promotion.

'The Green, Green Grass of Home'

Song by Tom Jones. 1967

One positive aspect of the pandemic was a renewed appreciation of how important junior clubs and sports were in supporting local communities and enhancing social cohesiveness. However, the prolonged restrictions exerted an economic toll. Sporting organisations, large and small, feared for their financial survival and the security of people whose livelihoods depended upon their existence. Pre-lockdown, sport contributed £24 billion to the UK economy and employed 400,000 people full-time.

Many sports proved flexible and proactive enough to ensure their own survival. They were aided by the goodwill of countless grassroots participants and volunteers. Inevitably, much of the adverse effects would be felt by the young as they missed many months, at vital times of their development, in the acquisition of sporting skills and experience.

Initially, people were forced to indulge in the simpler, isolated forms of exercise like walking, running and cycling. Indoor recreation venues suffered. Team sports would take longer to recover. As a result, there was a pivoting of people's recreational choices. Whether this would remain permanent, whether the population's overall fitness would suffer and what would be the financial consequences on grassroots sports were questions to be answered as our national sporting landscape settled in the years to come.

Chapter 11

One Skin, One Ball

'Land of Hope and Glory'

Song by Edward Elgar and A.C. Benson. 1902

For cricket, the crisis broke as professional clubs were in final preparation for the new season. There was a lot to look forward to. Increased media coverage following the exhilarating 2019 England World Cup win and exciting Ashes series would surely promote the sport to young and old alike. The Hundred competition for male and female cricket would launch in July and swell the game's coffers.

All hope lay in tatters.

Most of the 18 county club grounds resembled the *Marie Celeste*. Many clubs could not afford to pay the salaries of the players simply to keep them training. They did not know if a season, and hence income, would follow. Gloucestershire announced 'early in the piece' that they would survive 2020 without any cricket if they furloughed players and cancelled overseas players' contracts. Most would follow. Only Lancashire and Surrey had the financial wherewithal to avoid furloughing players and staff. At Northants, only five people were gainfully employed – CEO Ray Payne, physiotherapist Barry Goudriaan, two senior groundsmen and chief medical officer Bill.

Before the end of March, the ECB released £61m. The 18 counties shared £40m and £21m was made available in loans to grassroots clubs. By mid-June, the ECB pumped a further £37.5m into the system. This included £30m to the counties – equivalent to the anticipated income from the cancelled Hundred campaign.

Larger Test venues probably had more cause for concern. The likes of the Oval, Lord's, Old Trafford and Trent Bridge had developed as venues 'beyond cricket'. Without providing hospitality for dinners and hosting conferences, staff and bills were hard to pay. Surrey projected that 2020 revenues would fall from £45m to £13m. Comparatively 'little counties', like Northants, could become 'lean and mean' very quickly.

In early May, ECB CEO Tom Harrison fretted that 2020 losses could reach £380m. Discussions in the media started. Might the entire domestic season be abandoned? Ironically, it was a scenario made more likely after Rishi Sunak announced, on 12 May, that the furlough scheme would be extended beyond the end of the cricket season. It took some pressure off the ECB and clubs. Players remained concerned for their livelihoods. Especially the 134 players out of contract in October.

November's second lockdown and the furlough scheme extension until March 2021 proved too much of a temptation, even for a club like Surrey. Their staff and players would be furloughed across the winter, saving £100k monthly. Other clubs had no option but to re-furlough players and staff across the 2020/21 close season.

Doctors 'open the batting'

Doctors involved in all sports began to organise and liaise quickly and widely.

In cricket, the ECB-convened weekly Zoom meetings fostered a 'COVID cricket clinical community'. Priorities and problems altered as the pandemic developed and the government announced its progressive strategies.

Links needed to be established with specialists in public health and microbiology, who traditionally had little to do with sport. Bill's first-hand experience, and colleagues' recollections, indicate that these medics gave up their time and knowledge fulsomely even when working ridiculous hours to manage the national crisis. Help came from both senior medical experts (frequently found flanking politicians in Downing Street press conferences) through to medics working locally to individual clubs. After 40 years in orthopaedic surgery, Bill had to rapidly reacquaint himself with the minutiae of virology and public health strategies.

The number of doctors involved within sports medicine nationally was relatively small. This helped as colleagues from different sports provided support and exchanged experiences, problems, plans and policies. Major medical journals, such as the *British Journal of Sports Medicine*, fast-tracked well-researched articles that helped foment our knowledge.

'The best laid plans of mice and men'
Quote from 'To a mouse' by Robert Burns. 1785

Like other sports, cricket digested the government's roadmap for elite sport's return. From 13 May, county clubs pored over the document and their own ground plans. Could it comply? For Bill, what exactly were the responsibilities of a COVID medical officer, a role to which he had been unwittingly appointed? Bill and the Northants CEO spent days developing policies and going over site plans. It takes time to work out the safest way to flush a toilet and the order of cleaning the lid and basin afterwards. PPE, sanitisers and thermometers had to be sourced at a time of scarcity. Detailed risk assessments had to be documented for any activity within the ground. Later, these would be inspected on-site by ECB officials before the go-ahead was given.

By mid-June, the expectation was that training would commence on 1 July. Clubs could not afford to un-furlough players before. It was not until 29 June that the ECB confirmed that a truncated season would commence on 1

August. Late June was hectic behind the scenes. Players and staff were screened for health risks for themselves and their families. All had to watch an ECB educational programme. Bill delivered online presentations to explain training arrangements and spent one weekend undertaking 1:1 calls with staff and players to discuss individual concerns. Many players seemed to conduct these consenting interviews from local golf course fairways. Everybody had to return signed opt-in statements if they wanted to train.

Cricket ball manufacturer Dukes called Boris Johnson's remarks that the cricket ball 'was a natural vector of disease' inexplicable. They believed that if hands were regularly sanitised, balls cleaned and no saliva put on it, the risk of disease transmission was minimal. All these processes were actioned for the new season.

At Northants, the first day of training was surreal. Players, coaches, staff, clinicians, groundsmen and cleaners met, socially distanced, in the car park. From there, they were walked through one-way systems, zoned areas and sanitisation points. Players had daily checklists to complete before leaving home. Each had their own set of personal balls – to comply with the ECB's mantra of 'one skin, one ball'. Even so, for players arriving at the ground, it was a novel experience to be greeted by a physiotherapist in PPE pointing a thermometer gun at their foreheads through an open car window. Players arrived alone, fully changed, and departed similarly to undertake their ablutions at home.

Typically, after glorious spring weather, it seemed to rain nearly every training day for the first week. Bill spent part of the first training morning checking that various loos' hand dryers had been decommissioned (for fear of spraying the virus widely) and gel bottles were operational. Sometimes our jobs can be very glamorous.

Despite swab-testing all international cricketers, the ECB decided not to test the rest of the first-class game. Contrary to Boris Johnson's view, the ECB assessed that the game carried minimal risk. Different measures for international and domestic cricket caused some consternation from county players. A cynic would conclude that it was all financially driven.

Like other sports, the duration of pre-season was uppermost in people's minds. Many county players had had no competitive cricket for ten months. Fast bowlers were most at risk of injury. Spinal stress fractures from sudden workload increases are feared. A pre-season time of 10 to 12 weeks is considered ideal. These concerns should have guided both designated preparation time and the intensity of cricket on restart. Bill made his views known to the ECB via a letter from the Northants chairman. In the end, Test cricketers returned with less than seven weeks' training and first-class cricket with just over four weeks. The dangers were clear. To counteract the risk in domestic first-class cricket, reduced limits were placed on total overs bowled per day and overs bowled per player.

Players were back in training one week before the domestic season's structure was released. The one-day 50-over game was jettisoned for the year. It would leave two formats to be played: Twenty20 (T20) and the County Championship. Test cricket would start first followed by recreational cricket three days later. County cricket would be another three weeks behind.

The normal two-division County Championship was abandoned. In its place would be the Bob Willis Trophy, named after the great English bowler and captain, who had died in late 2019. Three regional divisions of six were formed to minimise travel and hotel stays. A Lord's final would be played in late September. The whole condensed and anaemic red-ball season was over in seven weeks. Regional divisions would remain for 2021. After that, the two-division system would be restored for 2022. Teams in each league would be determined by their finishing positions in 2019 – three years before.

The T20 competition was held back. It was hoped that some crowds would be admitted. It started in late August and ran into October. All done and dusted in five weeks.

'I'm playing all the right notes, but not necessarily in the right order'

Eric Morecambe to André Previn. BBC TV. 1971

English cricket needed money to stop haemorrhaging from its bank account. The solution? Prioritise men's international cricket. West Indies, Australia, Pakistan and Ireland were slated in various formats. Amazingly, they would all appear but not in the order expected.

First up, Windies agreed to travel but delayed their arrival by three weeks until 9 June – the first overseas sporting side to arrive in the UK – albeit without three players who declined to travel. The ECB paid for their visitors' flights and lent Cricket West Indies £2.4m. The team would see little of the English countryside during their seven weeks' sojourn of which four-fifths would be spent in Manchester. Their first two weeks were spent in quarantine.

Two bio-secure bubbles were developed, one at Old Trafford (for the visitors) and the Ageas Bowl in Southampton (for the hosts). Both had hotels on-site. The tight security would have done justice to Fort Knox. COVID-19 testing machines, at a cost of over £80,000, were installed at both grounds. Players' temperatures were checked daily, and they were fitted with Bluetooth tracking systems. The tight planning was justified. The ECB was able to report zero positive tests from several thousand undertaken before cricket recommenced. Officials and media underwent the same deprivations. Like football stadia, only 300 people were granted entry to the sanctum sanctorum, which itself was zoned to prevent mixing of groups. BBC Radio's *Test Match Special* listeners were advised that commentators could not receive cakes from grateful listeners.

England's priority was their fast bowlers' lumbar spines, which needed gradually reintroducing to the rigours of bowling. This process started on 21 May under tight precautions at seven grounds nationwide. This was expanded later to a squad of 55 players training at 11 grounds. Thirty players would eventually unite in Southampton where they were introduced to eating at separate tables, travelling back-to-back in lifts, and their own box of balls. Both sides warmed up with intra-squad matches.

One month after the visitors arrived, the Test series commenced on 8 July at the Ageas Bowl. The final two Tests would be at Old Trafford.

The 2020 summer of cricket was set to recoup the ECB £200m. The fragility of the project was highlighted by a misjudged pitstop. England players were allowed to travel from Southampton to Manchester under their own steam after the first Test. Fast bowler Jofra Archer decided to take the scenic route via his apartment in Brighton. He reportedly came into contact with one undisclosed person, who subsequently tested negative. When the misdemeanour came to light, Archer was dropped from the second Test, fined and confined to his hotel room. England cricket's managing director Ashley Giles said, 'This could have been a disaster.' A contrite Archer apologised profusely. The speed and seriousness of the sanction underscored the ECB's determination to complete the series without any health scares.

Stuart Broad declared the visitors 'the heroes of the summer'. Visiting skipper Jason Holder commented, 'Mentally, some of the guys are worn out.' The West Indies hoped that England would repay their magnanimous gesture by touring the Caribbean before the end of 2020. Circumstances would make this impossible.

Australia were scheduled to arrive in July for a white-ball series but didn't leave until late August. Their government only gave them clearance to travel ten days before departure.

As different Australian states had dissimilar restrictions in place, some Aussies could train unfettered while others could not practise as a group. Their 19-hour journey came courtesy of a small French airline as Qantas was grounded. They arrived at East Midlands airport and onwards for three nights in a Derby Travelodge while they practised at the County Ground. Their six-game series was completed in 12 days in September.

Sandwiched between the Windies and Aussies came the Ireland and Pakistan tours. This was to be Ireland's first full white-ball series in England. Australian prevarication led to the Irish being invited to play the series at Southampton in the 'bubble' six weeks earlier than planned. They accepted with alacrity.

Pakistan's tour was next – or nearly wasn't. The tourists were due to leave home on 28 June. Five days before, the squad and staff underwent pre-travel testing. Ten of the 29 were positive. The infected members had to stay behind until clear. Like the Windies before, Pakistan would spend four weeks in isolation in Derby and Worcester playing intra-squad games. Like the other three visitors that summer, their six games were spread between Lancashire and Hampshire. As thanks to the visitors for putting up with numerous impositions, England agreed to play in Karachi in October 2021. One month before the games, England pulled out on 'player welfare grounds'. Even if England players were feeling bio-secure bubble fatigue, it was felt that a team of understudies could have been sent. The decision was met with general condemnation.

Women's cricket

The top women cricketers gathered in Australia for the 17th T20 World Cup in early 2020. Ten teams were whittled down to two – India and Australia – for the final in Melbourne on 8 March. Under floodlights and in front of 86,000 spectators, the hosts cruised home by 85 runs. Millions watched on television. It was described as 'the greatest moment in the history of women's cricket'. It would be the Aussies' fifth global title and the last meaningful women's international cricket for months.

The 2020 English summer was looking good. Visits from India and South Africa for T20 and one-day internationals promised 12 high-class white-ball games bookending women's participation in the inaugural Hundred competition. Women's cricket would get extensive exposure at grounds and on television.

The two visiting sides declined to travel. The South African withdrawal came a fortnight before their first game on 1 September. The irony of the 'Boks men's players preparing to travel at the same time to the UAE for the IPL was not lost on commentators. Women's cricket faced the first barren English season without international matches for a quarter of a century. The ECB had prioritised the more lucrative men's game. A harsh reality check was acknowledged by Clare Connor, women's cricket managing director, 'For the whole game to survive the financial necessity rests on many of these international men's matches being fulfilled.'

Like their male counterparts earlier, the West Indies women's team flew in to rescue the season. Ensconced in a Derby bio-bubble, the English women triumphed 5-0 in the T20 series behind closed doors. Neither side had played any cricket for seven months. Meanwhile, men's domestic county cricket teams were travelling around the country to fulfil fixtures. The women's domestic summer season was rescued as autumn approached. A one-day competition, labelled the Rachael Heyhoe Flint Trophy, was contested by eight regional teams over one month in parallel with the West Indies series. It finished on a chilly Wednesday in late September. The Northern Diamonds beat the Southern Vipers. The competition returned in 2021 with the 2020 final result reversed.

Things were worse in India where no women's cricket was played in 2020. Australia, South Africa and New Zealand managed some cricket towards the end of the year. However, an early decision was made to delay the 2021 New Zealand-hosted 50-over World Cup for a year.

The year 2020 had placed a major dent in the aspirations and financial security of the women's game.

Taking guard

The long-awaited domestic season started on Saturday, 1 August. Opening games at Edgbaston (Warwickshire v Northants) and the Oval (Surrey v Middlesex) were designated as pilot spectator events – along with Goodwood racing and Sheffield's World Snooker Championship on the same day. Several thousand fans were expected at each game. The audience was 'called off' the day before by the government as COVID-19 cases started to rise. The hosts incurred considerable expenses in staffing and catering costs. It was particularly galling for Surrey, who had successfully hosted the first live spectator sport in the UK only a week before. One thousand fans had attended the 'friendly' between Surrey and Middlesex.

Fans reverted to watching games using online streaming services. They watched in their thousands and clubs realised the potential of this medium for future seasons. Throughout the shortened domestic season only one game admitted fans. Surrey were allowed 2,500 fans in early September when they entertained Hampshire for a T20 match. The trial would not be repeated.

T20 cricket was televised to secure much-needed revenues for the sport. However, TV crews were not allowed to travel the country and remained rooted to the spot at predetermined grounds. Northamptonshire hosted Glamorgan in Birmingham.

Bill spent an unusual evening at an empty Edgbaston. Glamorgan were housed on one side of the vast ground and

Northants on the other. Ne'er the twain should meet except on the centre square.

Having been made a 'training bubble', Derbyshire received successive overseas travelling teams to prepare for international fixtures. The hosts would become nomads. It would be the first time in 60 years that the club had played no games within their county boundary.

COVID cancels cricket

Northamptonshire were responsible for the only 'first-class game' to be abandoned because of COVID-19 in 2020.

The virus had stayed away until the final round of Bob Willis Trophy divisional matches on Sunday, 6 September. Five days earlier, a non-selected Northants player had watched a T20 game from the stands. Two days later, he developed vague symptoms. Bill advised him to get tested and isolate. Swabs nationally were in short supply. The NHS had a 185,000 backlog of tests at the time. Non-international players had no access to tests via the sport. Instead, the NHS offered him a return journey of several hours and no prospect of a result for days. The positive result eventually arrived after the four-day game between Gloucestershire and Northants in Bristol had started. Queue panic. Two of his 'housemates' involved in the game were deemed close contacts. Risk assessments were undertaken remotely and in Bristol. The match was abandoned. Gloucestershire were 66/6 in their first innings at the time. The game was drawn.

Ramifications from the incident spread. Glamorgan contacted Bill to discuss the risks following the 'very socially distanced' T20 game at Edgbaston on 3 September. One symptomless and contact-free player involved in the original 1 September game had travelled to play in Ireland. His opposing team cancelled the game. Nobody tested positive subsequently. The wheels came off Northants' T20 campaign. Unbeaten before the incident, they lost their next four matches.

Elsewhere, everybody was being careful. A Kent player had to self-isolate after posing for a selfie with a fan. Hampshire and Yorkshire lost players during the white-ball competition. The virus was back with a vengeance.

Drawing stumps on cricket 2020

COVID-19 reminded cricket where everybody's meal ticket came from. The domestic season was partially rescued fixture-wise. However, it was men's international cricket that drove the game financially and represented the 'cavalry coming over the hill'.

Amazingly, all the 18 scheduled international fixtures for the 2020 English summer were fulfilled. Just not necessarily in the right order. All games were split between Old Trafford and the Ageas Bowl behind security doors. While the English team had been asked to sacrifice much, so had our visitors. They saved the ECB from potential ruin. In May 2021, the ECB could announce that losses had been kept to £16m for the financial year 2020–21.

Chapter 12

Let's Go Racing

March 2020 – stuck in the pit lane

In 2019, Formula 1 celebrated its 70th instalment. Over four million fans would attend the 21 races spread across four continents. Over a third of a million watched the Silverstone Grand Prix alone. The season lasted for 37 weeks. The sport's annual worth had grown to an estimated £4 billion.

The year 2020 planned to be even grander with one extra race and another fortnight added to the season – rubbing up against the Christmas holidays. Vietnam would host its first-ever Grand Prix and the Dutch Grand Prix would return for the first time in 35 years. Germany would miss out. February pre-season testing had been completed in Barcelona.

The 14/15 March weekend was a calamity for Formula 1. Its season would be four races 'light' before Sunday was out. The debacle of the abandoned 2020 season's opener in Melbourne was described earlier. The April Chinese Grand Prix had been cancelled more than a month before. Both the Vietnam and Bahrain races were postponed indefinitely. Only a week before, the Bahrain Grand Prix had announced that the second race on the calendar on 22 March would continue as a fan-free event. Reality was dawning. The nascent season's schedule was in chaos even before the vapour trails of the thwarted drivers' and senior executives' private jets had disappeared out of Australian airspace.

However, only two days after the planned Melbourne race, F1 English-based race-car manufacturers would be turning their brain power and hands to making a significant contribution to the treatment of the critically ill, described in chapter 5. Their efforts balanced the imbecilic attempts by the aforementioned Red Bull manager to organise 'COVID-camps'.

Like all sport, it soon became apparent that F1 was facing a lengthy closure. Within a week of Melbourne, five other Grands Prix would be shelved including the iconic Monaco event. It would be the first time since the 1954 season that Monte Carlo's famous street circuit would not feature.

F1 had major problems as a truly international sport. An F1 season needs to complete eight races to constitute an official championship. Air and land travel was badly disrupted. Team staff had expressed reservations already about travelling. Personnel were domiciled across the globe. Many of its favoured venues were imposing strict conditions on visitors. Incoming personnel could not escape quarantine. Some countries had effectively closed their borders. Two of the major bases for F1 teams – Italy and Britain – were amongst the most seriously compromised COVID-19 countries with strict and prolonged initial lockdowns. The teams invest huge amounts to make their cars competitive. In 2019, Ferrari and Mercedes each had annual budgets of over £400m. The less-well-resourced teams were likely to be even more vulnerable to financial streams being turned off. The money needed to keep rolling into the coffers. However, F1 would have to watch, wait, plan and negotiate.

If the F1 season were to be rescued, various criteria needed to be met. Bio-secure bubbles within venues and teams needed to be established. Various sports were wrestling with how this could be done. Circuits needed to be secure for protocols to work. Street circuits, such as Monaco, Singapore and Azerbaijan, were difficult to control and increased problems if public mobility and social-distancing regulations remained 'in situ'. Travel needed to be kept to a minimum. Effective and regular testing had to be available at a time when globally such technology was in short supply, even for essential emergency staff.

July 2020. Under starter's orders

The initial hope was that racing could recommence in May. After many false dawns, a new starting date was agreed on 2 June with the first eight venues announced – thus 'ensuring' a legitimate season. The strategy included double-headers – a tactic used in English international cricket and some American sports. Additionally, the plan was to keep the racing in western Europe until late September while hoping that the global position would improve.

The Austrian Red Bull Ring would host the first two races, on 5 and 12 July. Silverstone would welcome another double-header in early August. Gradually more events and dates were announced. Eventually, 17 races took place with the last three taking place in Bahrain and Abu Dhabi ending in mid-December. However, 13 of the original 22 races were cancelled.

Events in the Americas, Australia and the Far East were scrapped. Only the Austrian, Belgian, Italian and Russian Grands Prix kept their original dates. Germany got a reprieve using the historic Nürburgring circuit last used in 1976. Portugal returned for the first time in 14 years. Two one-off events were added in Italy – the Tuscan and Emilia Romagna Grands Prix.

The COVID-19 crisis required inevitable changes to protocols, budgets and time-honoured traditions. Bubbles and regular testing became de rigueur. The teams' annual two-week summer break was brought forward to the spring. It was scheduled to last three weeks, but the factory shutdown eventually extended to nine weeks.

Changes to the sport's governance, car designs and sporting rules due to be introduced for the 2020 season were deferred for two years. The first eight races were run behind closed doors. The rest of the season proceeded with very restricted crowd numbers or locked gates again. The condensed calendar increased the costs of competing and its longer-term budgetary plans will be returned to later.

On restart, the normal drivers' parade, and pre-race assembly to hear the host's national anthem was scrapped for race days. Fewer personnel were allowed on the start grid. The planning to recreate bio-secure bubbles repeatedly in different countries and race circuits was huge. Each team formed bubbles. Strict isolation for contacts was followed. F1 undertook 80,000 tests in the five-month season; 93 positive results were returned – 0.1 per cent. Around £8m was spent on testing.

All were tested 72 hours before entering the paddock and again on the Friday and Saturday. This needed 'beefing up' after Racing Point's Canadian driver Lance Stroll had tested negative despite symptoms, withdrew, flew home and tested positive subsequently after the Germany Eifel Grand Prix October weekend. As a result, another test was added 24 hours after entering the paddock with a further test required on Sunday race day.

Other drivers did miss races because of positive tests. Another Racing Point driver, Sergio Pérez, missed both Silverstone's Grands Prix in August. He had flown home to Brazil after the Hungarian race and blamed the chef on his private plane for the transmission. Lewis Hamilton tested positive again and missed the penultimate race of the season in Bahrain. Eight months later, the world champion feared he was suffering from long COVID with dizziness and fatigue.

Despite the upheavals, the phrase *'plus ça change, plus c'est la même chose'* is apt. Mercedes won their seventh consecutive constructors' championship and Hamilton successively defended his drivers' world title.

2021. The brakes are off?

It was clear in early January that the 2021 calendar could not return to normal.

An original schedule was announced in November 2020. Surging cases and deaths around the world post-Christmas meant further amendments. Once again F1 had to be agile, its published diary regarded as no more than a moveable feast. An ambitious 23-race schedule (with room for additions) was announced on 12 January extending out to mid-December. After that the game of musical chairs started. Varying quarantine restrictions, local caseloads and vaccination rates amongst F1 personnel and venue populace would be crucial factors.

Even pre-season changes had to be made. Testing was moved from Spain to Bahrain in March. The hosts offered to vaccinate the entire F1 village, which was declined on behalf of the sport by Stefano Domenicali, the F1 president. He refreshingly said that 'the priority is the most vulnerable. We don't want to jump the line of vaccination.' At the time, vaccination programmes in most countries were not being offered to the young and fit. However, several teams availed themselves subsequently of the Bahraini offer.

Australia was pushed from the March opener to November because of quarantine requirements and low vaccine uptake in Victoria. F1 had to 'war game' for the eventuality of even one person testing positive in Melbourne, which would mandate a city lockdown and race abandonment. In early July, the race was cancelled altogether as tight border controls were likely to remain in place until beyond the race weekend.

The Far East remained problematic. The Chinese Grand Prix was cancelled in early January because of travel restrictions. With rising cases between the Tokyo Olympics and Paralympics, the Japanese Grand Prix, scheduled for October, was scrapped. Four months ahead of the scheduled October Singapore Grand Prix, F1 announced its cancellation for a second year. The local authorities refused to relax their tight immigration restrictions for the thousands of motor racing personnel arriving. Vietnam, having failed to make its debut in 2020 because of the pandemic, was removed permanently because of corruption charges to key officials. F1 would not be visiting the Far East in 2021.

The Turkish organisers must have wondered if they were coming or going. The Istanbul race had been left off the original schedule – having ridden to the rescue in 2020. Like Singapore, the Canadian government refused to drop its 14-day quarantine for visitors for the June Montreal race. Turkey was asked to substitute but, two weeks later, removed when the UK government added Turkey to the red list in May – preventing many of the English-based personnel attending. Turkish patience was rewarded in late June when they agreed to substitute for Singapore.

Intended only for the 2020 emergency contingency, the Portuguese, Imola and second Austrian races were retained to plug the 2021 gaps. Racing returned to the American continent in Texas, Sao Paulo and Mexico. Qatar (benefitting from Melbourne's misfortunes) and Saudi Arabia made their Grand Prix debuts, increasing the Middle Eastern venues to four. Holland finally made its long-awaited return having been cancelled in 2020.

The remaining pack of F1 circuits were shuffled several times to fill in gaps and allow late additions to 'seamlessly' fit in. The season started two weeks later than originally envisaged in Bahrain. However, F1 did remarkably well to complete 22 races in the end.

To ease financial pressures on teams, there was a limit to component modifications for the cars. The normal four-day race weekend was reduced with Thursdays media and promotional events removed for 2021.

French quarantine restrictions prevented F1 personnel from entering the country for testing and caused problems for Brixworth-based Mercedes in June. However, exemptions would be granted for the main event in June when 15,000 spectators attended the Circuit Paul Ricard. A similar number attended the Styrian Grand Prix at the Red Bull Ring in Austria one week later. The Formula 1 circus took root at the same track for the 4 July Austrian Grand Prix when restrictions were relaxed to allow 100,000 fans to be admitted. It must have felt like Independence Day in the south-east of Austria. However, the Austrian euphoria did not last. Four months later, the country would be placed in its fourth lockdown with less than two-thirds of the population jabbed.

Better news followed in Britain. On 24 June, the government signposted that the Silverstone Grand Prix three weeks later could be watched by a capacity crowd of around 140,000. It was scheduled the day before the country's restrictions were due to be lifted. It followed closely on the announcement regarding other major July sporting events. The Wimbledon final would have full capacity on Centre Court, golf's Open Championship could have 32,000 spectators per day, and the Euro 2020 football final would be watched by 60,000.

Not everybody was pleased. Lewis Hamilton felt the decision was 'premature' amid the rising Delta-variant cases in the UK. Over the three-day weekend 356,000 fans attended Silverstone. Later, the government announced that 343 attendees were likely to have been infected already and 242 more became infected as a result.

F1's strict regulations and testing regime worked well despite the large numbers of personnel, many countries, and vast distances and logistics involved. By the end of June, 44,000 tests had been undertaken with 27 positive cases, a rate of only 0.06 per cent. It was a further improvement from 2020. By the end of 2021, eight Grand Prix drivers (out of 27) had contracted the virus since the start of the pandemic – Pérez, Stroll, Hamilton, Norris, Leclerc, Gasly, Raikkönen and Mazepin. Leclerc caught it twice in 2021.

Fittingly, the F1 World Championship ended in thrilling and controversial fashion in Abu Dhabi on 12 December as

Max Verstappen overtook Lewis Hamilton on the final lap to take the Briton's title. Ten months later, the new champion's team, Red Bull, would be fined $7 million and lose testing time in the 2023 wind tunnel for breaking the cost cap.

2022. From grid to chequered flag? No jab, no grid walk

The 2022 edition of F1 would be the first for three years with unrestricted travel for teams, media and fans. Twenty-two races were planned and completed – once Russia had been removed after the invasion of Ukraine. Not a withdrawal, addition or change of date in sight. Technical regulations that had been held over from the pandemic could be introduced.

While many sports were jettisoning COVID-19 regulations, Formula 1 maintained strict protocols for 2022. A truly international sport with personnel crisscrossing the world, it imposed strict rules on the paddock. Only the fully vaccinated were allowed within its environs wherever it landed in the world. Ex-world champion Nico Rosberg was part of the Sky Sports commentary team. He had been infected but not vaccinated. No grid walks for him. Instead, he commentated from the comfort of his Monte Carlo home.

After the excitement of 2021, Max Verstappen 'walked' his Red Bull to the Drivers' World Championship and retained his title with four races to spare. F1 thrives on adrenaline, noise and petrol fumes; 2022 must have felt like a welcome relief after the turmoil of the previous two years.

After the season was over, F1 moved quickly to cancel the April 2023 Chinese Grand Prix. China's continuing 'zero tolerance' policy towards COVID-19 with frequent lockdowns meant that the sport was unwilling to risk its travelling personnel becoming isolated in the country.

The view from parc fermé

Formula 1 receives spades of bad press on account of its perceived financial profligacy, exclusivity, frequent processional racing and lack of eco-credentials. COVID-19 caused it to face daunting challenges. The global fixture list was its major obstacle. Some of its initial responses in March 2020 did it no credit.

As befits a sport attracting space-age technology and some of the brightest minds, it thought its way through the problems with flexibility and pragmatism. It even managed to importantly assist the health effort in the UK. It produced two World Championships in 2020 and 2021 without any last-minute postponements after Melbourne. It did not stand on sentiment as when Monaco was ejected for the first time in 66 years. Like elite football, its wealth allowed a rapid introduction of testing and bio-bubble establishment. To its advantage was the fact that drivers and staff could be socially distanced from rival teams. When full crowds were reintroduced in 2021, vaccination programmes were well advanced, and most spectators could be accommodated outside. However, the teams bought into the draconian protocols resulting in low positive rates across the two years – when taken in the context of the amount of travel required. Mindful of accusations of privilege, the sport's leaders eschewed early vaccination offers in 2021 and were quick to insist on mandatory vaccinations in 2022. It attempted to trim its very rich cloth according to the needs of the crisis and no team went bust.

Overall, F1 emerged from this crisis with more credit than most sports and national governments.

Chapter 13

Large Hooves, Small Balls and Saddle Sores

PROJECT RESTART was not all about getting 22 footballers back on the park, even if media attention was seemingly fixated on the beautiful game. Every sport and athlete worldwide were wrestling with the same problems and fears. How did five other sports surf the tidal wave of the 2020 coronavirus pandemic?

Four-legged friends

Greyhound racing was first out of the traps as elite British sport returned on the morning of 1 June 2020. Horse racing would be hot on canine heels only hours later. That afternoon's Newcastle meeting was the first for 76 days.

British horse racing employs 20,000 people directly. The British Horseracing Authority (BHA) had furloughed most of its staff with others taking pay cuts. It saved the BHA one third of its £3m monthly operating costs. A further 46,000 people are employed in the betting industry. The sport adds an estimated £4.1 billion to the economy.

The Cheltenham debacle and its contribution to viral spread was fresh in people's minds. However, racecourses' wide-open spaces made it an obvious choice for an early return behind closed doors. Furthermore, the horses were ready to race. During lockdown, stables were entrusted with maintaining their charges' fitness as part of essential equine welfare. European racing had started earlier, in the first half of May, in Germany and France. Ireland followed the UK one week later. Meanwhile, further abroad, horse racing had continued unabated in Australia, Hong Kong and the USA.

The season restarted with maximum fields of 12 horses piloted by senior riders. This arrangement was hoped to minimise accidents and prevent piling up pressure on the NHS.

The five classic races are highlights of any British summer. Delays to the Flat racing season meant traditional dates for the first four races needed revising. All were delayed by a month. The Newmarket 1000 and 2000 Guineas ran on the first weekend after June's resumption. The Epsom Derby and Oaks were in July. Being staged on a course with open access via public footpaths and bridleways, permission had to be granted to render the venue bio-secure. Only the St Leger survived its original date.

The Royal Ascot June meeting is one of the centrepieces of the English season. Usually awash with luxuriant gowns and top hats and tails, it took place with no crowds. Instead, people were requested to dress up in front of their televisions. Jockeys wore PPE masks that occasionally misted up their goggles. Waivers were given for horses to be flown in from America, France and Ireland. It would be the first time in the 68 years of her reign that Queen Elizabeth II was absent. Like many meetings, extra races were added to compensate for weeks of inactivity. However, total prize money for the five-day meeting would be halved to less than £4m.

Betting and the equine industry enjoy a symbiotic relationship. The April Aintree Grand National was the first major casualty. Normally, it generates £250m in wagers. Instead, it was run as a virtual race involving 40 runners and riders. Five million punters laid bets with a share of proceeds contributing to NHS charities. The Jockey Club promised 10,000 tickets for NHS staff for the 2021 National. Sadly, it would also run without spectators. On-course bookies and caterers had no customers to serve. The Ladbrokes Coral betting company announced a 50 per cent drop in betting in the first half of 2020. By August 2020, William Hill bookmakers permanently closed 119 high street shops. One third of punters reported trying different pastimes to gamble on during lockdown. Activities like online poker gained in popularity.

Now you see them, now you don't

Getting crowds back on to the courses was frustrating. The Glorious Goodwood meeting intended welcoming back 5,000 members on 1 August as part of the government's pilot events. Normally 20 times that number attend. It would have been the first course to have spectators on-site. Over £100,000 was spent getting ready. The prime minister cancelled the plans the afternoon before as cases rose, leaving meeting organisers 'gutted'. Racing continued behind closed doors with only horse owners present.

It would be another five weeks before a further 'test event' was tried. The early September Doncaster St Leger meeting planned to welcome back 20,000 people over four days. On the eve of the meeting, the government revised its COVID-19 advice. Two thousand, five hundred fans were admitted for the first day and, then, the meeting reverted to behind closed doors. Later in the month, small spectator meetings at Warwick and Newmarket were allowed. However, cases were rising nationally and, by November, the country was back in lockdown for a month. Fans were back watching the gee-gees on telly. On 1 December, limited numbers were allowed back into courses in Tier 2 regions. Cheltenham welcomed 2,000 fans to its International Meeting early in the month. However, it was all false hope. By early January 2021, racing was spectator-less once more. Another four months passed before the turnstiles turned again. Horse racing endured 14 months with minimal contact with spectators.

As in other sports, not all jockeys were angels in silks. In April 2020, Australian jockey Luke Tarrant found a new way to breach social-distancing guidelines. He head-butted fellow rider Larry Cassidy during a post-race fracas in Brisbane and was banned for six months. That autumn, Irish jockey Oisin Murphy went on holiday. He told the world he was in Italy when he was sunning himself on a 'travel red-listed' Greek island. It took until February 2022 for his misdemeanours to catch up with him. He was also found guilty of two alcohol breaches and had his licence to ride removed for 14 months.

Snookered

The professional snooker season runs May to May, culminating in the World Championship played at the Crucible Theatre, Sheffield ever since 1977. Final frames take place over the early May Bank Holiday weekend. For 2019/20, 47 events were planned across ten countries in Europe and the Far East. The Chinese Open in Beijing was the last planned ranking event before the Crucible and the earliest casualty.

On 13 March, the tour had reached Gibraltar. Many players and referees had withdrawn because of the deteriorating situation. Only 100 spectators were admitted that day. The tournament was completed two days later behind closed doors. One week after that, the World Championship was officially postponed. Professional snooker ceased for 11 weeks.

Cabin fever

Snooker was one of the first elite sports to return on 1 June – alongside horse and greyhound racing. The ten-day-long Championship League moved from Leicester to the Marshall Arena, Milton Keynes. The venue was chosen for its on-site hotel and ability to provide bio-security with swab-testing beforehand. With so little live sport, games were broadcast around the world. Players remained within the complex until eliminated. The event's success led to a second tournament, the Tour Championship, to be played at the same venue under similar arrangements nine days later.

On Friday, 31 July, snooker returned to the Crucible for the delayed World Championship. Eleven days before, it was announced that a limited number of fans would be admitted. It was part of the government's stress-testing of plans for spectators to return to live sport – alongside Goodwood horse racing and Edgbaston cricket.

Anthony Hamilton withdrew before playing. As an asthmatic, he objected to spectators being present. One hundred and twenty-five people attended the opening frames before Boris Johnson announced a U-turn that evening and suspended the pilot events. The cost for all those sports involved was considerable in administrative, catering, staffing and ticket revenue losses. A limited number of spectators were eventually admitted a fortnight later for the last two days of the event. Ronnie O'Sullivan beat Kyren Wilson 18-8 in the final.

The three-month-late finish to the 2019/20 season meant a rescheduling of the 2020/21 calendar. Compared to years gone by the fixture list looked very parochial. All tournaments would be played in England and Wales. The first 11 events, through to February 2021, were played in Milton Keynes under the same claustrophobic conditions. Frames continued throughout the second November lockdown watched by television viewers. The Gibraltar and German Opens (plus many more) were hosted in Buckinghamshire.

The Masters was scheduled for Alexandra Palace, London on 10 January. Six days before, it was deemed not bio-secure and reverted back to Milton Keynes. Two days before it started, Judd Trump and Jack Lisowski tested positive and withdrew.

Snooker had done well to maintain its tournaments in 2020 and early 2021. However, it had to be pragmatic and nimble to rearrange venues in the light of external events.

However, arrangements affected participants. Ex-world champion Shaun Murphy spoke of the psychological toll of being isolated for long periods in hotel rooms away from family and friends: 'The lasting damage to players' and everyone's mental health during this pandemic over the last year, we will see the results of it for a long time to come.'

Anyone for tennis?

Elite tennis revolves around the four grand slam tournaments, the quadrennial Olympics and Paralympics, and team events like the men's Davis Cup and women's Fed(eration) Cup finals – 2020 promised much from each but in the end had to settle for less.

The Aussie Open had successfully completed in early February but would not hold another 'normal' tournament for three years. The first casualty would be the Fed Cup finals scheduled for Budapest in mid-April. The Hungarian government took early action against the virus, leaving the organisers no choice but to postpone on 11 March. The event would not be rescheduled until November 2021 and switched to Prague. In the interim, the entire enterprise was renamed the Billie Jean King Cup. Next 'double faulted' would be the Tokyo Olympics and Paralympics events shelved in late March and completed in summer 2021.

The Wimbledon postponement announcement soon followed. It was its first cancellation since World War II. Presciently, the All England Club had taken out an insurance cancellation policy, which covered infectious diseases. It recouped £100m in compensation and removed the pressure felt by many sporting events to try and continue behind closed doors. It was the only one of the grand slam tournaments to have such a policy in place. The £1.5m premium was instigated after the 2003 SARS coronavirus outbreak. Normally, Wimbledon would gross £250m but would make considerable savings by cancelling the event. The payout allowed the club to distribute £10m to the players.

The men's Davis Cup finals were due to be played in Madrid at the end of November. In late June, they were postponed and rescheduled for a year later. In the interval, the finals were expanded from six to 11 days and spread between Innsbruck, Turin and Madrid with the semi-finals and final retained by the Spanish capital.

The earliest attempt for tennis to return was the ill-judged Adria tour in the Balkans in May. Its rise and fall will be reprised in chapter 27.

An American an' Paris

The US Open in New York found itself in the unusual position of being the second rather than fourth 'slam' of the year. It went ahead behind closed doors, keeping its scheduled opening slot of 31 August. It became the first major tournament to be played without spectators in the 143-year history of grand slams. No player quarantined on arrival but they had to stay in designated hotels or private accommodation and subject themselves to regular testing. Trips to Manhattan were banned. There would be no qualifying tournament opportunity for the young wannabes. Protocols in the grounds were strict. Players had to wear masks when not playing, had limited time in changing rooms, and could not ask ball boys or girls for towels at the end of points or games. Twenty-four of the top 100 women were missing. The defending men's champion and world number two Rafael Nadal and number nine, Gaël Monfils, withdrew with COVID-19 concerns. The Frenchman Benoît Paire tested positive during the tournament and took with him into exile the top-seeded women's doubles players, Tímea Babos and Kristina Mladenovic, regarded as close contacts.

After Djokovic was disqualified for inadvertently hitting a line judge with a ball, the second seed, Austrian Dominic Thiem, took his first major title. Japanese Naomi Osaka took her third women's slam.

The French Open at Paris's Roland-Garros survived by shunting its tournament away from its customary late May slot to an early June position. This would be its first break with tradition for 73 years. Unlike Wimbledon, it had no insurance policy to invoke and faced losing £230m in income in the event of complete cancellation.

The clay court competition was rescheduled twice and, finally, took place from late September. Earlier that month, the organisers expected 23,000 spectators daily across four show courts. However, the resurgence of French cases eventually limited numbers to 1,000. Precautions were tight. Ticket holders were balloted daily with the unlucky ones refunded. Spectators with face masks sat in socially distanced family groups. Competitors were regularly tested and given a choice of only two hotels. They were only allowed into the grounds when playing. Neither of the eventual champions, Iga Świątek and Rafael Nadal, dropped a set in the tournament, creating history for the open era. However, like the US Open, no room was found for the mixed doubles tournament.

It had been a tough year for top tennis. Both global team tournaments and the Olympics and Paralympics were postponed until 2021. Wimbledon was cancelled, the French Open delayed by four months and the US Open played without fans. Unfortunately, early 2021 would be no better.

Under par

Like tennis, men's golf had its four majors, the Tokyo Olympics and the biennial men's team event, the Ryder Cup, scheduled for 2020. The women professionals had their five majors and Olympiad, while British and American female amateurs would compete in the Curtis Cup.

On the men's American PGA tour, golf returned after three months at the Charles Schwab Challenge in Texas on 11 June. Despite early hopes, the PGA announced that the rest of the season's tournaments would be played behind closed doors because of continuing worrying levels of US virus cases.

Initially, overseas players and caddies were required to quarantine for 14 days on arrival in America. Although the requirement was lifted in late July, it was not enough to tempt some foreign golfers back. English golfer Lee Westwood declined to play on the rearranged PGA tour citing travel worries, lack of motivation and the boredom of hotel confinement.

In late May the European PGA announced a new schedule starting in mid-July. The remnants of the season were compressed, dates changed and some tournaments cancelled. To ease travel and safety, after the first two tournaments in Austria the next six events would be played in the UK. It would be September before the tour stepped back on to the European mainland.

The four men's golf majors have their traditional annual diary dates in neat order. The Augusta Masters is in April, the US PGA in May (although proior to 2019 it was normally the last major of the year, being held in August) , the US Open in June, and the Open Championship in July. COVID-19 changed all that. The Masters announced an immediate postponement on 13 March – the same day that the Sawgrass committee drew flagsticks in Florida. The PGA was pushed back to August, the US Open to September and the Masters rescheduled for November.

The 149th Open Championship, due to be hosted by the Royal St. George's, Sandwich in Kent was scrubbed. Only World Wars had seen it scratched before. Like Wimbledon, the Open had a 'complete' cancellation policy in place. The problem for the Royal and Ancient (R&A), the body that organised the Open, was who to award the 2021 and 2022 editions to. St Andrews had been accorded the honour of hosting 2021's 150th edition. The answer was to slide the venues back by a year. Sandwich would be n the menu in 2021.

The August PGA would be the first major for over a year. Irishman and former winner Padraig Harrington joined

Westwood in declining to travel to California. The US Open in New York state would be the first held in September for over a century and the Masters' beautifully manicured course exchanged its normally azalea-adorned backdrop for red, yellow and gold autumn foliage.

The Ladies Professional Golf Association (LPGA) Tour has a truly global schedule with tournaments across four continents. It would be 31 July before the tour restarted in Ohio. The first major, the Evian in France, was lost, but the other four majors survived, including the AIG Open in Scotland in August. The tour was heavily rescheduled with the US Open (originally due in early June) played two weeks before Christmas. The Curtis Cup – scheduled for Conwy, Wales – was moved to summer 2021.

Hooked into the long grass

The 43rd edition of the Ryder Cup was keenly anticipated. Europe had trounced the Americans in France in 2018. The 2020 event was due to take place at Whistling Straits, Wisconsin in late September.

The disruption to the elite golfing calendar meant that other major tournaments needed shoehorning into the autumn. The US Open was scheduled to finish only five days before the Ryder Cup. Traditionally, teams gather early in the week, practise together and allow team captains to determine optimal pairings for the first two days of foursomes and fourballs. Getting everybody from New York to Wisconsin and familiar again with the less-oft-played formats was going to be a challenge in those times of bio-secure bubbles and testing regimes.

Added to those logistical challenges was the issue of spectators. Over the previous 30 years, the Ryder Cup had been increasingly popular for live audiences. The team structure and huge galleries have given the cup almost a gladiatorial atmosphere. Whistling Straits had intended to welcome 40,000–45,000 spectators daily – many of whom would need to travel from Europe. Huge amounts of people needed to be health-screened and kept safe during their stay. Despite encouraging words from the respective American and European PGAs and team captains, Steve Stricker (USA) and Padraig Harrington (Europe), it became increasingly difficult to imagine the event proceeding. On 8 July – 11 weeks before the event – the American PGA bowed to the inevitable and announced its postponement for a year. It meant that future Ryder Cups would slip back a year and other biennial golf events, such as the President's Cup (USA versus the Rest of the World), would have to fall in line.

The Solheim Cup – competed for between US and European professional women golfers – was played in 2019. It alternated years with the men's Ryder Cup. With the latter slipping back a year due to COVID-19, the Solheim went back-to-back with it beinbg contested in 2021 and 2023. To 'uncouple' the events again, it was announced in November 2020 that the Solheim would throw in an extra edition in 2024 to avoid clashes.

'Hell' of a different kind

Professional cycling peddles its wares around the world. Thirty-six races were planned for 2020 by the UCI (Union Cycliste Internationale). Events ranged from classic one-day races to the blue-riband three-week jewels – the Giro d'Italia, Le Tour de France and the Vuelta d'España.

In late February, the tour had reached the UAE and abruptly halted on the fifth stage when two Italian staff members tested positive. The entire entourage, including the media, were impounded in their hotels and some quarantined for over two weeks. Undeterred, the teams moved on to Europe.

The eight-day Paris–Nice race started in early March. Several teams elected not to compete. On Friday 13th one bike team withdrew, and five other teams voted to stop the race. The previous day, French schools had closed, and its government banned gatherings of more than 100 people. The organisers announced that the final Sunday stage was cancelled. Australian Richie Porte commented, 'No one really knows whether we should be here or not.'

There would be no more competitive elite road racing for four and a half months. Fifteen of the 36 races were eventually cancelled, including RideLondon–Surrey (the only event on British soil) and the 'hell over cobbles' from Paris to Roubaix. The UCI produced a truncated programme from August to November, but the precarious finances of the sport were laid bare. The programme survives on the largesse of teams' and events' sponsors. The perilous global economic times meant that the sport would suffer if major sponsors' businesses wilted. Some sponsors withdrew and individual teams sank. The McLaren car racing team announced the end of its sponsorship of the Bahrain–McLaren bike team at the end of 2020.

The three grand tours were postponed and, on return, operated a 'two strikes and you're out' policy. Any team with two riders testing positive within one week would be expelled en bloc. French government strictures on sports and spectators would affect all three grand tours.

The Tour de France was delayed for over two months from its original start date of 27 June. The event took place amongst the tightest security and testing regimes. In the circumstances, it was ironic that race director Christian Prudhomme tested positive mid-event. The race turned out to be a classic with the long-time race leader Primoz Roglic dramatically dethroned by fellow Slovakian Tadej Pogačar on the penultimate day's mountain time trial. The race did not lose any of its lustre for finishing in late September with different climatic conditions from the traditional scorching summer heat. It was just in time as French cases rose.

The Giro is usually the year's first grand tour in May. The revamped calendar meant that the Grande Partenza would be in early October and the race overlapped with the Vuelta. Teams had to split forces to compete at both.

The Giro's start was switched from Hungary to Sicily after the Magyar government refused permission for the race. Mid-race, two teams, Mitchelton–Scott and Jumbo–Visma, withdrew following multiple positive tests. The former had already lost its team leader, Simon Yates, to the virus two days earlier. Other teams carried on despite staff members contracting the disease. The penultimate stage was shortened only three days before it happened when new French regulations prevented it crossing the border for its mountain stage. At the end, British cycling had a new hero when Tao Geoghegan Hart unexpectedly won.

The Vuelta is usually the finale of the racing season. It started two months late at the end of October. The original plan was to spend its first three days in Holland. These plans were an early casualty in late April, shortening the race from 21 to 18 stages. In pre-race testing, two team staff members tested positive, but the event started on time. Fans were banned from lining the mountainous narrow roads and distanced from stage starts and finishes.

Like the Giro, the Vuelta was due to have a mountain-stage finish atop the French Col du Tourmalet. Seventy-two hours before, French government decrees meant re-routing the day. The extreme precautions taken by the organisers appeared to pay off. No positive tests were returned once the event commenced. Primoz Roglic successfully defended his title to make up for the bitter disappointment of the Tour de France.

There was an unusual end note to the Vuelta. One hundred and fifty of Spain's national police force, the Guardia Civil, were deployed to ensure race safety. Post-race they were swabbed in Madrid and 45 tested positive. They had all returned to their hometowns before the results were known, causing consternation at the risk of significant spread.

With the loss of the Tokyo Olympic cycling programme, the other main road races for men and women were the 2020 Road World Championships. The Swiss-hosted event was cancelled in mid-August when its authorities would not allow events greater than 1,000 people and required visitors from abroad to quarantine on entry. It was relocated to Imola in Italy for late September. Juniors and Under-23s events were scrapped.

Competitive mileage was severely restricted, teams and competitors fell by the wayside, but the carnival limped beneath the *flame rouge* to the end.

By hook or by crook

The five sports had global reach and seemingly deep pockets and lucrative television contracts. It did not immunise them from the ravages of the virus. However, all managed to cobble together something of a programme from the embers of their 2020 schedules. With a few exceptions, the sports would ply their trade in glorious isolation divorced from the paying public. However, there is a vicarious pleasure and pride in the knowledge that two of Britain's major summer sporting summits, almost alone, had the foresight to insure themselves against such an eventuality.

Chapter 14

A Tale of Two Codes

Rugby union and rugby league in 2020

Rugby union and rugby league parted ways in 1895; 125 years later they would find themselves back in the same boat. Courtesy of coronavirus.

The two oval ball codes shared similar issues in struggling to survive COVID-19 both on and off the field. By 2020, the elite ends of both games were fully professional with all the financial headaches that entailed. The bodily intimacy involved in their respective codes risked increased contact time between players and the potential for viral spread. However, the timing of their respective seasons meant that the impact differed in certain ways. Additionally, the two sports in England would come to different decisions about game and fixture modifications while attempting to complete their respective seasons.

Rugby union

International sanctions

The 2020 Six Nations Championship began on 1 February and was due to conclude on 14 March. As explained previously, the earlier pandemic impact on Italian soil caused a rapid abandonment of their country's fourth-round match in Dublin scheduled for late February. The tournament's final round was also subsequently postponed – albeit with the Wales–Scotland game halted only 24 hours before kick-off. The women's parallel competition folded simultaneously.

Four months elapsed before a solution was announced. The remaining games would be played in October. The six unions' reliance on tournament revenues meant that there was zero chance of the competition being canned. The rareness of postponements in the tournament was reflected in the fact that 2020 witnessed the first games to be postponed for eight years and the first multiple adjournments since foot and mouth disease ravaged UK livestock in 2001.

Rugby around the world contributed to the humanitarian effort. At home, both Twickenham and Cardiff's Millennium Stadium were repurposed – for a testing centre and field hospital respectively.

RFU CEO Bill Sweeney was examining plans B, C and beyond if the pandemic continued. One option was playing the 2021 Six Nations as a ten-game home and away tournament if travel restrictions prevented playing internationals in the autumn. He wanted lockdown to be a period of reflection on the existing global rugby calendar. Sweeney told BBC Radio's *Today* programme, 'The opportunity here to align a global and domestic calendar which works in the interest of the game is a huge opportunity.' It would take until October 2023 for World Rugby to confirm a realignment of global fixtures with the addition of a biennial Nations Championship to begin in 2026.

The RFU announced that the English game would lose £107m and the WRU £50m if their four autumn internationals did not proceed. Before that potential doomsday scenario, World Rugby announced the inevitable. All summer internationals and the World Sevens series were cancelled. The ramifications were being felt into 2021. The British Lions tour to South Africa was considering moving from July to autumn 2021 to accommodate calendar modifications. The £20m loan taken out by the WRU and passed to its four regions to keep the game afloat in Wales would have major ramifications in the years to come.

The premier product postponed

The 2019/20 English Premiership season would have been notable and controversial without the impact of a global pandemic.

On 18 October, the season started seven weeks late courtesy of the Japanese-hosted World Cup. Leading players already faced a compressed fixture list. On 5 November, the Saracens scandal first surfaced. The club was fined £5.3m for irregular player payments. Having accumulated a total of 105 penalty points for multiple transgressions, the north London club was condemned to relegation to the Championship for the 2020/21 season. It was an astonishing fall from grace for the reigning champions. At the time, it was called 'the biggest story in English club history'. Arguably, it was about to be trumped just four months later.

The Premiership season had reached unlucky round 13 by early March. The league announced its suspension on 16 March with initial hopes for a 24 April restart. This optimism was quickly dissipated. On 8 April, the season was put into hibernation.

April and May was a period of firefighting and looking for what could be rescued on the national and international front. Most Anglo-Welsh players agreed a temporary pay cut of 25 per cent. The RFU senior executive team and England coach, Eddie Jones, agreed similar. Later in the summer, the RFU announced widespread redundancies including the loss of staff supporting the community game.

As plans for the restart approached, relationships between the clubs, the players and their representatives became increasingly fractious. Players complained of being delivered ultimatums to sign permanent contracts at lower wages. The Premiership announced a reduction in each club's total wage bill from £6.4m to £5m for three years starting in season 2021/22. A few players could not agree new club contracts. Six Leicester Tigers players, including England international Manu Tuilagi, left the club after refusing to accept a 25 per cent pay reduction for the 2020/21 season. It was not the optimal backdrop for players to return to Stage 2 training – contact work.

Preparing to perform

As various government groups and sports doctors began to look at restarting, it became apparent that rugby union had specific problems. The close nature of the game with tackling, rucks, mauls, scrums and lineouts meant that it would be difficult to ensure social distancing during games and training. Rugby union did not have the finances that allowed Premier League football to rapidly enact measures for their 17 June return.

In late May, a group of sports doctors and scientists, including the RFU's head of medicine, called for a six-week period of training before games commenced. They examined the specific nature of rugby, considered the key physical attributes required to return to a collision sport, and the effect of a prolonged period of relative inactivity. They also considered the compressed second half of the season and the players' inability to rest and recover. After the players returned to contact training, they would get 40 days before the league resumed. Somebody had listened. The time allowed was greater than that afforded to footballers. Players needed to be 'battle hardened' and reacclimatised to absorbing collisions. Chris Ashton, the Premiership's all-time leading try scorer, remarked, 'Normally we have eight weeks maximum without contact but this has been getting on for four months … it takes the body a long time to get used to it.'

In early June, Premiership Rugby announced it hoped to restart in mid-August. Their counterparts in France, the Top 14, followed the Gallic football route and abandoned their season. There would be no champions or relegated clubs.

However, three French clubs re-emerged in September for the quarter-finals of the European Champions Cup.

Nine rounds of the English season, league play-offs, the final of the Premiership Rugby Cup, and three outstanding rounds of the European Rugby Champions Cup remained. Exeter Chiefs had the prospect of 15 games in ten weeks. Players' welfare needed consideration. Clubs faced schedules that included three games in eight days. Workload and mental health were to be monitored.

The players started contact training in early July. In advance, the COVID-19 testing regime started in earnest. The testing programme for the 12 clubs was costing £100,000 weekly. Ten cases were revealed in that first trawl. In total, 39 players and staff would be identified prior to the league's resumption – a rate of 0.6 per cent (1:160) – a higher count than football on its resumption. However, once the games began, the rate of positive cases dropped significantly – until the final round of matches.

The Premiership returned on 14 August with scrums, mauls and rucks as normal. They did not modify as rugby league would. Referees were given guidelines around the breakdown and rucks to minimise contact time. World Rugby introduced several voluntary law trials to reduce viral transmission risk. Research suggested that eliminating upright front-on-front tackles reduced high-risk exposure by 20 per cent. The RFU and other unions around the world chose not to adopt them.

'It's my party, and I'll cry if I want to'
Lyrics from 'It's My Party' by Lesley Gore. 1963

The Premiership had been away for 159 days and successfully negotiated nine of the ten rounds required to complete the season. Unfortunately, it fell apart at the 'last knockings'. The usually admirable Exeter Chiefs director of rugby, Rob Baxter, called for an end to COVID testing on 28 September. It was not the best-timed intervention.

Sale Sharks had beaten Harlequins in the Premiership Rugby Cup Final on 21 September and eight days later won in the league at Northampton Saints. However, 19 people at Sharks were incubating the virus at the time. Saints were furious when several players were forced to isolate as 'contacts' of Sale players and had to forfeit their last league match at Gloucester.

Rumours swirled in the media that Sharks players had partied with students in Manchester after the final. COVID-19 cases were rising fast again, especially in the North West. People were getting jumpy. On 26 September, 1,700 Manchester students were incarcerated in their accommodation for two weeks. Sale vehemently denied any wrongdoing. The RFU ordered an inquiry.

Sale were due to play Worcester Warriors in the last round of games. They had to win to qualify for the play-offs. The game was postponed for three days. Sharks claimed that they could still field a team, thus avoiding forfeiting the game and their title ambitions. Commentators complained at the inconsistency. Northampton, as innocent close bystanders, had lost a game while Sale wriggled.

Eventually, no decision had to be made. Sale forfeited the Warriors game when another eight tested positive – making a total of 27 at the club. It circumvented another potential banana skin. If the Sharks had triumphed at Worcester, they could have been required to contest the play-off semi-final three days later. There would have been no guarantee that they could have fielded a full-strength team and, accordingly, jeopardised the competition's integrity. Seven weeks later, the RFU cleared Sale. The Sharks' version of events – that their players partied at the own training ground – was accepted. However, the RFU made recommendations about contact tracing and social distancing.

Finally, on 24 October, Exeter triumphed in the Premiership final to complete a double with the European title in the bag the week before. It was a monumental effort.

The Celtic cousins

The Pro14 rugby competition had additional headaches to contend with in 2020. Its 14 teams came from five different countries – Ireland, Wales, Scotland, Italy and South Africa. It served up all the headaches that international travel brought. The league restarted on 22 August and conjured up a neat solution. With eight of the scheduled 21 rounds of matches incomplete, the organisers rearranged the fixture list, leaving only two more games for each team. Each side would play teams in their own country and the two South African sides would not participate. The two Italian sides were not in the hunt for the semi-final places. In three weeks, the competition was sewn up and Leinster completed an unbeaten season, winning their third consecutive title.

Rugby league

The devastating effects of COVID-19 on community and academy rugby league has been described in chapter 10. But how had the elite end coped? The Betfred Super League (BSL) embarked on its new season on 30 January 2020 – a nine-month season with 29 league matches followed by play-offs culminating in a Grand Final in Manchester on 10 October. Super League began in 1996 when the sport abandoned its normal winter season for a summer schedule.

Running in parallel with the BSL, the Challenge Cup involves clubs from all strata of the game. Traditionally, the denouement of the tournament had taken place at Wembley since 1929. It was staged in May until 2004 but then moved to the August Bank Holiday weekend. However, for 2020, it was planned to move it forward to mid-July in response to falling attendances during the popular holiday period.

Calling for a Canadian Canis

Since the BSL's inception, it always had a crusading mission to spread the game beyond its northern English heartlands.

Outpost clubs in London, Wales and France had all been admitted to BSL. Except for the French outfit, Catalans Dragons, admitted in 2005, all other attempts had fallen by the wayside by 2020. Undaunted, BSL prepared for its most ambitious project yet. The Toronto Wolfpack side had worked its way through the leagues over three seasons and was admitted to the 2020 BSL.

The early seven BSL rounds proceeded as planned. However, the harsh Canadian winter meant that the Wolfpack had to play 'home games' at Leeds, Warrington and York. Leeds Rhinos refused to travel on Friday 13th to play Catalans Dragons in Perpignan following a Rhinos player testing positive. The last BSL game took place on Sunday, 15 March – later than most professional British sports. Castleford Tigers beat St Helens at home. At that stage, Toronto had lost all six of their games and propped up the table. The next day, the Rugby Football League (RFL) announced a temporary suspension of the sport. Nine days later, the RFL suspended the sport indefinitely at all levels.

On 1 June, the much-anticipated Australian 'Kangaroos' tour to England in the autumn was cancelled. It would have been their first tour since 2003 and swelled the coffers of the English game.

Below the BSL, all leagues and other competitions were declared null and void in late July. Women's league competitions had not started at the time of lockdown and were abandoned until 2021.

In late June, BSL announced a resumption on 2 August, but the Canadian representatives would not get that far. On 20 July, Toronto Wolfpack withdrew from the BSL and Challenge Cup. They cited 'overwhelming financial challenges' posed by COVID-19 and the inevitable visa and travel problems from Canada. The BSL board voted to expunge their record. The remaining clubs had brought their players and staff in 'off furlough' and into training in July for a three-week pre-season period.

No scrums. No spectators

When the BSL restarted, modifications were required on player welfare grounds. Like other sports, regular COVID-19 testing was introduced for players and staff. Kicking out on the full was punished by a ball handover to the opposition instead of scrummaging. PHE regarded scrums as a 'microclimate' with increased risk of disease transmission and they were removed from the game. The scrum would not return until 2022 and only then for a reduced number of infringements. The BSL adopted a rule change that the Australian NRL had adopted when they became one of the first global sports to resume games in late May. This was known as the 'six again' award following a defensive ruck infringement, such as holding down the player. The attacking side restarted their possession for a maximum of six plays.

No British crowds were allowed to attend but Catalans Dragons hosted three games in front of a maximum attendance of 5,000 spectators. The number of regular season games was reduced eventually to 20. It was decided that league position would be determined by 'win percentage'.

The Challenge Cup needed to adjust. By the suspension of play in March, the first five rounds had been completed. With no rugby below the BSL taking place on restart, the remaining six teams below the elite level (including the doomed Wolfpack) had to withdraw from the competition. This required a redraw of the sixth round with only ten sides left.

The Cup resumed on 22 August with its restricted field. It would be another month before Wembley would confirm that it could accommodate the new final date of 17 October – a behind-closed-doors event for the first time in its illustrious history. In a tight game, Leeds Rhinos beat Salford Reds 17-16. The appetite for the match saw TV audiences increase by 50 per cent compared to 2019, making it the most viewed final since 2012.

Seasonal shrinkage

The BSL August restart was significantly affected by COVID-19 cases within the clubs. Games were postponed and rearranged at short notice. There were pulses of downtime followed by a rash of games for players.

The original intent was for all clubs to complete a minimum of 15 games in the WSL season. This looked ambitious and then forlorn when Hull Kingston Rovers announced on 3 November (just two days before the second national lockdown) that they could not complete the season because of outbreaks at the club. The BSL scrapped the rest of the league fixtures. Of the 11 remaining sides, Catalans had completed 13 games while Salford and Huddersfield had played 18. Chartered flights to maintain a bio-secure bubble for the Perpignan-based side cost £50,000.

Wigan were top of the pile with a 76 per cent win rate and declared winners of the League Leader's Shield – the award to the team leading the table at the end of the regular season. Play-offs for the top six were brought forward and the venue of the Grand Final changed. Old Trafford was discounted due to concerns about the heavy fixture schedule for Manchester United and the risks of postponements and rescheduling. Accordingly, Hull's KCOM Stadium hosted a spectator-free final where St Helen's beat Wigan Warriors 8-4 on Friday evening, 27 November. The losers in the first two play-off rounds were retained on standby in case a victorious team had to withdraw with positive tests. Fortunately, all passed muster.

Toronto Wolfpack applied to be reinstated for the 2021 BSL but were expelled at a meeting on 2 November. The Canadian outfit announced that they would disband. COVID-19 had struck out another attempt to widen the BSL club base and its overseas appeal.

On 14 December, Leigh Centurions were awarded the Wolfpack's place in the BSL. Leigh had been ramping up for potential promotion in 2020 and had a large wage bill to service when COVID-19 ended their season. They remained afloat courtesy of the government's furlough scheme and 90 per cent of fans and sponsors not requesting their money back. However, the late confirmation of their BSL slot caused problems. They received only £1m in central funding for the 2021 season rather than the £1.5m received by the 11 incumbent clubs. It meant they had to scramble to assemble a competitive squad. Not surprisingly, they finished bottom by a country mile in 2021 and were relegated.

'... and finally the whistle blows for no side'

The completion of rugby union and rugby league's seasons in 2020 never ran smoothly. How could it? Both codes restarted later than football because of economics and sport-specific perceived risks. The financial toll to stay afloat would reverberate throughout the coming years.

The English Premiership decided to complete the season in its entirety. It eschewed the Top 14 and Pro14 decisions to either abandon or concertina their remaining fixtures. It meant a season that extended to late October. The players hardly had time to draw breath before the next season started 27 days later. It was scant time for bodies to mend. Intriguingly, and faced with the same evidence and PHE advice, it chose to retain scrums at the elite level, unlike rugby league, while outlawing them in the community game for 16 months.

Rugby league with a 'tweaked' format still had to duck and dive as COVID-19 cases took their toll and shortened its already truneated fixture card. The BSL lost 47 per cent of its season's games – including the Wolfpack's expunged fixtures. Unlike football, cricket and rugby union, it had no international fare to help refill coffers and was the only one to lose a member of its elite league in 2020.

Both codes returned higher rates from COVID-19 testing than Premier League football. Did this reflect the fact that the sports were intrinsically riskier than soccer or indicate more widespread societal issues surrounding the sports? It is a question that will be returned to later in the book.

Most importantly it revealed financial fault lines. Neither sport was as fiscally robust to withstand the viral buffeting as it would have liked.

It had been a sobering experience.

Chapter 15

Going Viral Stateside

FOR SPORT worldwide, the impact of the coronavirus in spring 2020 depended upon several critical factors. These included activity location (such as indoors/outdoors settings), participants' ability to socially distance, financial robustness and the season's timing when normal competition takes place.

Stateside, NFL American football had completed its season in early February. The Kansas City Chiefs won Super Bowl LIV in Miami. NBA basketball and NHL ice hockey were in the middle of their regular seasons which were scheduled to end in April before commencing play-offs through to June. For MLB baseball, the franchise teams were all closeted in Florida undergoing spring training before starting their regular season in late March. Soccer's MLS was a fortnight into its new season.

Decision time for stopping 'in season' sports took place at the same time as in Britain – that fateful week beginning 9 March 2020.

Gridiron looks for a touchdown

By mid-March, the 32 NFL franchise teams were well advanced in planning for the 2020 season opener in September.

One of the major jigsaw pieces is the arrival of new players following the annual spring draft. The circus lasts three days. Las Vegas would host the late April edition. Set in front of Caesars Palace, the red carpet would be placed on a floating platform. The cream of college football would be transported to and from proceedings via boat. Only in America. By 16 March, it was all off. Instead of orchestrating events in front of the spectacular Bellagio fountains, NFL commissioner Roger Goodell announced the 'picks' from the basement of his house in Bronxville, New York. Would-be NFL superstars, coaches, fans and owners watched on TV. Dallas Cowboys owner Jerry Jones watched from his luxury yacht in lockdown isolation.

The year 2020 was posted for a 17-week campaign ending in January 2021. Each team would play 16 games to determine play-off qualifiers.

Major changes and sacrifices were required. Teams returned to pre-season camp in August. The NFL, the owners and the Players Association (NFLPA) worked closely together. Labour relationships had not always been cordial between the three groups. Eight lockouts had been recorded since 1968. The NFLPA's assistant executive director, George Attallah, remarked 'how incredibly frustrating it is that we have to have a global pandemic to make the NFL and NFL owners realize that they need us to do this'. Many players chose to live apart from their families for months. Players could opt out without contravening their contracts. Sixty-six players took this route before August.

Pre-season games were abandoned. Teams started the season with only in-house 'contact' beforehand. Overseas games in London and Mexico City were cancelled. The prestigious Pro Bowl game, played the week before the Super Bowl and featuring the 'best of the rest', was replaced by a virtual event on YouTube featuring such luminaries as Snoop Dogg.

Pre-season testing started on 1 August and continued daily during the season – except game days. In 17 weeks during the regular season, there were only 618 positive results.

An average of one case per franchise per week. Strict protocols of behaviour at training, at stadia and socially were expected. Touchline adherence to mask wearing seemed better than English Premier League football. Coaches approaching a match official without a face mask faced a 15-yard team penalty for 'unsportsmanlike conduct'.

Only seven of the scheduled 256 games in the regular season were postponed because of COVID-19. All were replayed within the planned season. Players and TV schedules had to be flexible.

Breaches of protocols were dealt with harshly. On 30 September, the Tennessee Titans had an outbreak affecting 24 employees and were subsequently fined $350,000 for poor compliance – including 'lax mask-wearing'. On 29 November, the Denver Broncos played New Orleans Saints without a recognised quarterback (QB). All their QBs had attended a meeting without masks and one player had subsequently tested positive. They lost 31-3. Their opponents were fined $500,000 for failing to wear masks when celebrating after a previous game. In December, Washington QB Dwayne Haskins was filmed partying without a mask. Some media reported he was with strippers. He was fined $40,000, stripped of the captaincy and, after a lacklustre performance during Christmas week, fired.

Some players reacted badly to the virus. A Jacksonville Jaguars running back missed the entire season with viral complications requiring two hospital admissions, and a Buffalo Bills tight end developed myocarditis (heart muscle inflammation), missing the second half of the season. A Denver Broncos coach was hospitalised but survived.

Only 19 of the 32 teams welcomed fans during the regular season. Permitted crowds were reduced to allow social distancing and mask wearing was mandatory. The NFL enforced the playing of compulsory crowd noise for attendances of less than 2,500. Cheerleaders and mascots were banned. Only four teams had fans to all eight home games and one team, Minnesota Vikings, had fans at one game only. On 28 November, Santa Clara County, in California, banned all contact sport – including practices. The San Francisco 49ers had to relocate their final three home games to Arizona.

The Super Bowl is a national event and drew 102 million television viewers in 2020. The Tampa Bay game on 7 February 2021 would be different. Media passes would be restricted, and interviews undertaken remotely. The crowd would be limited to 22,000 – one third would be vaccinated healthcare workers. However, the pre-match flyover with USAF bombers and half-time music survived. In the end, Tom Brady led the home team, Tampa Bay Buccaneers, to a 31-9 victory over defending champions Kansas City Chiefs. He received his tenth Super Bowl winners' ring. It was a moment of history to crown an incredibly difficult season described by Attallah as a '24-hour stress cycle'.

Nearly normal service would resume in 2021. The annual draft was held in Cleveland at the end of April. Pre-season, the NFL got tough on unvaccinated players and staff. A game lost because of COVID-19 involving unjabbed players would require match forfeiture and full financial compensation for the other side. Unvaccinated players would be subjected to $14,000 fines for COVID-19 protocol breaches and subjected to daily testing – compared to weekly for their jabbed team-mates. Before the start of the season, 93 per cent of players were vaccinated. The NFL had mandated all team coaches and executives to be jabbed and wanted all players similarly protected.

Games returned to London for the first time since 2019. In late 2021, like the UK, cases were seeping into US sport as Omicron infections surged.

In November, the Green Bay Packers' star QB, Aaron Rodgers, tested positive and missed the Kansas City game. In August, Rodgers claimed that 'I've been immunised'. It transpired that he was not vaccinated. His side lost 7-13. On the weekend before Christmas, the first NFL games had to be rescheduled. Cleveland Browns had 20 cases – mostly in asymptomatic and vaccinated players. At new year, Tampa Bay Buccaneers sacked wide receiver Antonio Brown for refusing to take the field in a game. He had been suspended for violating COVID-19 protocols earlier in the season. The NFL and players' union decided he had 'misrepresented' his vaccination status.

Super Bowl LVI was held on 13 February 2022 in Inglewood, California. It was won for the second year running by the host team, Los Angeles Rams. A capacity crowd was admitted but not before they had shown their vaccination passes and a negative test result. The media had to go further with proof of a booster dose!

The decisions, difficulties and solutions would be mirrored by the other great American sports.

Skating on thin ice

The National Hockey League (NHL) had difficult problems to surmount as the coronavirus crisis deepened. Ice hockey is an indoor activity and, like other great American sports, requires teams to traverse the country on a weekly basis. Seven of its 31 teams were based in Canada – a country with different pandemic regulations to its southern neighbour and creating obstacles for cross-border travel. The border remained closed to non-essential travel until 21 June.

The 2019/20 season was in full swing in March 2020. It was over four-fifths of the way through its planned 82-game regular season. As a health precaution, all media had been banned from the locker rooms earlier that month. Planned overseas games in the Czech Republic and Sweden were cancelled.

Although the league was suspended and players sent home on 12 March, scattered cases began to be reported amongst the teams. As early as 22 May, it was agreed to scrap the rest of the regular season and a formula for organising the play-offs developed. Teams in each of the two (Eastern and Western) conferences would be ranked according to their mid-March positions – determined by win percentages. The top 12 teams in each league would advance to the play-offs. Two hubs would host all the games. Many cities either side of the border were proposed.

Eventually the Canadian cities of Edmonton (Western) and Toronto (Eastern) were named as the play-off hubs. All 130 post-season games would be played with no spectators. The teams required special Canadian government dispensation to travel from the USA. Training, testing and protocols were progressively ramped up. Players returned to staged training from 8 June. From 13 July, testing became daily and, a week later, increased to three times every 48 hours.

The teams arrived at their designated 'hub' cities on 26 July; 7,000 tests were performed in that first week of 'return to play' – all negative. Hotels and playing areas were designated as secure zones with access only to essential personnel to comply with the Canadian Quarantine Act exemption accorded to the sport. Rule-breakers would have to self-isolate for 14 days and teams faced fines and loss of future 'draft picks'. There were no positive tests from players or staff once they had entered the 'hub bubbles'. Some players spent 64 days in quarantine.

Games were played inside these bubbles from 1 August until the concluding sixth game in the Stanley Cup Final on 28 September. Tampa Bay Lightning beat Dallas Stars 4-2 in Edmonton to lift the title.

The 2019/20 season finished only a week ahead of the original start to the 2020/21 season. Players rested while the NHL worked out what to do next. The NHL draft had already been postponed. The sport expected to lose billions during the new season as half of its revenues were derived from ticket sales. Some owners wanted the season abandoned.

Ten days before Christmas, plans were not cemented. A return to bubbles in restricted hubs was mooted. However, the NHL did not think it reasonable to quarantine players for six months. Players agreed.

On 20 December, the decision was unveiled. Four divisions would be created specifically for the season – including one comprising the seven Canadian teams to avoid cross-border travel. The number of regular season games was reduced to 56. Fixture lists were created so teams could play each other two to three times consecutively to reduce travel – a system traditionally favoured by baseball. 'Taxi squads' were introduced – extra squad members available to play in the event of viral outbreaks. Overseas games and the annual All-Star Games were canned.

The season started finally on 13 January and the Stanley Cup finals were delayed for a month until July. The Dallas Stars closed their training camp and postponed their first game because of cases. Before January was out more games needed postponing because of outbreaks at the Carolina Hurricanes and Vegas Golden Knights. Many more games would be postponed because of COVID-19 before the truncated season ended.

Like the NFL San Francisco 49ers, the San Jose Sharks fell foul of the Santa Clara County ruling and went on an extended road trip at the beginning of the season. During the regular season, no Canadian teams could admit spectators. Three American sides allowed very restricted numbers at the start but, by the end, the remaining 21 teams followed suit albeit with none exceeding half capacity. By the June play-offs, Canadian teams were allowed to admit small numbers of fans.

On 7 July, the Tampa Bay Lightning won the Stanley Cup in five games by defeating the Montreal Canadiens and winning their second consecutive title during the pandemic.

The 2021/22 season began on time in October. However, at Christmas, a 'circuit breaker' was introduced because of rising Omicron cases. Numerous games had been lost at that point. The postponements continued into the new year in Canada. Having started the season with large crowds, Canadian franchises saw restrictions reintroduced in December and maintained variably for many months.

In the end, the Tampa Bay Lightning could not make it three titles in a row and were defeated in the final by the Colorado Avalanche in June. It had been a bruising two years on and off the ice for the sport.

Dealing with unexpected curveballs

Major League Baseball (MLB) franchises migrate south to warmer climes in Florida and Arizona for spring training. In late March, the 162-game marathon regular season starts. On 16 March 2020, the MLB announced the season was postponed indefinitely, and all international games cancelled.

For three months, the MLB, owners and MLB Players' Association (MLBPA) failed to agree on restart plans. Players started testing positive as they continued to train for the restart. Finally, on 19 June, training camps were closed for deep cleaning. Most teams returned to their home cities. On 30 June, Minor League Baseball (the level below the MLB) was abandoned for 2020.

A reduced 60-game season was announced on 6 July as players returned to 'Summer Camp'. Twenty-four players chose to take some, or all, of the season off because of COVID concerns.

The season began in earnest on 23 July. Many changes to the game were required including increased size of the dugout to allow social distancing. Like in hockey, 'taxi squads' were introduced. Teams exchanged line-ups with the opposition using the MLB app rather than on paper. Five days before the season commenced, the Canadian government refused permission for the Toronto Blue Jays to play at home because of the need for cross-border travel. They relocated across the border in Buffalo. Over nine weeks, the 30 sides tried to complete 60 games. It was a punishing schedule. Double-headers (two games per day) and reduced travel helped ease the burden. Forty games were postponed because of COVID-19 – all but two were rescheduled.

Sixteen sides made it to the play-offs at the end of September; an expansion from the normal ten. Alcohol was banned post-games. All celebrations were to be on the diamond (pitch) and two metres distanced. The final three rounds – the Divisional Series, League Championship and World Series – would be played at neutral venues – like basketball and hockey. The American League played in California and the National League in Texas.

Thankfully, the last act of the season was not the first. The season finished on time on 27 October when the Los Angeles Dodgers defeated the Tampa Bay Rays 4-2 in Arlington, Texas.

In the dramatic World Series sixth game, the MLB were informed in the eighth innings (out of nine) that one of the Dodgers' tests from earlier that day was positive. The asymptomatic player, Justin Turner, was summarily pulled from the game. The reason was not made public, but the player was told to self-isolate. At the end of the game, his team celebrated on the diamond as Fox News announced the positive result on live television. Turner ran on to the field, hugged his team-mates and removed his mask for a team photograph. Public reaction was unsurprisingly negative. National numbers were rising with 76,000 new cases announced the day before. A subsequent MLB investigation applied no sanctions to player or team. However, there were reported to be five further positives amongst the LA Dodgers' organisation. If the World Series had required a 'winner-takes-all' seventh game, it may have been delayed because of the problem.

The 2021 season saw a return to the full regular season. However, international games remained banned. Teams were allowed to ease protocols if over 85 per cent of players and staff were fully vaccinated. By mid-June, 22 of the 30 sides had reached that threshold.

By early July, nearly all baseball stadia had capacity crowds. However, the Toronto Blue Jays started the season in Florida, migrated north to Buffalo and, finally, in late July, were given a Canadian government exemption to return home for the first time since 2019 – but with a crowd limit of 15,000. The Atlanta Braves took the World Series in early November.

The 2022 season should have seen calm descending on the choppy waters left by the virus. However, in December, the team owners voted to lock out the players following the expiration of their collective bargaining agreement (CBA). It took nearly 100 days to resolve, players returned late to spring training and the season was delayed by one week. However, the season finished on time with the Houston Astros crowned World Series champions in November.

Only fully vaccinated people could travel from the USA to Canada during the season. Thirty-six visiting players from ten teams could not go to Toronto. Instead, they were put on the temporary 'restricted' list and not paid during that time. Philadelphia's catcher, J.T. Realmuto, was happy to lose $250,000 in salary in exchange for not having 'Canada tell me what to do'. The overall MLB players' vaccination rate of 91 per cent in mid-summer 2021 mirrored that of the whole US population.

Slam-dunked by a microbe

By 11 March 2020, the 30 teams of the National Basketball Association (NBA) had played between 63 and 67 of their scheduled 82 'regular' season games. That day, Utah Jazz versus Oklahoma City was pulled shortly before the game when a Jazz player tested positive. The same night, the New Orleans Pelicans and Sacramento Kings game was postponed before 'tip-off'. A referee had officiated a Jazz game a few nights before. The NBA announced that the rest of that evening's games could be completed but then the game would shut down. Just 38 days before the play-offs were scheduled, the sport lay dormant.

College basketball was cancelled as it was reaching its climax – known as 'March Madness'. The games, involving the 68 best college sides, are watched by millions. Television companies annually paid $891 million for the rights. It would be the first time since its inception in 1939 that no champion team would be crowned. The women's competition followed suit.

A plan was hatched to 'point guard' the NBA season – sporting superstars and science working together. It would provide everything that was needed to observe human behaviour, sporting endeavour and social policy in unison.

In late May, the NBA was negotiating with The Walt Disney Company to use the Orlando complex for a behind-closed-doors single bio-secure hub. Plans were signed off on 4 June with a start date of 30 July.

Only 22 of the 30 teams would be involved – those that retained a reasonable play-off berth 'shot'. A six-phase return to competition play was hatched, which was comprehensive and tough. The NBA reserved the right to examine and exclude any player or staff member deemed high-risk individuals. Testing and graduated training began in the teams' home cities before they started convening in Florida on 7 July.

Unlike a holiday in Disneyland, this controlled setting was more Mickey Mouse than Snow White with players living, training and playing in isolation. Rooms needed redesigning. A six-foot bed might be ideal for would-be sleeping beauties. However, at 6ft 9in (2.06m), LeBron James and his mates needed bedding of another dimension. The NBA spent $190m on the project, which allowed it to recoup an estimated $1.5 billion in revenues.

Teams would be confined to hotels and no mixing with other teams allowed. No spitting, no hand licking, no guests in their hotel rooms, and compulsory face masks. Miami Heat player Jimmy Butler started selling $20 cups of coffee to his team-mates using the espresso machine and El Salvador coffee beans that he had taken into the bubble. Post-pandemic, he built this into a business – the BIGFACE brand.

Quarantine was enforced after both leaving and re-entering the bubble. Negative test results were required as players and staff arrived. A violation hotline was established for anonymous breach reporting. Players could opt out but would lose a proportion of their annual salary.

The regular season finished in the bio-bubble with each team playing eight games to determine which 16 teams would make the play-offs. Los Angeles Lakers beat the Miami Heat to take the title on 11 October. The season lasted 11 days short of one year – the longest in the NBA's 74-year history. The finalists spent three months cocooned in the Florida bubble.

The bubble games never burst. No crowds. Just cameras from five major TV partners. There were no positive COVID-19 test results throughout the process and only four players were asked to leave because of rule-breaking.

Players and staff appeared to buy into the Magic Kingdom ethos. This experiment in infection control, epidemiology and behaviour modification while undertaking elite sport could act as a model for decades to come. The results will be revisited in chapter 31.

The 2020/2021 NBA season started two months late just three days before Christmas. The regular season was cut by ten games and planned to finish by late July – over a month later than normal. By the end of February, 31 games had been postponed for COVID-19. On occasions, teams could not field the required minimum of eight players. Only seven sides admitted any spectators at the beginning of the season. By the end of the season only Oklahoma Thunder had not allowed fans into home games. Like the Toronto Blue Jays in hockey, the Toronto Raptors played the whole season in Tampa, Florida because of Canadian government restrictions. Milwaukee Bucks took the title by defeating the Phoenix Suns.

The 2020/21 college basketball season was similarly disrupted. Many events were postponed, cancelled or relocated. The start of the season was pushed back two weeks until the end of November. In early 2021, it was announced that both the men's and women's 'March Madness' would take place in restricted locations. The men would play in the state of Indiana with the final games in Indianapolis. The women's tournament would be confined to Texas with most games held in San Antonio.

The 2021/22 NBA season returned to its regular 82-game fixture list. Over 90 per cent of NBA players had been vaccinated ahead of the mid-October season opener. This was much higher than the overall national percentage of 65 at the time. At the same stage, only 35 per cent of English Premier League football clubs had achieved a vaccination rate greater than 50 per cent.

Pre-season, the cities of Los Angeles, San Francisco, New York and Toronto required all spectators to have had vaccinations. This affected six of the 30 teams. Unvaccinated players in those teams could not play home games and would have to forgo salaries for those matches. Illogically, visiting unvaccinated players could play subject to a strict testing regime. In early January, Philadelphia announced similar restrictions, adding the 76ers to the list. By the end of 2021, 97 per cent of players were vaccinated and only ten games lost because of COVID-19 – all before the turn of the year. Dallas Mavericks' Luka Doncic from Slovenia missed five games with COVID-19. On his return, he scored 14 points and said, 'My chest was burning.'

Around 30 players across the NBA remained unjabbed. Shaquille O'Neill, the ex-NBA star, said, 'If you're on my team and you can't play home games, I don't want you around. Get your ass up outta here.' As well as being tested more frequently, unvaccinated players were banned from high-risk environments like restaurants. It could have been worse for the recalcitrant players. All coaches, staff and referees had no choice. Get vaccinated. Canada was even tougher on the unjabbed. All unvaccinated visiting players were subject to regular testing and could only leave their hotel rooms to play and train. Breaching the rules could lead to heavy fines and even a six-month jail sentence.

The effect that these restrictions had on players is revealed in chapter 27.

Eight months after the season began, Golden State Warriors landed the title by defeating the Boston Celtics 4-2 in the final.

Soccer on the defensive

Soccer, as the Americans refer to it, had been trying to establish itself as a rival to the 'Big 4' sports for over half a century. Major League Soccer (MLS) appeared to have been the most sustained bid. In 2020, it was celebrating its 25th season. Three Canadian sides participated, based in Montreal, Vancouver and Toronto.

Twenty-six clubs were split into Western and Eastern Conferences with the top teams from each entering the play-offs. The season was less than two weeks old when games were suspended on 12 March. There would be no further fixtures for four months.

The competition on its return was split into several phases with complex arrangements rooted in player and staff welfare and following varying American and Canadian government guidelines.

The initial phase would be like the NBA – with which it overlapped. It was a behind-closed-doors bio-secure event at Florida's Walt Disney World beginning on 8 July – called the 'MLS is Back Tournament'. Both FC Dallas and Nashville SC clubs withdrew without playing a game after multiple positive tests.

Each remaining team played three games in a mini group. The results counted for both advancement to the 'final-16' knockout part of the tournament and for regular season standings. On 11 August, the Portland Timbers were crowned champions of this one-off tournament. The knockout games did not count for the regular season.

After leaving Florida, the regular season restarted with the intention for all clubs to play a 23-game season instead of the original 36. Each club played six matches against opponents in their own 'conference'. Canadian teams stayed north of the border, playing their own mini-tournament. Dallas and Nashville played each other an extra three times to make up for their Floridian withdrawal. The 'second phase' started on 11 September. Three more games were played while avoiding excessive travel. The Canadian trio travelled south to host home games in neutral venues to circumvent their own government regulations. However, not all teams reached the 23-game landmark, because of COVID-19. The MLS decided that final positions would be determined on a points-per-game basis instead.

The play-offs began a month later on 20 November and expanded to 18 teams. Three weeks later, Columbus Crew SC beat defending champions Seattle Sounders FC 3-0 in the final.

The year 2020 was catastrophic for women's soccer. It was suspended on the same day as the MLS. The National Women's Soccer League (NWSL) top division has nine clubs and is heavily dependent financially upon the United States Soccer Federation (and to a lesser extent the Canadian Soccer Association) who sponsor their leading international players' salaries. The 2020 season was scheduled to commence on 18 April and finish with a Championship game on 14 November.

The season started two months late at the end of June with the 2020 Challenge Cup hastily organised. Orlando Pride had to withdraw after multiple COVID-19 cases. For safety, an 'NWSL village' was formed in Salt Lake City. The teams were quarantined for the entirety of the competition and only two grounds were used. After a series of matches, Houston Dash were crowned winners one month later. However, it had the accolade of being the first US professional sports team event to restart after the first lockdown.

A novel Fall Series was organised to provide more game time. To reduce travel, each team played four matches against two local rivals. The overall winners, Portland Thorns FC, were determined by the best results from these games and received the Verizon Community Shield. The teams played little competitive football. Houston and Chicago played the most (11 games) and Orlando the least (four games).

Because of the ongoing viral crisis, the 2021 MLS start date was delayed from late February to early April. A further fortnight's delay occurred following a contractual dispute between clubs and players. As for other sports, the three Canadian teams moved south to host matches. However, with the lifting of Canadian government restrictions in mid-July, matches started to be played north of the border. At that stage, 95 per cent of MLS players were fully vaccinated. New York City FC took their first MLS Cup two weeks before Christmas.

After the devastation of the 2020 season, the NWSL managed to start 2021 a week before the MLS. It announced a restructuring of the season. The Challenge Cup was retained as a stand-alone season hors d'oeuvre. In mid-May, the regular season commenced, and the play-offs finished in late November with Washington Spirit lifting their first title.

Is there more than the Atlantic Ocean that divides us?

The great American sports came to different decisions at important times compared to their British cousins. Where do American sports' accomplishments sit against the often-criticised English football Premier League? The players in all these sports command huge salaries and enormous media attention akin to European footballers.

All US sports came back later than European football. Each sport took its time and involved the three important components in decision-making – the governing body, the owners and the players. The latter, via their associations, appeared at the top tables and had more influence than was apparent in Britain. The power of individual municipal authorities to insist on sport following local vaccination protocols seemed to be accepted without demur. Except for the NFL, other sports had to come to terms with different regulations between American and Canadian governments and provide solutions for meaningful competition.

All professional American sports managed to bring their seasons to a conclusion. The NFL had the advantage of beginning six months after the global pandemic started. It could observe how other sports had planned and enacted protocols. It spent time on player education and only had to cope with 16 games per franchise during the regular season.

The teams and sports showed flexibility. The English Premiership would not countenance neutral venues, bio-secure bubbles or isolation from families for months; American sport showed itself more ready to embrace such 'hardships'. Basketball, ice hockey and soccer accepted moves into single, locked-down facilities. They were willing to introduce different formats and competitions rather than insisting that the season should be completed as intended – albeit late. Intriguing innovations like 'taxi squads' in baseball and ice hockey were introduced.

Their protocols were fiercer than in Europe. Penalties and restrictions were harsher. Sideline protocols, like mask wearing and player celebrations were more strictly regulated. Testing regimes were more frequent. Positive test numbers were not insignificant. However, team player and staff rosters for many of the sports were large. Only 2.7 per cent of NFL games in 2020 needed rearranging because of COVID-19.

Vaccination levels were much higher than in English football. The game made life uncomfortable for the rump of refuseniks and different protocols were applied regarding testing, travel and socialising for the unjabbed. Seemingly, more athletes 'opted out' for the 2020 season than in Britain and unvaccinated players seemed content to pass up on huge amounts of salary to adhere to their principles.

Chapter 16

Fall Guys

Autumn 2020

Like the rest of the global community, sport was emerging from its worst nightmare. Months of lockdown, restrictions and financial terrors.

The last quarter of 2020 had to be better. Unencumbered training, certainty of competition, re-established revenues and the re-admission of fans to live sport. Wrong, wrong, wrong and wrong. Instead, the period would be played out against a tide of rising cases, hospital admissions and deaths. A new viral strain's emergence would be superadded to a second lockdown. Sport would try and continue with inadequate funds for the most part. It would compete without vaccinations, and before lateral flow tests made testing cheap and rapid. Spectators would mostly follow their heroes from the safety of their lounges.

By the year's end, professional sport would once again be taking a standing count but not yet laid out on the canvas. However, people would be questioning whether the towel should be thrown in to safeguard its participants' health.

English first-class cricket had declared an end to its summer innings in early October and promptly re-furloughed its players. Rugby league continued until late November, limping to its Grand Final during lockdown, its fixture list littered with COVID-19 cancellations.

The old and fresh challenges facing sport during 2020's fall are examined through the immune systems of cricket, rugby union and football.

Cricket moves camp

Since it was founded in 2008, the Indian Premier League (IPL) had become the world's leading T20 cricket competition. Attracting the very best of global white-ball players, its central importance to the whole sport was clear. By 2020, the IPL generated one third of all the game's income. It was a matter of whoever pays the piper when dealing with its demands and politics.

Despite the postponement of its spring 2020 seven-week edition, its organisers were not prepared to let something like a global pandemic derail it.

Indian infection rates remained stubbornly high. What was a possible solution? Move it 1,600 miles to another country and start in September. International calendar dates became fallow after the men's T20 World Cup in Australia was postponed. It meant 'IPL game on' in the United Arab Emirates (UAE).

Players flew in using chartered aircraft and straight into luxury hotel 'homes' for eight weeks. Abu Dhabi required one week's room isolation. Hazmat-suited men sanitised training facilities. The holders, Chennai Super Kings, had 17 positive tests after emerging from a week's quarantine! They would finish last but one in the competition.

Games were played to a wall of canned noise and cheering spectators' images on large screens. It was atmospheric but barely replicated a joyous night at Mumbai's Wankhede stadium.

Still, audiences around the world got their IPL 'fix' and the organisers their media money. The final was played on 10 November. Little did the teams know that they would be back in less than one year to complete the Delta-interrupted 2021 version.

Bubble pressure

By the end of 2020, Cricket South Africa's finances were critical. Its board had resigned following mismanagement accusations. Their team had not played for nine months. TV revenues from an England mini-tour could net the hosts £3.5m.

In mid-November, the England squad flew into Cape Town to begin ten days' quarantine. Intra-squad matches and socially isolated golf were allowed to break the boredom. Both teams stayed at the same luxury hotel. South Africa had players isolating before entering quarantine and still lost a warm-up squad match when a further cricketer tested positive. The squads were separated inside the hotel until all returned virus-free results. Hotel staff were not allowed out of the premises. Three T20 games would be followed by three one-day internationals (ODIs). Only two venues would be used – Newlands and Paarl.

The first half of the mini-series went well. Then the virus struck. First a home player's positive test caused the first ODI to be scrubbed. It baffled those entrusted with security. A Sherlock Holmes-type investigation failed to reveal the breach.

As the visitors were en route for the second ODI, news filtered through of cases among hotel staff, including one allocated to England's area. Additionally, England were accused of breaching protocols by using the wrong practice nets. The local police threatened charges against the visitors. Two of England's squad tested positive – later these proved erroneous. The game was rescheduled and the 'all-clear' signalled beforehand. Indeed, since early summer, the England group had undergone over a thousand tests without a single positive result.

It was all too much and getting very messy. The England team had had enough and doubted hotel security efficiency. Despite efforts to broker an agreement, there would be no more cricket. Recriminations began. South Africa's doctor,

Dr Manjra, was reported as being 'devastated'. There was a view that England were simply fatigued from months of isolation and protocols. Eleven of the English players had been involved in the recent UAE-hosted IPL and had had less than two weeks at home. Even before arrival, the visitors were openly talking about mental well-being issues within bio-secure bubbles. The ECB supported its players with the view that their well-being – physical and mental – was paramount.

The hosts believed that the last two games could have been rescheduled and played. Aspersions were cast in the direction of England playing golf. England picked up the £400,000 hotel bill. The fact that England didn't check out immediately after the abandonment of matches was viewed cynically by some of the hosts.

'Twickers' open for business?

The culmination of the delayed 2019/20 domestic rugby union season would act merely as an hors d'oeuvre to the main *plat de saison automne*. International games would return after a seven-month hiatus. Like cricket, it was Test matches that mattered financially.

For English-based players (particularly the all-conquering Exeter stars), it would be a case of out of their club's fire into the nation's pan with only six days in between to put their feet up. Players' already exhausted bodies would be required to tackle and scrummage over at least five punishing weekends.

First an 'audition'. It didn't go well. England were due a run out against scratch outfit Barbarians at an empty Twickenham on 25 October. The game was abandoned 48 hours before. Some Baa-Baas players had gone 'walkabout'. More precisely, two unauthorised nights in Mayfair hostelries. Having compounded matters by giving false statements, the unlucky 13 were variably banned from playing, fined and made to do community service. It cost the RFU £1m that it could ill afford. England coach Eddie Jones claimed that rugby had become a 'laughing stock'. Astonishingly, the Baa-Baas would repeat the feat in 2021.

Next up was the small matter of the final four games of the 2020 Six Nations to reschedule. The outstanding fourth-round match between Ireland and Italy would be played on October's penultimate weekend. All six nations would play their final games a weekend later in front of echoing empty stadia.

Traditionally, Europe hosts a series of internationals in late autumn involving southern hemisphere powerhouses ably supported by 'second tier nations'. However, continuing global infection rates, travel restrictions and quarantine rules meant that no 'big beasts' would voyage north. Plan B was required. The Autumn Nations Cup was dreamt up.

The Six Nations, plus Fiji and Japan, were inked in for two pools of four sides followed by a weekend of ranking play-offs from mid-November to early December. Amazon Prime reportedly paid £20m to screen the tournament – described as a financial lifeline for cash-strapped northern unions. Only the first/second-place final between the eventual winners, England and France, at Twickenham admitted spectators. Two thousand attendees included NHS and front-line services personnel.

Edinburgh's Murrayfield and the Dublin Aviva Stadium acted as hosts. Cardiff's Millennium Stadium had been seconded for COVID-19 purposes – aka the Dragon's Heart hospital – and was not ready to host rugby. Llanelli's Parc y Scarlets stepped into the breach. France named Vannes and Stade de France, Paris as their venues. Italy avoided Rome and scheduled games in Ancona and Florence.

An early casualty was Japan, who withdrew in August. Their team could not train, and foreign nationals were not allowed into the country, including the Cherry Blossoms' head coach, New Zealander Jamie Joseph. Japan had not played for a year after exiting the World Cup they hosted. Georgia substituted.

Governments had to agree to the games, the travel across countries, testing regimes and strict bio-secure environments. Their acquiescence would be sorely tested.

After Fiji's warm-up game against Portugal was cancelled because of COVID-19 cases, matters deteriorated for the South Sea islanders. All three of their pool games were axed. During several days, over 30 positive tests were returned from the Fiji group. With many more isolating as contacts for ten days, the nation could not train or field a team. France, Italy and Scotland were each awarded 28-0 wins. It was claimed that strict isolation procedures had been followed but it sounded like a case of 'closing the stable door after the virus riding the horse had bolted'.

The integrity of the competition was threatened. A quarter of the pool matches had been lost. Would Amazon Prime hold back some of its investment? After three weeks of hotel isolation, illness and lack of preparation, Fiji took on Georgia in Edinburgh on 5 December. Amazingly, they won 38-24 in the seventh/eighth-place play-off game.

The game to determine the winners looked a foregone conclusion; 813 English caps would take on 68 French *capuchons*. England won, but only after a 22-19 'sudden death' overtime victory. The Top 14 French clubs would not release 25 senior players as it breached their agreement with the national team.

Staggering to the next scrum

English domestic rugby union restarted during the second lockdown and international series, and only four weeks after the previous year-long season had completed.

Lasting 32 weeks, 2020/21 would be seven to eight weeks shorter than normal and finish in late June. It would be gruelling for players – especially those touring South Africa with the Lions afterwards in July. However, the jeopardy of relegation was removed, condemning the Premiership to expand by one team for 2021/22.

By the end of the year, four rounds had been completed. It would be Boxing Day before the first two games were cancelled, because of COVID-19. On 5 December, Worcester welcomed the first Premiership fans back for their clash against Bath. Only a quarter of scheduled games before New Year would entertain spectators. After that the doors were locked again.

The Pro14 had wrapped up their previous season in mid-September. It started 2020/21 three weeks later and before the 2019/20 European Heineken Champions Cup Final was played. Trying to embrace clubs from five different countries was immediately problematic. Neither of the two South African sides could play – one because of COVID-19 and the other had gone bust. However, despite the challenges of air travel and lockdown, the first nine rounds pre-New Year were completed without a game being cancelled.

'I Guess That's Why They Call It the Blues'
Song by Elton John. 1983

On a weekday afternoon in early December, thousands of undergraduates descended upon west London for the annual Oxford–Cambridge varsity rugby union matches at 'Headquarters'. Twickenham and the universities took an early decision in July 2020 to postpone the iconic fixtures scheduled for 10 December. At that stage, there was no certainty that the students would even be back in lectures, let alone training on a rugby field. As amateurs, they would have to follow non-elite sport's guidelines. Eventually, the students were given the green light to hold their games at Welford Road, Leicester on 4 July 2021 – Independence Day for student rugby. Community rugby would not be able to start scrummaging or mauling for another two weeks.

Back on the treadmill all too soon
On 12 September 2020, English Premier League football kicked off five weeks later than scheduled and only seven

weeks since the previous season had concluded. Ten weeks had been sliced from a normal off-season in the haste to get going again. The concertinaed late-summer break did little to let weary limbs recover, injuries to mend, and new players to be integrated into teams and tactical systems.

Fatigue concerns were held, particularly for those English clubs still involved in European competitions when the shutters came down in March 2020 – Chelsea, Wolves and the two Manchester clubs. Not surprisingly, all were granted an extra week's preparation. Manchester City would play 61 domestic and European games from September 2020 to May 2021; 250 days, averaging one game every four days.

The hard-won 'winter break' to reduce injuries and finally introduced in the winter of 2020 (after 25 years of discussion) would be scrapped for 2021. The season would finish on 23 May 2021 and only one week later than originally planned pre-pandemic. It would allow 19 days of preparation time before the postponed Euro 2020 commenced. The domestic season was being squeezed into a four-week-shorter season than originally envisioned.

After the first nine Premier League rounds, a 23 per cent increase in muscle injuries was being reported. Muscles were beginning to complain.

Fans' hopes spring eternal

'Hope springs eternal' by Alexander Pope from *An Essay on Man*. 1732

Surely fans would return to grounds in the new season? Test events had taken place. In late August, Brighton had entertained Chelsea in a pre-season friendly with 2,500 fans present. Several Chelsea players were quarantining with COVID-19 after holidays. It reminded everyone of the continuing challenges ahead. In mid-September, two Championship games admitted 1,000 fans. It would lead nowhere fast.

The COVID-19 national situation was deteriorating. Schools had returned and undergraduates were heading for university. These were Petri dishes preparing to incubate microbes. Soon cases would start rising alarmingly. It was too much for NHS systems, which were unable to handle demand. Results were taking an eternity and people were travelling hundreds of miles for available testing appointments. Baroness Dido Harding, who headed Test and Trace, was forced to publicly apologise.

'Get those turnstiles ticking'

It would only be towards the end of 'Lockdown Mark II' that the first glimpses of normality returning were espied.

From December, limited crowds would be permitted into grounds located within Tiers 1 and 2. Elite sports had planned and practised their risk management strategies and wanted to safely welcome back spectators after nine months. However, the extra expenditure on stewarding, signage and health checking of attendees meant that it wasn't the equivalent of a lottery-winning ticket.

Tier 1 regions could welcome back 4,000 fans outside – however, the Scilly Isles had never been a hotbed of Premier League football. Half of Premier League and EFL clubs, and eight WSL teams fell on the right side of the Tier 2 boundary. They qualified for 2,000 fans. The rest found themselves in Tier 3 and would remain playing home games in front of empty terraces. However, such boundaries proved fluid.

At the time, Germany was only allowing fans to return in areas where infection rates were below 35 cases per 100,000 of population. Within the Premier League, only Brighton played in an area where cases were below 200 per 100,000.

On Wednesday, 2 December, football fans returned 'properly' after 266 days' absence. That honour would not fall to grounds like Old Trafford or Anfield. Carlisle hosting Salford City were first to welcome back 2,000 fans. Another 8,000 fans attended four further EFL games later that evening. Yes, fans were masked, herded and temperature-checked – but they were back!

Unfortunately, fans' bio-bubbles were about to be burst just after they had been blown. The lesser-spotted football fan was in danger of becoming extinct. Again.

The next day, Arsenal played in front of fans against Rapid Vienna in the Europa League. The first Premier League fixture to be played with supporters present was West Ham versus Manchester United on 5 December. It was not supposed to have been the first. The previous night, Aston Villa's game against Newcastle was postponed because of infections in the visitors' camp. It was the first COVID-19-related postponement of the season.

Less than a quarter of Premier League games scheduled for December would admit crowds. Four teams – Aston Villa, Burnley, Leicester City and Newcastle United – would not see any spectators home or away. None of the 'fan-less four' would see home supporters until their last games of the season – late May. Over 14 months without hearing your home support roar you on in a league fixture.

By mid-December, Tier 3 would expand and swallow up clubs. Two days before Christmas, Bournemouth on the south coast stood alone as the bastion of live fan participation in the Championship.

On Boxing Day, only Cornwall and Herefordshire were in Tier 2. Forty-three per cent of England would be in Tier 4. Of the 30 Premier League games scheduled across the Christmas–New Year period, only one fixture (Liverpool versus West Ham) would provide festive cheer for fans. This was an astonishing achievement for Liverpool given its dire coronavirus numbers a month or two earlier and a degree of success for the mass testing regime established in the city.

By 30 December, the whole of England was either in Tier 3 or 4. The gates of all grounds in the Premier League, EFL and WSL were finally slammed shut. The last elite game to admit fans was at Plymouth's Home Park on 29 December. Two thousand supporters witnessed Argyle lose

2-3 to Oxford United. It seemed like we had returned to 23 March. Little gained and an awful lot lost.

'The haves and have nots'

From the start of the 2020/21 season, clubs' differential financial clout was re-accentuated when it came to decisions on regular COVID-19 testing. EFL Leagues One and Two still could not afford to test. The consequences were inevitable. Clubs argued that 99 per cent of tests during summer's Project Restart were negative and that £5,000 per round of testing was unjustified. Instead, they intended to rely on careful health screening and strict protocols. The Premier League were testing weekly. Most Championship sides tried to test regularly but were vulnerable to testing not being available. Bristol City's New Year game at Brentford was postponed as their local lab had closed for the festive weekend!

The third round of the Carabao League Cup potentially matches Premier League and EFL sides. At times, it appeared like cases of the 'unwashed' meeting the 'holier than thou' crowd. Some elite clubs took umbrage. West Ham's co-owner David Sullivan asked, 'Why are we in a competition where we're playing teams who have not been checked?' Some lower league clubs bit the bullet and funded testing, some took up opposing Premier League clubs' offers to pay for testing, others declined.

Problems arose early when most of Leyton Orient's League Two squad tested positive in mid-September. It resulted in their home Carabao Cup tie against Spurs being awarded to the visitors. Sky was due to pay Orient £125,000 for televising the game.

Pre-November lockdown, no Premier League or Championship games became viral victims. Only eight EFL League One and Two games succumbed. It would all change in December. The issues of appearing and disappearing fans was paralleled by the problems of getting a virus-free team on to the park. League One clubs appeared particularly attractive 'breeding grounds' with 18 games biting the dust in December.

More slowly, COVID-19 would take its toll on Premier League and Championship games – seven in total across December. The Premier League doubled its testing rate and the EFL reintroduced compulsory testing from New Year. The latter asked the PFA to pay the estimated £5m bill. Football's case levels were far higher than in the summer. The Premier League's Project Restart produced 20 positive tests over ten weeks. The first 12 weeks of the autumn revealed 78 cases and weekly numbers would further double in December.

The virus was more than fighting back.

'All the leaves are brown, and the skies are grey'
Lyrics from 'California Dreamin'' by the Mamas and the Papas. 1965

Historians of previous pandemics know that few episodes finish with a single wave. Politicians, sport and the rest of us hoped that 2020 would be different. It wasn't. Viruses only 'change their spots' to produce new variants and will take their leave slowly.

The autumn promised so much in sport. However, once elite sport restarted, it would continue through 'hell or high water' – otherwise known as lockdowns and lockouts. The public was weary and wary. Our sports people must have felt at times like performing circus acts, obeying their ringmasters' commands. Through it all, our rugby players reminded us that footballers do not have a monopoly when it comes to committing selfish acts.

Chapter 17

Christmas Covidiots, Cuddling and Cup Ties

AS THE nation prepared for a festive period of restricted fayre, a few professional footballers looked for ways of carrying on regardless.

Arabian night(mare)s

The WSL had pre-planned a three-week break across Christmas and New Year. It was a sage move. Aston Villa's last game at West Ham was postponed as the hosts harboured COVID-19. One in 25 WSL players tested positive that week.

Some WSL clubs forbade players from seeing families over Christmas. It forced some to spend the holiday period alone having not seen loved ones for nine months. Other players decided to travel to Dubai for a festive break.

London-based players were in Tier 4 and only allowed to travel after producing evidence that the trip was for bona fide business purposes. Arsenal's Katie McCabe posted pictures of herself sunbathing on the beach. She claimed the UAE trip was for a meeting with her brother-in-law agent who lived near her in London. The UK government advised against such travel and later removed the UAE from the safe travel corridor as cases rose by 52 per cent at New Year.

After New Year, Manchester City and Arsenal reported that five of their Dubai visitors had tested positive. Their respective games against West Ham and Aston Villa on the second weekend of January were postponed. Neither club could name a minimum of 14 players for the fixtures. Overall, five of the six WSL games were cancelled. Each postponed game had COVID-19 as a contributory factor.

The recriminations began. West Ham's skipper, Gilly Flaherty, asked the girls who had travelled to apologise for the disruptions. She posted, 'I really don't like the arrogance that the money and wages have brought into it [the professional game]. Players need to be humble.' The Arsenal women who went to Dubai relied upon their manager to apologise for them. Manchester United's boss, Casey Stoney, apologised for allowing her players on the Dubai trip, 'It was a poor error of judgement from me.' How refreshing.

Players were reminded of the increased scrutiny of their actions following the enhanced exposure that the women's game enjoyed. Naive players were encouraged to learn from the ill-fated Dubai trip. The FA's head of women's football, Baroness Sue Campbell, was 'personally disappointed'. Everton boss Willie Kirk commented that 'there was probably more important things to focus on during that period than going on holiday to Dubai'. The antics of a few WSL players were compared to the number of players in the Championship who had part-time key worker jobs in supermarkets, teaching and the health sectors.

Of course, WSL players were not the only ones Dubai-bound.

Glasgow Celtic and Scottish First Minister Nicola Sturgeon locked horns after the men's club's Hogmanay trip to Dubai. She felt Celtic had questions to answer about their winter training break. She commented that 'I've seen comments from the club that it's more for R&R than training' and added that 'all bets are off' if those involved in Scottish professional sport do not respect extra privileges.

Celtic retorted that the trip was fully authorised. Shortly after their return, 13 players and their manager were forced to self-isolate after a case amongst the party. Manager Neil Lennon claimed the decision was more political than a public health one.

From the outbreak of the pandemic, Sturgeon appeared to have been 'one foot ahead of the game' compared to south of the border. She had previously issued a stern 'yellow card' caution to Scottish football following breaches in August.

The Tiers of a clown

'Tears of a clown' by Smokey Robinson and the Miracles. 1970

Back in Blighty, government prohibitions on mixing outside your domestic bubble in Tier 4 London escaped the ears of a few Premier League footballers.

After the appearance on social media of festive japes, Jose Mourinho was forced to admit that three Spurs players had breached COVID-19 regulations and attended a Christmas party along with a West Ham player. This was particularly embarrassing for the 'Special One'. Only a day before, he had called the Premier League 'unprofessional' after Spurs' game against Fulham was postponed following cases at Craven Cottage.

Mourinho expressed 'disappointment'. He had presented one of the partygoers, Sergio Reguilón, with a Portuguese piglet to offset the player's dismay at being 'home alone' at Christmas. Was the Spanish full-back's contribution to the celebration bacon sandwiches? Tottenham included the player in the team's squad to play Leeds United that day. West Ham closed their training ground for deep cleaning as another squad member tested positive.

The same day, Fulham's Aleksander Mitrovic, fellow Serbian and Crystal Palace's Luca Milivojevic and seven others were revealed to have attended a New Year's Eve party. At the time, Fulham could not play because of COVID-19 cases in their club. Manager Roy Hodgson condemned his actions.

Forty-eight hours later, Manchester City's Benjamin Mendy was revealed to have hosted a New Year's Eve party. An earlier chapter had identified that the French defender had 'previous' on similar matters. Guardiola, Mendy's boss, felt that it was unfair to expect footballers to be role models and described the player as 'one of the good guys'.

Rod Liddle in the *Sunday Times* scorned the players' premeditated actions and subsequent attempts to seek redemption by donating money to charities, 'It galls [the public] to see these pampered dimbos from stage and screen and football pitch cavorting around without a care in the world.' Ex-Premier League striker Tony Cascarino believed such transgressions should have led to three-match bans.

The Premier League and FA appeared dismayed but allowed clubs to deal with matters internally. The Metropolitan Police declined to act. Clubs reminded players of their responsibilities. The media reported fines of one to two weeks' wages. The Premier League announced a record number of weekly cases but declared confidence that the show must go on.

The breaches must be viewed in context. The nation had just had its Christmas plans seriously disrupted at a few days' notice. For some it was cancelled altogether. New Year went uncelebrated, and the Hogmanay weekend finished with Boris Johnson announcing a third indefinite national lockdown.

People were told to stay at home and only essential shops opened. Access to exercise facilities was severely restricted in the middle of winter. National cases were soaring. There were more COVID-19 patients in hospital than during the first wave. People were losing their lives in their hundreds every day. NHS staff and essential workers were on their knees physically and psychologically. Millions had been unable to take holidays or travel abroad since March.

Cuddling, carousing and cup ties

The first weekend after New Year is FA Cup third-round time. Will one of the Premier League 'sharks' be drawn against a non-league tiddler? Such ties can ease small clubs' finances for years. January 2021 had the added frisson of the COVID-19 lottery. Would clubs be laid low with players self-isolating?

The draw did not fail us. Marine in Liverpool faced a home tie against Spurs. Marine were 161 places below Tottenham, the biggest gap between two teams in FA Cup history. Marine sold 32,000 virtual tickets and raised £300,000 for the fan-less match. Their tiny ground backed on to neighbouring domestic gardens. Each property had its street number nailed to the mesh fence. In the absence of ball boys, Harry Kane would know which bell to ring to get his ball back. In the event Kane didn't turn out and Spurs still won 5-0.

However, Chorley (sixth tier) versus Derby County (second tier) and Crawley (fourth tier) versus Leeds United (first tier) provided greater pickings. Derby were seriously depleted by COVID-19. Their entire first-team squad, manager Wayne Rooney and many under-23s were confined to barracks. Chorley triumphed 2-0. Crawley went one better and destroyed Leeds United 3-0.

Hot on the heels of the covidiots' antics came concern over non-adherence to behaviour regulations in and around matches. The PFA had reminded clubs of their responsibilities in the week leading up to the cup weekend. The advice was ignored.

The question of professional footballers cuddling in celebration before TV cameras became heavily debated. Some on-field hugs would not have looked out of place in an ancient Roman brothel. Not a socially distanced salutation in sight. Players continued spitting and swopping shirts. Mask use for non-combatants seemed haphazard and illogical. Managers were elbow-greeting and then proceeding to embrace like long-lost siblings.

The crescendo of approbation peaked after the cup weekend. Videos of changing-room sing-songs at Crawley and Chorley hit social media. The FA warned the clubs to behave in future. It was too late. The EFL's reinstated testing returned 1:31 positives. The Premier League recorded 40 weekly cases. Aston Villa had such a large outbreak they was forced to play 'the kids' against Liverpool in the cup and lost 1-4.

Nine days after beating Leeds, Crawley postponed their fixture against Stevenage because of a COVID-19 outbreak and delayed their fourth-round cup tie against Bournemouth.

Football claimed that it was hard to stop hugging and that mass celebrations were natural and spontaneous. People signposted regular testing and the outdoor setting for these perceived peccadillos.

Sports medics commented that regular testing was not bulletproof and that footballers' behaviour outside of their clubs was leading to rising cases. Professor James Calder, orthopaedic surgeon and independent chairman of the government's committee on elite sport's return, believed players should refrain from 'any type of celebration'.

Some players did not appreciate that the rest of the country was making large adjustments. Millions had been denied the opportunity to embrace loved ones for months. Football just didn't get it.

Not a hair out of place

Attention turned next to footballers' neatly coiffured pates.

The rest of the population was resembling tropical castaways again. Elite footballers' hair never seemed to grow. Either they had found follicle-arresting cream or had broken lockdown rules and been to the barbers.

For Newcastle's Brazilian, Joelinton, the answer was clear. He went to 'celebrity crimper' Tom Baxter, who labelled his customer an 'idiot' for sharing an image on Instagram. The hairdresser said that he could have claimed it was a legal photoshoot for his business but was still expecting a call from the 'boys in blue'.

Infringements were not confined to British-based footballers. Cristiano Ronaldo ignored Italian travel laws by heading to the mountains with his family. The Juventus star shared images on social media of his frolics in the snow and celebrating his partner's birthday.

Blue January

January is the gloomiest month of the year in the best of times. The third Monday in January is known as Blue Monday, when most people admit to feeling depressed. This year it was Blue January. People were frightened for their health and finances. Elite sport was getting out of touch with the national mood in the early weeks of 2021.

Like summer 2020, the government believed that a daily diet of televised games would keep the populace indoors, reduce crimes like domestic violence and bring a semblance of normality into people's lives. A sporting sop for the masses. However, it seemed that even the government was losing patience.

Some people within football were scratching their heads and wondering why it was continuing. Newcastle manager Steve Bruce thought it was morally wrong for football to continue. Two of his players had developed long-term COVID-19 complications. Football authorities issued graphic pictures for footballers to understand what social distancing looked like. The images would not have looked out of place in a primary school classroom.

Elite football appeared to be completely detached from reality, seemingly uncaring of the risk that 'out of control' players posed to the public and NHS as vectors of viral transmission. It appeared unwilling to place standards of personal discipline above concerns that the sport's financial 'gravy train' was heading for the buffers. The English soccer response was in stark contrast to American sports' reactions to protocol breaches described previously in chapter 15.

Football escaped being locked down with the rest of the country. Just.

Chapter 18

The New Dawn or More of the Dark Ages?

Will 'old acquaintance be forgot?'

The year 2020 had become everybody's *annus horribilis*. Hopes that 2021 would see society turn the corner and put the pandemic, and all its consequences, behind it had been extinguished even before New Year had begun.

Brits were entering their third lockdown. They had no idea of its length. No conception of the scale of the wave of viral destruction that would be wrought in 2021. In 2020, 72,178 people died from COVID-19 in the UK; 78,128 more would lose their lives in 2021. English hospitals treated 242,000 people for COVID-19 in 2020. January 2021 alone would see 102,000 patients admitted; 2021 was not meant to be like this.

The vaccination programme had started in early December. There were reasons for cautious optimism. England's Deputy Chief Medical Officer Jonathan Van-Tam predicted that the first vaccinations could reduce UK hospitalisations and deaths by 99 per cent. However, that was before the world was assailed by new viral variants: Alpha (December 2020); Beta (January 2021); Gamma (January 2021); Delta (May 2021); and Omicron (November 2021).

However, the genie was out of the bottle. Sport had come back from spring 2020 with no appetite to be closed down again. Science and sport were learning how to negotiate the microbial minefield. Even if it meant taking tough decisions, such as further internment periods in bio-bubbles, modifications to rules of sporting engagement and periods of play in echoing, eerie and empty stadia. The financial viability of many elite sports and organisations depended upon it. Even if a price would be paid in other ways.

So much sport needed to be packed into 2021. Certain events deserve their own spotlight within this account: the early 2021 covidiots' antics; Australia's and America's Open tennis tournaments; cricket's IPL and England's international programme culminating in the Ashes; the delayed 2020 Olympics, Paralympics and football's Euros; the Boat Race; the autumn vaccination football fiasco and World Cup qualifiers; and rugby's British Lions and Cape Town captives.

However, so much more sport soldiered on. This is the 2021 story of some of their toils.

Sport on trial

On 4 April, the government announced nine events would be designated as initial trials to test mitigation strategies in combatting the pandemic.

Test events would commence at a comedy club in Liverpool 12 days later. Five would be sports events, including a 3,000-participant fun run, the World Snooker Championship in Sheffield, and three football matches at Wembley culminating with the FA Cup Final on 15 May. The results would be closely analysed. Overall, 58,000 people would be tested with only 28 positive cases. Naturally, the results were trumpeted by government and other agencies. Others criticised the study as too reliant on the less accurate LFTs and the low numbers of attendees who bothered to return 'mandated' post-event tests. LFTs had become available to the public in early April and eased financial pressures on sporting organisations unable to afford PCRs. Gradually, more sporting events would be added to the 'trial list'.

A further easing of restrictions from 15 May allowed football fans back in reduced numbers to grounds for the last two rounds of the Premier League season.

Dangers lurk indoors

Just as the UK was hunkering down for its third month in its third lockdown, the four-day European Athletics Indoor Championships were held in Poland in early March. Shortly after, one of the support staff told the authors that it was a 'car crash'. Great Britain won the most medals of any country, but all its athletes and staff had to isolate on their return home following a positive case. The hosts' men's relay team pulled out because of COVID-19 and a female hurdler had a positive test and withdrew before returning negative on subsequent testing. It was a shot across the bows for the Olympics less than five months away.

Four-legged friends back in the parade ring

The 2021 Cheltenham horse-racing festival was run behind closed doors in mid-March to ensure no repeat of the 2020 virus-spreading event. The festival's leading jockey would be a woman for the first time: Rachael Blackmore.

The Aintree Grand National returned the next month having been run as a 'virtual race' in 2020. The entire Liverpool meeting was held behind closed doors despite requests from the equine industry to delay the event until betting shops had reopened – which happened only two days after the big race. Total prize money for the National was reduced from £1m in 2019 to £750,000. The race was memorable as Blackmore added to her Cheltenham triumphs. She became the first-ever female to win the race, in its 173rd running, riding home Minella Times at 11/1. What a shame that her historic moment was not cheered home by packed race stands. Fortunately, she would receive her rightful ovation a year later when she became the first woman to win the Cheltenham Gold Cup.

The two principal June Flat race meetings would be able to welcome back restricted crowds. The Epsom Derby returned to its normal diary date of the first Saturday in June after its month's delay in 2020. Restrictions allowed only 4,000 spectators to attend on the Downs.

The five-day Royal Ascot meeting in mid-June was designated as a test event. Twelve thousand spectators attended daily – so long as they returned negative test results. It would be the biggest UK horse-racing crowd since Cheltenham 2020. It appeared that the sporting world was returning to a semblance of normality with the Queen in attendance and ladies' fashions to the fore.

Anyone for tennis?

The French Open was pushed back a week to 30 May as the country's third lockdown was easing. However, a national 9pm curfew remained in situ, causing the capped 1,000 fans to be ushered out of the door at the witching hour – whatever the state of play. Players were only allowed outside of their hotels for an hour except when playing.

By the middle of the second week, the curfew was raised to 11pm and 5,000 spectators welcomed. However, Paris traditionally runs late. The Nadal–Djokovic semi-final threatened to overrun into the Friday night air. To avoid *une émeute* amongst the fans, the French prime minister had to telephone personally, granting spectators an exemption from prosecution. A French waive had replaced a Mexican wave.

Wimbledon returned after a two-year hiatus to its normal mid-summer 'slot'. With the French Open late, it left only a fortnight between tournaments. Nadal pulled out of Wimbledon (and the Olympics), announcing 'two weeks … didn't make it easy on my body to recuperate'.

The original release of English pandemic restrictions was scheduled for 21 June. However, one week before, Boris Johnson announced a four-week delay. Wimbledon started on 28 June and needed test event status to allow 50 per cent capacity; 21,000 daily across the entire SW19 campus. Fans were banned from ticket queuing and had to prove vaccination status or negative tests. Vacated seats could not be resold for charity. Players were banned from renting houses in SW19 and stayed in allocated central London hotels. Three people could stay with each player. Britain's number one star Johanna Konta nominated her coach, who tested positive subsequently. It cost Konta a minimum of £48,000 – the prize for a first-round loser. It would be the start of a summer of misfortune for the 'ace'. Konta missed the Olympics when she caught COVID-19 herself and withdrew with a leg injury before the US Open started at the end of August. She lost her six-year reign as the British number one and retired three months later. Her career deserved a more fitting ending.

Wimbledon's first week's success meant that crowd plans were accelerated. Full crowds were admitted from the quarter-finals onwards. Centre Court could accommodate 15,000 fans. However, Wimbledon had problems shifting tickets. Ground tickets were left unsold. Court One had 2,000 empty seats midweek and tickets for the women's singles final were available only days before. The population simply didn't realise what was on offer. Djokovic would take his third 2021 major title. His quest for a calendar grand slam in New York in September will be returned to later. Ash Barty took the women's title.

Un-snookered

The difficult 2020/21 professional snooker tournament came to an end at the World Championship at the Crucible, Sheffield on May Bank Holiday weekend. Only 19 tournaments had been held compared to 54 in the last full pre-COVID-19 season of 2018/19. Prior to Sheffield, two tournaments had ventured across the Severn Bridge to Newport. The rest were held in Milton Keynes without spectators. The World Championship would act as another of the indoor activity trials. Beginning with one-third capacity on 17 April, it would be increased to full capacity for the final 17 days later.

Back on the fairway

The normal start to the major golf championships annually is the Augusta Masters. In early April, the tournament returned to its traditional slot only five months after the delayed 2020 version. Spectators were admitted in reduced numbers and witnessed the first-ever win by an Asian-born golfer, Japanese player Hideki Matsuyama.

At the early June Ohio Memorial, perhaps the most personally expensive positive COVID-19 test in sport occurred. Jon Rahm walked off the 18th green at the end of the third round in Dublin with a six-shot lead. A half-decent round on Sunday would win him the £1.18m first prize. It was at this point that an official told him he had tested positive. Exit one 'very disappointed', tearful Spaniard. It was only the fourth positive test amongst the players since the PGA tour restarted almost one year and 50 events earlier. To be fair, Rahm was aware pre-tournament that he was a 'close contact' but was allowed to participate so long as he tested daily. His bad luck would not end there.

Finally, the Open Championships made it to Royal Sandwich 12 months late in mid-July; 32,000 fans were allowed to attend daily. Players were warned about disqualification if protocols were breached. They stayed in approved accommodation and did not visit pubs, restaurants or shops. Several leading golfers withdrew because of having COVID-19, self-isolating as contacts or recovering from the disease. A drop-in centre was on course for spectators to be vaccinated.

One American, Collin Morikawa, was glad he made the trip. He became the first debutant to win the oldest major for

19 years. One Spaniard probably had regrets. Rahm tested positive again in late July – along with Bryson DeChambeau. They had shared a practice round together at the Open the week before. Both withdrew from the Olympics.

It's all waffle

Rugby union's 2021 Six Nations began only three months after the interrupted 2020 version finished. With countries in lockdown and health services under pressure, none of the 15 games in February and March admitted any spectators.

The competition only got the go-ahead four days ahead of the first round of matches when the French government exempted squads from one week's quarantine on entering the country. The wizard Welsh winger Josh Adams didn't make it to the first match. He had attended a family gathering and was banned for two games.

On 25 February, Scotland's third-round match in France was postponed. The French had had 12 players and several coaches test positive. It transpired that French head coach Fabien Galthié had left the team bubble to attend his son's rugby match in Paris, and permitted the national team to visit a Rome restaurant to eat waffles. Bernard Laporte, the French rugby president, stated that 'obviously, zero risk does not exist'. A subsequent investigation cleared Galthié of any wrongdoing. France's sport minister had threatened to withdraw the team if the inquiry was not thorough enough. The tournament continued and the postponed match rescheduled for the week after the tournament officially ended. France finished second behind Wales.

Local difficulties

Rugby's 2020/21 English Premiership started during the second lockdown and spanned the third. In the 19th of its regular season's 22 rounds, small 'trial' crowds were introduced in mid-May. However, some clubs, like Northampton Saints, did not play in front of a home crowd all season. Ten out of 132 regular season matches were cancelled because of outbreaks at clubs. There would be no rearranged fixtures. The games were officially recorded as 0-0 with four points to the innocent party and two to the guilty.

The 26 June Premiership Final featured Harlequins and Exeter Chiefs. A 20,000 audience was hoped for as part of the government's 'test pilot' status policy. The request was denied. The RFU had to refund 10,000 tickets. Communications between sport and government was not clear and decision-making not strictly obvious at times. The Harlequins CEO said he was 'at a total loss as to the logic or rationale to live sport at the moment'. Exeter chief coach Rob Baxter asked why rugby was being treated differently to other sports?

The aftermath of Quins' final triumph saw the team go on a three-day celebratory 'bender'. England prop Joe Marler decided to seek sanctuary one night in a Harlequins Stoop Memorial hospitality box rather than pay for a 120-mile Uber ride home. The next morning, a woman in a nurse's uniform appeared in his makeshift dormitory. Having established that he was not dreaming, Marler realised that the club had repurposed his 'bedroom' as an NHS vaccination centre.

Summer sojourns

For those rugby players not booked on the Lions' South Africa tour, other summer internationals beckoned. However, the rising tide of cases stymied all three of Scotland's planned games. This included cancellations on the morning of the match against England 'A' and the Tbilisi game – when the Georgians cried off following their own outbreak during their South Africa travels which had left their coach in ICU. Wales and England did at least get to play. The former welcomed fans back to the Principality for the first time in 14 months. England had additional worries. With senior players on the Lions tour and many more rested, the summer squad had a callow feel. By the time England beat Canada on 10 July, ten players had been injured during their period together. Matt

Proudfoot, an England coach, blamed the toll on fitting one and a half seasons' games into 11 months. The psychological effects on players of living within the bio-secure bubbles were recognised.

In a league of their own?

The BSL kicked off in March – two weeks late. The first five rounds of matches were played behind closed doors. For the rest of the season, a 25 per cent capacity cap (or 10,000 fans) was in force. The 2020 rule amendments remained, and table positions were decided on a win percentage basis rather than accumulated points. The sport did well until the first 'COVID cancellation' in June. One tenth of games were lost to COVID-19, a vast improvement on 2020. Only Wigan Warriors achieved a full fixture list. The RFL Women's Super League returned in April after missing a year. It achieved this by being granted elite status by the government. Accordingly, they returned to training during lockdown in March. Like the men, some games were forfeited because of COVID-19 and others cancelled as medical cover was not available.

There was a ray of sunshine: the Rugby League Challenge Cup. Some teams in lower leagues did not participate, but the competition proceeded through five rounds until Castleford Tigers and St Helens qualified for the July Wembley final. In late June, it was announced that the showpiece game would form part of the government's Events Research Programme (ERP) on 17 July and 45,000 saw St Helens triumph.

The good news about the cup final was needed. The World Cup was due to be held in England starting in late October 2021. It was planned to simultaneously hold men's, women's and wheelchair competitions. The game badly needed the revenues after Australia cancelled their autumn 2020 tour. It would have been their first for 17 years.

Five days after the Wembley occasion, Australia and New Zealand withdrew from the World Cup – £40m of anticipated profits gone. There were angry words. Rugby

League chairman Simon Johnson called it a 'selfish, parochial and cowardly decision'. Both countries were sending athletes to the Olympics, the Wallabies rugby union side coming to Britain in the autumn, and the UK had held Wimbledon, the Open golf and the Euro 2020 competitions. It was rumoured that Antipodean players were weary of bio-secure bubbles. Several of the ANZAC players were not citizens of the countries they represented and might be denied re-entry to Australia and New Zealand. The tournament was held in autumn 2022.

Bleak House

Book by Charles Dickens. 1853

English professional football continued behind closed doors during the first four months of 2021. Mirroring the national crisis, numerous games were lost because of COVID-19. December and January would see 56 matches postponed across the top four divisions and FA Cup. Several clubs faced a significant fixture backlog. Sunderland would lose five matches in just over three weeks. They would play eight fixtures in April and win only one – denting their promotion hopes.

When the EFL season finished in early May, no spectators had been admitted to any of its 72 grounds in 2021. With the Premiership season extending for two further weeks, the lifting of certain restrictions meant that all clubs admitted reduced crowds for their final home match. The FA Cup did not receive fans until it reached Wembley Stadium. The second semi-final, between Leicester and Southampton, admitted a paltry 2,728 fans as one of the early pilot events. All spectators were invited, lived locally and included essential workers.

The Carabao League Cup Final between Manchester City and Spurs was played in front of 7,737 one week later. It would be the first time that rival fans would congregate in the same stadium for over a year. On 15 May, Leicester beat Chelsea in front of 18,720 spectators in the FA Cup Final, the first time that more than 8,000 football fans had assembled together.

Matters were worse north of the border. Not a single Scottish league or cup match would admit fans for the whole of the 2020/21 season. Below the fourth tier of Scottish football, all leagues were suspended in mid-January. Strathspey Thistle in the fifth tier Highland League did not get to kick a ball in anger all season. A month later, all men's English football below tier five was abandoned. English women's football only survived in the top two divisions beyond New Year.

An even bigger headache would be cross-border European club competitions. Like in 2020, the final of the Champions League was moved to Portugal. However, Porto rather than Lisbon would welcome the finalists: Manchester City and Chelsea. For the second year running, Istanbul would have the game removed from it as Turkey was on the UK red list in May 2021. The competition was played with five substitutes per team to compensate for fixture congestion and fatigue. Unlike 2020, when all games from the quarter-finals onwards were played in one location, the competition was played home and away until the final.

Fourteen thousand fans arrived in Porto to watch the game at the end of May. In the health crisis, it had not occurred to anybody at UEFA to switch the game to Wembley. Local Porto inhabitants were less than impressed as protocols were relaxed for the English fans, allowing them to flood into bars and restaurants. Locals were still banned from attending matches. Back at home, fans travelling on five separate planes tested positive. Hundreds of fellow passengers were contacted by Test and Trace and asked to isolate or submit to daily LFTs. This included government minister Michael Gove, who had flown to Portugal with his son.

Euro 2020 was not the only continental football competition 'in town' in the middle of 2021. The quadrennial Copa América was, like the Euros, displaced a year due to

COVID-19. The joint hosts were due to be Colombia and Argentina. Three weeks before the tournament, Colombia was removed due to political protests and, a week later, Argentina lost its hosting rights due to rising COVID-19 levels in the country. Brazil stepped in despite suffering from a wave of contagion themselves and suffering 463,000 deaths. Jair Bolsonaro said that the decision to host was not up for discussion. The Brazilian Supreme Court gave the president five days to submit evidence behind the decision-making. The controversial politician might have regretted his decision. Bitter rivals Argentina beat Brazil in the final.

The scene was set, and fingers and toes crossed, for the delayed, upcoming Euro 2020 and its final scheduled for Wembley.

The unequal struggle for control

No politician, administrator or athlete could have foreseen the continuing carnage that COVID-19 would wreak on the sporting landscape in 2021. Vaccinations and the wider availability of viral testing kits could not come to the rescue of spectators fast enough. By late 2021, sport was far from back to normal. Disruption would be highest at the beginning of the third lockdown, when national deaths and cases were at their greatest and vaccination levels low in the young. Control was regained by extreme society restrictions before loosening again in mid-summer around the time of the Euros. Government and sport would continue to struggle to regain the upper hand before early 2022.

Chapter 19

COVID Calamity:
Australian Open Tennis 2021

'Parachuting' players

In early 2021, 37,000 Aussies were still stranded abroad. They were burning up savings, unable to work and outlasting visas in their host countries. Their anger was fuelled by restricted flights, eye-watering travel prices and quotas for weekly returnees limited by hotel quarantine numbers. Qantas did not restart international flights until the end of 2021.

Into this crisis, tennis players and their entourage, were planning to play in Melbourne. It would prove a logistical nightmare. The Open was delayed for three weeks from its scheduled 18 January start. Negotiations with the Victorian government continued as to how 1,300 people could safely be accommodated.

On New Year's Eve, Andy Murray announced that he would not play in a pre-Open Florida warm-up tournament because of COVID-19 fears. Instead, he caught the virus in London from what he believed to be lax precautions where he was training. Without special consideration from Australia to shorten his quarantine time on arrival, he withdrew.

For the first time in grand slam history, qualifying tournaments were held outside the host country. Fifteen chartered, sparsely occupied jumbo jets transported pretested players and their teams to Australia from America and the Middle East. Players would be released for five hours' daily practice from their hotel rooms for 14 days. Stars like Djokovic, Serena Williams and Nadal had seemingly superior separate arrangements in Adelaide, including hotel gym access and larger entourages. Fellow players complained of favouritism.

Don't feed the animals

Ensconced in hotels, ten positive tests were announced. Seventy-two players were banned from practice sessions. Social media was awash with clips of players using hotel walls as opposition for impromptu rallies. If it was not so serious, the whole event was turning into a pantomime with dozens of bored and fractious young athletes inside small hotel rooms.

Outside, the world waited for ill-judged messages to appear. They did not have to wait long.

Complaints from hotel rooms started. These included questioning the need to self-isolate, and the standard of sustenance and accommodation. Images of food trays on Instagram were posted. Aussie player Bernard Tomic's girlfriend, couped up with the volatile right-hander, complained that she was not used to having to wash her own hair or share toilet facilities with him. Reportedly, the relationship did not develop long term. Victoria's police minister pleaded with inmates not to feed rodents. A video was posted showing a mouse jumping out of a cupboard. Tournament director Craig Tiley was abused on conference calls by players regarding the quarantine period.

However, many players accepted their imprisonment with a degree of understanding, equanimity and appreciation of their good fortune in being able to travel and play sport. A week into the incarceration, one player, Paula Badosa, tested positive and was transported to a 'health hotel' for a further two weeks.

Into the controversy waded the co-leader of the Professional Tennis Players Association: Novak Djokovic.

He suggested that the 'isolated 72' could be moved to private houses with tennis courts and granted reduced quarantine time. Fellow player Nick Kyrgios labelled the Serb a 'tool'. The Victorian prime minister, Daniel Andrews, would not play ball. He insisted players should not receive special dispensation. The politician had had his fingers burnt in the aftermath of the March 2020 Formula 1 Grand Prix abandonment in his city. Most Australians agreed with him. Others supported Djokovic, explaining that he was merely trying to reduce training time inequalities.

Following their release on 30 January, various warm-up tournaments at the venue were organised. Within four days, the tournaments were suspended. A hotel worker tested positive, and 507 players and staff were put back into hotel quarantine as a precaution. All were released the next day.

The spectator 'hokey-cokey'

It was an enormous relief when the tournament finally started on 8 February. The venue was limited to half-capacity: 30,000. Even so, the locals were not flocking in. The next day, the organisers were offering free tickets as fans seemed reluctant to attend with all the restrictions in place. Spectators were split into zones to reduce mixing and aid any subsequent contact tracing. Fans had to pre-order food and drink and 'click and collect'.

Four days later, Victoria declared a statewide lockdown following 13 cases related to an infected Melbourne hotel worker. Fans were packed off home that evening – mid-Djokovic match. Fans were let back in during the second week.

Amazingly, the tournament finished on time. An imperious Djokovic claimed a record ninth men's singles title. Naomi Osaka triumphed in the women's competition.

Scars, loans and playbooks
Was all the effort worth it?

Would the players flown in weeks in advance and hotel-quarantined for 14 days only to be knocked out 'first up' want to repeat the experience? Badosa, who spent a total of three weeks incarcerated, called it one of the worst experiences of her tennis career. She promptly lost her first match. Djokovic believed that players would not carry on touring if they were required to suffer multiple periods of isolation.

Several players experienced injuries, including Djokovic, with an abdominal wall injury. This was partly ascribed to the less-than-optimal preparation. For a while it seemed to threaten the eventual winner's continuation in the event.

What of the Australian organisers and the public? The locals opposed the preferential treatment offered to players entering the country and the 'whingeing few athletes' received little sympathy from their hosts. Melbourne did not embrace the tournament – based upon paying spectators. Tiley spoke of the mental pressures of holding the event.

Pre-tournament Tennis Australia (TA) held reserves of £45m. The event made a £56m loss. Such a situation was clearly not sustainable. TA took out a loan of £25m to secure its financial viability.

On ethical grounds, should the players and their support staff have been awarded priority over beleaguered Aussies trapped abroad and desperate to be reunited with their families?

The sporting world looked on with interest. It gave other sports and tournaments a blueprint for what was required. Tournament director Tiley claimed to have 'a playbook that we can share with the rest of the world'. The Tokyo Olympic and Wimbledon organisers were amongst many who liaised with his team.

However, at enormous expense, the grand slam was completed. The measures ensured that the incoming players and teams were not responsible for a viral outbreak in Melbourne. The question going forward for 2021 was whether other sports had the finances, logistical skills and enthusiasm to follow their lead.

Chapter 20

Ashes to Ashes

IN THAT glorious cricketing summer of 2019, England and Australia battled to a 2-2 Ashes tie. The first drawn series for 37 years was exhilarating and compelling. It would be over two years before these old foes locked horns again down under.

No one could have foreseen the turmoil that would afflict the sport during that intermission. Elsewhere, this book examines the English game surviving the vicissitudes of 2020 and how the IPL waned and waxed in 2020 and 2021. There would be many more highs and lows before 2021 was out.

'Now is the winter of our discontent'
Richard III. William Shakespeare. 1594

Less than one month after high-tailing it out of Cape Town with seemingly scrambled heads, England embarked upon the new year with a highly ambitious 2021 international calendar.

However, there would be changes. The ECB had listened to the complaints.

With no obvious letup in COVID protocols, management embarked upon a policy of player rest and rotation to preserve mental well-being and family life. Without it, some players involved in the Sri Lankan and Indian tours, followed by the IPL, faced not returning home for five months. On-the-spot support would be beefed up. Starting with Sri Lanka, a COVID compliance officer (with an anti-terrorist background) and clinical psychologist would be added to the burgeoning support group.

And so it was to Galle, in southern Sri Lanka, that England reconvened to continue a tour they had abandoned in haste mid-match ten months previously. Quarantine requirements meant that no pre-test competitive matches could be undertaken. Both Tests would be played at the same ground.

Moeen Ali was touring hoping to reignite his Test career. No chance. He tested positive on arrival and spent 13 days in isolation. Chris Woakes, who shared a car to the airport with him, could not be considered either for the matches – despite testing negative. Without crowds, a lone Barmy Army trumpeter stood on the Galle fort walls belting out 'Jerusalem'. England won the series 2-0.

Next up, an Indian tour that had undergone multiple changes in timing, venues and formats since the onset of the pandemic. The final schedule would be a concentrated tri-format schedule across February and March. Only three venues would be used. Chennai hosted the first two Tests, Ahmedabad the last two Tests and all five T20 games. Finally, the circus would move to Pune for three ODIs.

Different squads were required for each format. Players needed resting. Some returned home for temporary relief from the psychologically challenging bubbles – the rest and rotate policy. The taboo topic was making players choose between representing their country and appearing in the lucrative IPL that followed. Moeen Ali, having not played in Sri Lanka, would play in the second India Test before flying home merely to return for white-ball cricket.

It would be a sterile and disappointing visit for the English visitors, both on and off the field. The serious second wave of the pandemic was sweeping across India as the tourists arrived. By March, India's total death toll stood behind only the USA and Brazil. Despite this, plans to play early games behind closed doors were jettisoned.

By the time the entourage arrived in Ahmedabad, over 60,000 fans would be present in the Narendra Modi Stadium. It is the world's largest cricket ground and named to honour the prime minister. Players spoke of their enjoyment of playing in front of an audience after nearly a year of largely empty grounds. But COVID protocols were hard to administer. Cases increased in the city. The Board of Control for Cricket in India (BCCI) went into reverse. The last six white-ball games would be played behind closed doors. England lost all three series.

The IPL was just around the corner and, in late March, one of Mumbai's most famous sons, the cricketing legend Sachin Tendulkar, caught the virus. He was admitted to hospital as a 'precaution under medical advice'. India collectively held its breath.

Back home

Back in Blighty, the international calendar was packed with hopes of replenishing the ECB's bank accounts.

First up would be New Zealand for a two-Test series in early June. The government was not ready to play ball quite yet. All fans had to agree to pre- and post-game testing. At Lord's, only 6,500 fans were allowed.

The second Test in Birmingham could admit 18,000. Unlike Lord's, fans were not required to socially distance. However, an app had been created allowing fans to order drinks and food from their seats. 'Heat maps' would show which parts of the ground were congested. The first day was a huge success with the Barmy Army in fine song. The Hollies Stand was a riot of colour with fancy dress, chants and beer snakes soon appearing. The media recorded, 'Edgbaston doubles up as the world's largest stag do.' It didn't stop the Kiwis dominating.

By late June, Sri Lanka had arrived for six white-ball games. They probably wished they hadn't bothered and didn't win a match. The UK government had awarded games pilot status for crowds as part of their ERP. Three visiting players lost their compasses and were sent home in disgrace for an unauthorised 'walkabout' in the hotbed of COVID-19 that was Durham. They were banned for one year for their northeast night out. Additionally, some match officials became infected and had to be substituted mid-series.

The mini Sri Lankan tour was a gift that just kept giving. The entire England squad was forced into isolation after the visitors had left. Seven positive 'home cases' were reported following mingling between the teams. Pakistan had been shoehorned into July. Two days before their start, an entire new England team had to be selected. Players were pulled from ongoing County Championship matches. The tyro squad, including nine uncapped players, was at best a third XI. For England to triumph in five of the six games was a remarkable feat.

An Indian summer

However, all of this was an appetiser for the summer's main course – five Test matches with India. Each game would add £25m to the ECB's coffers.

Pre-tour, Indian wicketkeeper Rishabh Pant went to Wembley to watch a Euro 2020 football match. Players had been advised to 'avoid crowded places' by the BCCI. He caught COVID-19 and took four others into isolation with him as close contacts.

During the fourth Test at the Oval, Indian coach Ravi Shastri tested positive. The bowling and fielding coaches and a physiotherapist subsequently followed suit. One theory was that the virus was caught at Shastri's own book launch in London, which was attended by many of the Indian squad. Masks were not worn at the event. Shastri stated that he had caught the virus in Leeds at the previous match.

Four days later, on 10 September, the fifth and final Test was scheduled to start at Old Trafford. India led 2-1. It had been a pulsating series. The day before, with another physio testing positive, the entire Indian squad had to isolate pending testing. All were negative. The Indian team did not want to play, while PHE and ECB doctors declared the game safe. Indian players feared not getting to the UAE for the restart of the IPL scheduled five days after the Manchester game's denouement.

Two hours before the start, the Test was cancelled.

Eighty-five thousand tickets had been sold. Hotel accommodation, food and travel had been arranged. Lancashire Cricket Club stood to lose millions. Stadium bars were opened to sell off beer at £1 per pint. Ex-England captain Michael Vaughan commented, 'The BCCI would have been scared to death that players wouldn't have been able to get over and play in the IPL ... It's all about the IPL.' Yes. The IPL was worth £360m to the BCCI. The ECB was not covered for direct match cancellation due to COVID-19 and released a 'clarifying' statement, 'This is not a COVID cancellation. It is a match cancelled because of serious concerns over the mental health and well-being of one of the teams.'

Initially, it was announced that India had forfeited the game, and the series would end 2-2. India disputed this. It was agreed to replay the game a year later. At Edgbaston. England won by seven wickets.

It was clear that a 'managed COVID-19 environment' – asking people to behave responsibly – had not been effective. It would inform Australian thinking for the upcoming Ashes series.

The Hundred and counting

A year late, the new Hundred competition started on 22 July. It divided the cricket community. Joe Root's father commented that The Hundred was 'just about as welcome ... as COVID'.

However, launching it in the middle of a public health crisis was not ideal. Coming as it did in the midst of a cramped international season amplified problems. Over 40 originally selected men and women players and coaches withdrew. Fatigue, injuries, clashes with other fixtures, bubble fatigue and quarantine restrictions figured prominently. Some South Africans isolated in Croatia en route to England. It seemed £80,000 to £100,000 for a month's work was not enough to tempt the new jet-setting white-ball exponents.

Inevitably, COVID-19 cases occurred but no games were lost or even postponed for the viral outbreaks. Disease-related problems seemed as rife in the ranks of the support staff as players. Birmingham Phoenix lost their head coach, Andrew McDonald, long before the tournament began for 'issues caused by the COVID-19 pandemic'. During the month's competition, Trent Rockets and London Spirit lost their head coaches, Andy Flower and Shane Warne. Both viral victims.

Domestic concerns

While the packed international programme attracted most attention, domestic professional cricket continued to try and recover from the difficulties of 2020. However, the surge in Delta-variant cases nationally meant that cricket disruption was inevitable. Accordingly, the first-class counties (FCCs) voted to continue the cobbled-together 2020 conference system for red-ball cricket.

The UK had a vaccination priority batting order according to health and age. By mid-June 2021, all adults were eligible for their first jabs. A lot of education was used to encourage young cricketers to take up the opportunity. However, except for designated games, crowd restrictions would remain in place until 19 July. With Wales having more stringent social distancing regulations – 2m rather than 1.5m separation – Glamorgan would suffer, more than most. At Sophia Gardens, one occupied seat required 11 empty seats around it.

LFTs became freely available from early April, just in time for the 2021 summer season. Players and staff were encouraged to test twice weekly. It would be the first time non-international professionals could test regularly. It would be a game changer.

In mid-July, Kent had to withdraw their entire squad before the start of a four-day game against Sussex after one positive test. One day later, the Derbyshire–Essex game was abandoned on the second day as one of the home team tested positive. With the game declared a draw, the visitors' hopes of defending their 2020 title disappeared. Derbyshire's loss of a team led to their withdrawal from their following T20 games against Northants and Yorkshire.

The only red-ball game to be completely lost occurred in late August. Surrey declared that they could not raise a team for their game at Durham because of one positive result. Durham were not amused. The fact that Hundred matches had been played despite positive cases and Kent had fielded a second XI in similar circumstances cut no ice. Government and ECB advice was that if a close contact was double jabbed, had a negative PCR and was asymptomatic, they did not need to self-isolate. The issue was lack of consistency in applying regulations.

The 50-over Royal London Cup between the 18 FCCs was due to start on 22 July. One week before, the competition was reported to be on a knife edge. Counties segregated senior and academy squads to mitigate potential COVID-19 effects. The national landscape meant more outbreaks were inevitable to add to the England ODI squad, Kent (17 players isolating) and Derbyshire (14 players isolating) situations. Clubs were worried about the unavailability of staff for catering, bars and stewarding. This would be compounded by the fact that The Hundred was due to start on the same day. The latter would eventually hoover up over 100 county players with ongoing Hundred withdrawals. The Royal London did proceed but with its standing diminished.

The T20 started in early summer and played the entire group game series with restricted crowds and the inevitable effect on county clubs' finances. The ECB had guaranteed each FCC 75 per cent of their 2019 ticket sales income – but not the considerable revenue from drinks and hospitality. The reduced numbers did not guarantee good crowd behaviour. After problems at Durham, Warwickshire's home T20 game against Derbyshire was disrupted by streakers and a post-match invasion from hundreds of drunk students who had been given cheap promotional tickets. The authorities investigated.

However, by Finals Day on 18 September, the crowds were allowed back in full throng and song at Edgbaston. Kent triumphed despite having to field emergency XIs for their final two group matches in late July.

Ashes scattered under the Southern Cross

Historically, only World Wars had interrupted Ashes tours. Coronavirus threatened another unwanted milestone.

By July 2021, concerns were rife that the end-of-year clash in Australia was in jeopardy. The hosts' zero-COVID-19 suppression strategy was under severe stress. During that month, almost half of Australia's population was in lockdown with a surge in Delta-variant cases. Melbourne had become one of the most locked-down global cities. Its country's vaccine rollout had been lamentable. Not until October would the target of 70 per cent of the population being jabbed be reached and some restrictions lifted.

Some England players faced four months away from home under COVID restrictions. The Ashes would follow white-ball tours in Pakistan and Bangladesh and the UAE-hosted T20 World Cup.

As early as the end of 2020, ECB's Chief Medical Officer Professor Nick Peirce revealed in relation to bio-bubbles that 'we saw there was a ceiling of probably three to four weeks and [then] you need time out'. By the end of July, England's

Ben Stokes announced an indefinite break from cricket. Ex-England skipper Michael Vaughan felt that it should be a wake-up call to the sport. ECB CEO Tom Harrison admitted 'players are just fed up with bio-security and bubbles'.

A year's Ashes delay would mean disruption to the global cricket calendar. Obstacles were removed when the two subcontinent tours were postponed – to much criticism. The T20 World Cup was sacrosanct.

Some English players wanted families to travel to Australia as part of their touring consent. There was a precedent. Some Indian team families had been given dispensation during an Australian Test series a year before. Everybody had quarantined for 14 days and families only given short notice. England wanted certainty in advance. However, thousands of Aussies remained stranded abroad, unable to return even for family funerals. A tour postponement would put significant financial strain on Cricket Australia.

Negotiations continued through the late summer. It would be the Australian government and individual states who would have the final say. The latter had different lockdown regulations and certain Test venues were in doubt – particularly Perth, which maintained tough COVID-19 protocols.

When the Australian team returned home in August from the West Indian and Bangladesh tours, they quarantined for a fortnight in an Adelaide hotel with no training facilities. Australian politicians did not want to appear too acquiescent or, equally, blamed for an Ashes cancellation.

Sections of the Australian media blamed English reticence. In early October, the 2019 Ashes Aussie skipper Tim Paine seemed to target certain undecided tourists, 'No one is forcing you to come … the Ashes are going ahead.' The hazards of playing sport in the middle of a pandemic were highlighted when Tasmania abandoned a domestic Sheffield Shield game in Brisbane before it had begun. They flew home because of only four new cases in Queensland, concerned they might be quarantined if a state lockdown was re-imposed.

On 10 October, and only eight weeks before the first Test, England announced that they would travel. Skipper Joe Root had been instrumental in persuading the waverers. A shadow 'A' squad would travel to act as quarantine-served replacements and practice fodder. Families could travel without having to suffer 14 days of wall-to-wall hotel-room incarceration. With coaches and support staff, the party could reach 80 personnel.

The overall situation in Australia was beginning to improve. In October, the 70 per cent vaccination target was reached, and lockdowns were phased out. In November, international travel resumed tentatively but visas would not be granted to the visitors' Barmy Army of supporters. In December, most restrictions were lifted as the target of 90 per cent of adults vaccinated was achieved. However, not all eight states and territories would move at the same pace. It would affect the structure of the tour, stadium capacities and players' decisions.

In early November, some members of the squad flew to the Gold Coast to quarantine, including their talismanic all-rounder Ben Stokes. He had finished his sporting exile recovering from the mental strain of bubble fatigue and damaged digits. However, T20 World Cup players only met up with colleagues four days before the first Test in Brisbane.

Eventually, the fifth Test was moved from Perth to Hobart. Western Australia insisted on quarantine even if arriving from other parts of the country. Crowds in each ground would vary between 60 and 100 per cent of capacity according to individual state laws.

England's only warm-up would be two intra-squad practice matches in Brisbane. Both were significantly affected by rain. The paucity of preparation meant that England did not select their premier opening bowlers, Anderson and Broad, for the first Test. BBC commentator Jonathan Agnew reported that it was all 'very demoralising'. Australia had only one intra-squad warm-up game but the fillip of winning the T20 world crown only three weeks beforehand. Additionally, they had left behind nine squad members playing red-ball cricket in the domestic Sheffield Shield competition.

The five-match series and Ashes were lost by England in only 12 days of action. England capitulated in the first three Tests. For every English fan it was excruciating to watch. By mid-January, England had slunk off home 0-4 down in the series. Only a rain-affected draw in Sydney prevented a total whitewash.

The series had not escaped scot-free from COVID-19 – despite the elaborate precautions.

The night before the second Test in Adelaide, Aussie skipper Pat Cummins went to a restaurant. A diner on an adjacent table tested positive and Cummins was forced into isolation, and out of the match, as a close contact. He found an ingenious means of circumventing the hardship of seven days of staring at hotel walls in Adelaide. He negotiated flying in a private aeroplane to his Sydney home. New South Wales restrictions were less draconian, and he would be allowed to train. The comparison with arriving England players isolating for 14 days was not lost on some. The double-vaccinated Aussie bowler had previously been forced into isolation as a close contact in Kolkata during the 2021 IPL – part I.

During the Adelaide Test, both BBC *Test Match Special* and host ABC TV commentators were barred from the ground following positive tests amongst crew members. British listeners followed the match with substitute Australian journalists working from a remote studio.

The 'Boxing Day' third Test in Melbourne plumbed new depths.

Substitute television commentators were needed while 'regulars' were tested following a positive case. On the second morning, England players were ordered off their bus when it emerged that four members of their party had tested positive.

The day started late. As *Wisden* commented, 'Had this not been the Ashes, they might have been on the first plane home.' After returning to the hotel in the evening, they were tested again. The next day, the Ashes were lost.

There were doubts whether the England team would want to move on to the fourth Test in Sydney when Queensland had harsher regulations than Victoria. Match referee David Boon and batsman Travis Head caught the virus in Melbourne and were forced to miss the next Test. Cricket Australia CEO Neil Hockley commented that the tour was 'a day-by-day proposition'.

By the end of the Christmas week, the England camp COVID-19 count had reached seven. Head coach Chris Silverwood remained in Melbourne in isolation. With no Silverwood, strength and conditioning coach, or spin or fast bowling coaches – all *hors de combat* – ex-England player Adam Hollioake was called on to provide expertise. He never made it. He was deemed a close contact and forced into seclusion at his Gold Coast home.

The recriminations and grievances began as soon as the series was decided. England bowler Stuart Broad eviscerated the preparations and COVID-19 chaos. He remarked how many of the players were saturated with quarantine impositions. He used a golf simile, 'Imagine Tiger Woods rocking up at the Masters having not played for four months, spending time in a bio-secure bubble, and then seeing his entire practice rained off. He hasn't played a single round of golf, yet he's still expecting to win. Would you bet on him in those circumstances? No, you wouldn't.' Ex-England skipper Alastair Cook noted that since the pandemic began, England had played 17 Tests inside bio-secure bubbles – the most of any country. Ashley Giles, England's director of cricket, commented, 'The amount of time that these guys have spent in bubbles is not healthy … they get pushed and pulled everywhere.' England's assistant coach Paul Collingwood felt that 'bubble living' had turned the team into 'sitting ducks'.

His view on the previous 18 months was, 'I've been scarred by what we had to go through in those places.'

Winning an Australian-hosted Ashes series is hard for the English at the best of times. However, the dice were loaded before the first ball was bowled in Brisbane. Bio-secure bubbles had been successful in securing cricket and revenues for the English game but in the end its players were mentally traumatised.

Innings declared closed

The year 2021 was when cricket's bio-bubble burst. International cricket and the IPL financially drive the sport globally. It had to get back to work. However, players and staff had hit the wall. Some decisions defied sense and certainly relegated player welfare to the depths. One international cricketer expressed the general concern felt by fellow players. They were told that restrictions were initially a public health matter but now seemed primarily a commercial consideration.

In 2021, the England setup would not repeat the success of the year before. Players and staff would test positive and not all matches would survive.

The Ashes capitulation caused much gnashing of teeth. Within weeks, the team's managing director, Ashley Giles, and head coach, Chris Silverwood, were sacked. No sector of English professional cricket was off-limits when searching for answers to the debacle. It led to the Strauss report, published in September 2022. However, the players had been sent into a 'virological warfare theatre' armed only with proverbial pea-shooters.

Chapter 21

COVID Calamity:
IPL Cricket 2021

It's simply not cricket

On 4 May 2021, the world's richest cricket tournament pulled up stumps. Less than half of its scheduled 60 fixtures had been completed. Its planning and execution had turned into a fiasco.

It was highly embarrassing for the acting CEO of the BCCI, Hemang Amin. The week before he had reassured all those involved that they were 'totally safe'. It was all hot air arising inside the IPL bubble. The new message was 'everyone goes back to their families in these trying times'.

The IPL organisers were desperate to stage a successful tournament. Not least because of the previous year's problems. However, they were facing widespread criticism. In late April, the leading newspaper, the *New Indian Express*, suspended tournament coverage, commenting that its continuation was 'commercialisation gone crass'.

Reality and mishandling trumps misplaced optimism

By mid-April, India was in the grip of its second deadly coronavirus wave. Despite poor testing and reporting systems, it had reached several dreadful milestones. There had been over 20 million officially confirmed cases since the pandemic began a year before; 400,000 cases and approaching 4,000 deaths daily were being reported. The wave was not expected to peak for another few weeks. Global media coverage relayed a national healthcare system in collapse – patients dying in hospitals when oxygen supplies were exhausted, breathless people searching for beds and relatives paying for gas cylinders on the black market.

Despite India possessing a huge capacity for vaccine production, its national rollout programme pace was funereal when faced with this deadly surge. The ruling BJP party and prime minister, Narendra Modi, faced mounting criticism for their inability to learn from the 2020 lessons at home and abroad. Complacency had crept in as cases dwindled in January and February following the previous September 2020 peak of nearly 100,000 daily cases. By early March, Modi had declared his country was reaching 'the endgame' of the pandemic.

There was a belief that India would avoid the second surge consuming the rest of the world. Large rallies addressed by leading politicians continued. An April religious festival on the banks of the river Ganges was reported to have led to 2,000 cases in the local region.

Relationships between Indian politics and cricket have always been intertwined. One of the key BCCI figures was the son of the Home Office minister. As the government's stock fell with its crisis mismanagement, the threat to India's beloved game was clear.

'Let them eat cake'

Marie Antoinette's advice to the starving French
population. 1789

The government encouraged the tournament to continue and provide a televisual distraction from the pandemic. It was the Modi government's 'Marie Antoinette moment'. Lack of oxygen and vaccines being substitutes for bread shortages.

However, instead of 'giving cake' to the stricken masses they prescribed wall-to-wall cricket.

It had all sounded so promising in January. The BCCI announced its confidence in safely hosting the tournament rather than returning to the UAE. By late February, concerns were surfacing. The IPL asked for help. Experts advised that to ease logistics only three venues in Maharashtra (around Mumbai) should be used. All journeys could be undertaken by road. No teams would play at home, and crowds would be locked out. The advice was rejected. Other cities wanted a 'piece of the action'. The concept of 'cluster caravans' was devised. The entire circus would be based at two venues for a fortnight and then move on to the next staging post.

Elaborate security precautions were made. Players and support staff were isolated from the outside world. They travelled in chartered planes. The Indian government sanctioned separate airport arrangements, including dedicated check-in counters and security corridors. Hotels and grounds were hermetically sealed from life beyond. Regular testing was the order of the day. Games required two fully staffed ambulances with full oxygen backup.

As the crisis in the 'real India outside' deepened, complaints intensified when people were dying for the lack of the same medical equipment and personnel sequestered for the cricket. The IPL retreated further into its own world of 'make-believe'. External food deliveries to the hotels were stopped and testing ramped up from every five to two days. However, the PR disaster of a pampered international sportsman receiving preferential hospital treatment for an injury sustained dropping a catch at mid-on was too awful to contemplate.

Players begin voting with their feet and wallets

As in other sports, the bio-secure arrangements were taking their mental toll on players. On 21 April, Rajasthan Royals announced that Englishman Liam Livingstone would be flying home as a victim of bubble fatigue. He had spent much of the previous ten months in various sporting 'cages', had not been selected for any of his team's three opening games and wanted to avoid ten days quarantining in a British hotel. India was due imminently to be added to the UK's red zone of travel restrictions. The other 13 English players remained.

Three Australian cricketers anticipated the problem and left the IPL four days later. One described the situation as 'harrowing' and felt that by being inside the bio-secure bubble he had 'lost touch with the outside world'. He added that he wanted to 'get home before I get locked out of the country'. However, 40 Australian players and staff remained. One local Indian cricketer, Ravichandran Ashwin, broke camp and returned to his family to support them. It was at this point that Amin had stepped in to persuade everybody else to stay.

Australia went further than the UK on 2 May. It banned its own citizens from returning directly from India, with potential prison sentences of five years for rule-breakers.

Aussie bowler Pat Cummins donated £37,000 of his £1.6m tournament fee to an emergency fund. He urged other players to follow suit, stating that he felt helpless watching the media coverage of the suffering. Many players did, including Jos Buttler and Ben Stokes.

Players choosing to leave the tournament early would forfeit the remainder of their contracts. Organisers and players were more likely to recoup losses if the Indian government cancelled the tournament, allowing insurance policies to 'kick in'. The stiff upper lip attitude of the English contingent to stay in their subcontinent bunkers was noted to be in sharp contrast to the speed with which they had brought to an abrupt end their South African series in December 2020.

The wheels fall off the IPL's 'caravan'
The final nail in the coffin was the revelation that, within the space of 48 hours, half of the eight teams had COVID-19

in their camps. Whole squads were in quarantine, some were refusing to practise, and even Chennai's CEO had caught the virus. The game was up. The tournament had descended into a farce and the much-vaunted bio-bubbles had burst. The virus was becoming rampant within. The tournament organisers could not wait for their government and suspended the competition.

A mass exodus of international players began. Cricketing authorities worked hard to ensure safe repatriation channels for their cricketing superstars. However, Cricket Australia confirmed that it would not be seeking special dispensations from their own country's regulations.

Quarantine refuges were needed. For the 11 remaining English players involved, a ten-day stay in a government-approved Heathrow hotel room was the order of the day. The Aussies did not have even that luxury. They had to serve their sentence elsewhere if they wanted to avoid time in the 'slammer'. The Maldives islands had become a favoured destination for potentially virus-infected cricketers crossing the globe in early 2021. Sitting in the Indian Ocean, it was conveniently located for sportsmen fleeing the Indian subcontinent and South Africa en route to England and Australasia.

What this little country had done to deserve this honour as a rinsing ground for coronavirus is not clear. Perhaps scattering sportsmen across its 1,192 islands reduced the risk of mass transmission. Those suffering the hardship of ten days on a *Robinson Crusoe* island could maintain their skills with beach cricket. The UK slammed the door shut on this escape route when the Maldives were added to the red list on 7 May. Sri Lanka and Kenya were sometimes selected as alternative venues.

One Aussie did not make it to his tropical island hideaway on time. Mike Hussey, the Chennai Super Kings batting coach, tested positive and endured ten days' isolation in a Delhi hotel bedroom.

Counting the rupees and plotting the second coming

The financial implications of a complete cancellation were major – a projected £200m loss from sponsorship and broadcasting. Enough to put a large dent in the BCCI's budget.

No sooner had the tournament been suspended than there were machinations about how the remaining 31 games could be played. However, the relentless schedule of international cricket made finding a suitable window problematic without downgrading already arranged major series and tournaments. A narrow window at the end of September was identified, after the conclusion of the English international summer series. Quickly the 'runners and riders' declared themselves. Several English counties threw their hats in the ring as potential hosts. However, the UAE always seemed to be the preferred venue.

On 19 September, teams reconvened in the UAE. As they had done in 2020. All had to quarantine for six days on arrival. Prior to its commencement, the postponement of the final England–India Test in Manchester nine days before was greeted cynically as a means of protecting the IPL. Vaccinated and mask-wearing fans were admitted to the games as long as they socially distanced.

Several English and Antipodean cricketers declined to play, preferring to rest ahead of the winter Ashes and T20 World Cup (which would follow in the UAE immediately afterwards).

Four days after the opening games of the resumed competition, the first case was announced. One of the Sunrisers Hyderabad players tested positive, taking six other members of the setup into quarantine. However, unlike previously, their game the same day against Delhi Capitals went ahead. It was an indication of a more relaxed approach to dealing with the virus.

Finally, on 15 October, the IPL finished; 1,828 miles away and 189 days after the 2021 edition had started in

Chennai. Appropriately, Chennai Super Kings beat Kolkata Knight Riders by 27 runs in Dubai to take the title.

No-balled

The 2021 IPL tournament was a tragic farce. Once expert advice had been ignored, the logistics of shunting an enormous sporting enterprise around that vast subcontinent in the middle of a catastrophic health crisis was always likely to end badly. The motivation appeared to be pure avarice. The decision not to cancel the event because of financial concerns and the government's hunger for a diversion was craven.

The *New Indian Express*'s contempt had nailed it.

Chapter 22

Messing About on the River

'Skippers and mates and rowing club eights all messin' about on the river'

'Messing about on the river'. Words by Tony Hatch
and sung by Josh MacRae. 1966

The first Boat Race took place in 1829 in Henley and annually on the Thames since 1856. Of all the Varsity clashes across the sporting calendar, it is the sight of the two student crews heading for Mortlake Brewery that most completely captures the nation's imagination.

Neither boat sinkings during six races nor a 2012 attempt by an Australian swimmer trying to entangle himself with the oars (protesting British society's shortcomings) could dampen spirits.

During the Second World War, four unofficial Boat Races were contested. They do not appear in the official records nor were 'Blues' awarded. In 1944, Oxford University Boat Club took on their Cambridge counterparts in their own backyard – or own backwater to be correct – on a section of the fenland river Ouse. A former light blue cox described the stretch of water between Ely and Littleport as 'bloody straight, bloody cold and bloody boring'. Nevertheless, in February 1944, and just over three months before D-Day on the Normandy beaches, crowds packed the Adelaide Straight ten-deep to watch Oxford beat their rivals by three-quarters of a length.

252

It is doubtful if modern oarsmen or women were aware of the river's part in the rich tapestry of the nearly 200-year-old sporting event. They would by 2021.

The 166th men's race and the 75th women's race were due to take place on 29 March 2020. There was a lot to savour for the anticipated 250,000 live audience and millions watching on television. In the history of the event, it would be the first time that both races were to be umpired by women and the first ever for the men's race. For the fifth time only, the two senior races and two reserve team races would be held on the Tideway on the same day.

The oarsmen and women train for race day from the start of the academic year in the previous September. Crew members fit their studies around several exhausting daily training sessions. Students come from all over the world for the chance to earn a rowing Blue. The year 2020 would be no exception. From the 36 men and women chosen for the two races, rowers would be flying the flag for 12 different nations from three different continents. For many months before the event, training would take place both at home base, in sunny climes abroad and on the Thames itself.

As final preparations for the event were being made, the pandemic sweeping across the world reached British shores. Following government advice to avoid all non-essential travel and the cancellation of most of British sport the previous weekend, the Boat Race was cancelled on 16 March. It would be the first time, except during wartime (1915–19 and 1940–45), that the event would not be held.

The crews who would have made it on to the start line at Putney were officially named and recognised on 29 March – the day the race should have taken place. Under ancient rules, crew members only earn a Blue when their boat passes the Mile Post on the Thames course. None of the selected men's and women's crew members would earn that accolade.

However, some university students did earn that distinction in 2020. But only from the Oxford boat house.

The lightweight race (70kg (11 stone) average for men and 57kg (9 stone) for women) had been run on Sunday, 15 March. In the 46th running of the men's event, it would be only the second to be contested from Putney to Mortlake rather than further down the Thames at Henley. Early in 2020, the University of Oxford decided to upgrade the award for participants in the lightweight race from a Half to a Full Blue. Cambridge had not reciprocated. Therefore, the only 2020 holders of Full Blues were the male and female dark blue lightweights.

On 13 June 2020, a virtual Boat Race took place for charity. The universities were represented by teams of eight rowing on ergos at home. Collectively, they completed 6.8km (4.25 miles) and Cambridge were declared the winners. The teams combined males and females and included para-athlete oarsmen.

The 2021 line-ups would contain 14 of the 18 women but only six of the 18 men selected for the 2020 race.

The risk of a super-spreader COVID-19 event along the banks of the capital's waterway coupled with the spectre of a recently declared unsafe Hammersmith Bridge falling on the crews was too much to contemplate. On 3 December 2020, the universities announced that the 2021 event would take place on the river Ouse in Ely, Cambridgeshire – the 'home track' of the light blue crew and where they do much of their training. Seeking to outdo the previous description, the stretch of water was referred, suitably theatrically by the 1980 ex-Cambridge Blue and multiple award-winning actor Hugh Laurie, as 'a blasted heath of physical torment'.

The torment for all crews would be different while preparing for the 2021 race.

The usually long and bleak hours on winter river stretches would be confined to just four weeks in the water because of COVID-19 restrictions. Even that was allowed only as a special dispensation. During the third lockdown from New Year, only elite sport could continue. While potential Olympic rowing hopefuls could train as normal, the university eights had to exercise in solitary confinement between December and early March. Sitting alone at home on their 'indoor ergos' having their efforts supervised, analysed and refined by remote coaches on Zoom requires a special masochism to endure. As befits an elite academic institution, Cambridge had wargamed ahead. From July 2020, they had put team members in household bubbles together in anticipation of further lockdowns. This allowed camaraderie to build up during the dark winter months.

Eventually, on 6 March, the rowers were let back on the water but stripped of the normal warm-up races against other crews and overseas warm-weather training. The Oxford trial crews threw themselves into the spirit of the pandemic with the naming of their trial boats. The women's crews favoured the vaccine route with *Pfizer* and *AstraZeneca*. Their male counterparts slugged it out aboard *Track* and *Trace* in homage to the NHS's much-criticised virus-chasing operation.

The 4 April race day was inevitably a different experience for all. Usually, the crews are greeted on the Tideway by thousands of onlookers several pints to the good with Young's ales on board. In 2021, the teams' riverside arrival in East Anglia threatened to be met with silence. The BBC stepped in and organised high-octane music and flamethrowers as each member stepped out of the boat house. It would have been enough to cause long-deceased ex-Blues to turn in their rowlocks.

The Cambridgeshire Constabulary had been out in force from early on race-day morning. Access to the river was closed off. Even homeowners whose back gardens had the Ouse as their boundary fence received letters telling them to stay inside and watch the event on telly. In one of the less concerning acts of COVID-19 breaches, defiant Littleport old-age pensioners sat in the cold on their garden furniture in splendid social isolation with nothing closer than Union Jack bunting for company. True British defiance.

The Times reported that the passage of the crews across the finishing line was greeted by the polite applause of '30 Cambridgeshire villagers and a family of ducks'. Slightly less raucous than the 5,000 spectators who cheered on the Ouse crews 77 years beforehand.

The men's and women's races were closely contested with Cambridge proving triumphant in both. Knowledge of the river's geography and how to find the fastest water and harness the crosswinds undoubtedly favoured the light blues. History was made a year late with both races umpired expertly by females.

One of the main post-race talking points was the negotiation by the boats of a clump of weed mid-river in the men's race. One false move could have rendered a rudder inoperable and a re-run inevitable. It is presumed that the weed was of a different type to that favoured by certain undergraduates?

On 3 April 2022, normal service was resumed. Thousands of spectators packed the banks of the Thames on a cold Sunday afternoon to see the Oxford men beat Cambridge for the first time since 2017. The Cambridge women extended their winning streak to five years.

And so ended a typical British sporting riposte to one of the most damaging episodes in recent British history. 'Rule Britannia, Britannia rules the waves' – or at least a stretch of water in East Anglia.

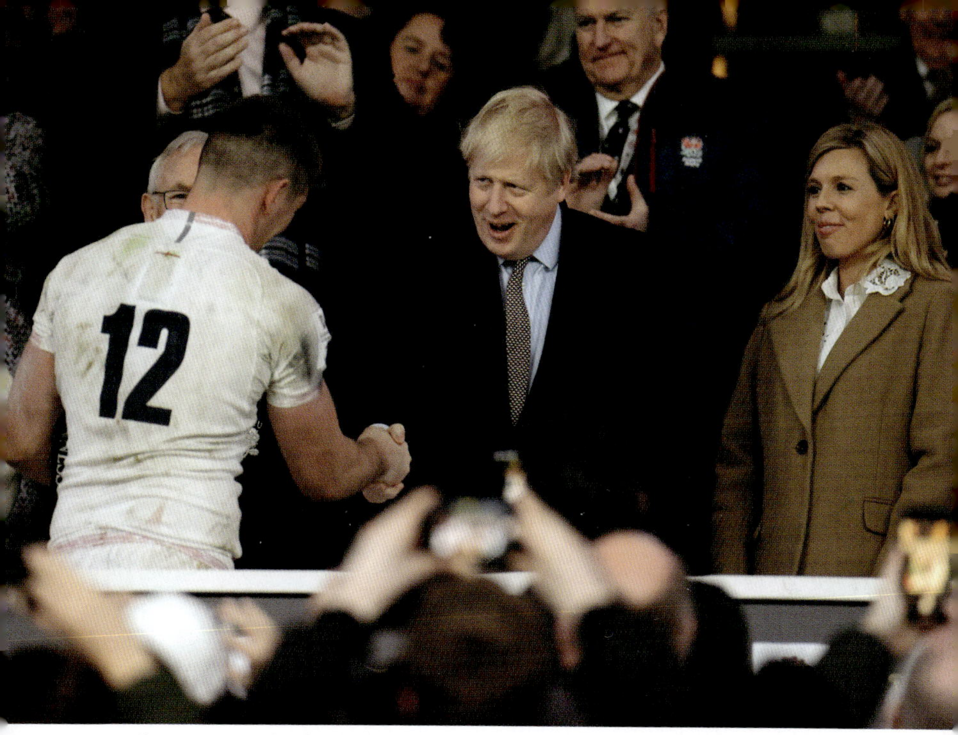

7 March 2020. Twickenham. Boris Johnson shakes hands with England captain, Owen Farrell, after the England v Wales game after his own scientific advisors warned against it.

11 March 2020. Anfield. Atlético Madrid substitutes sit in front of unmasked Liverpool supporters in the European Champions Cup match.

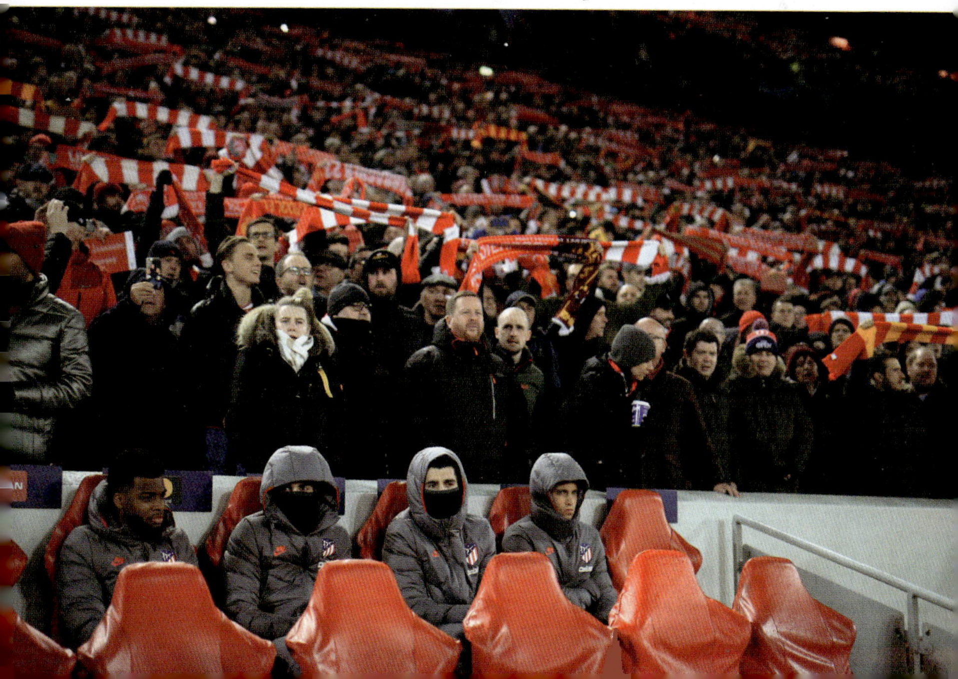

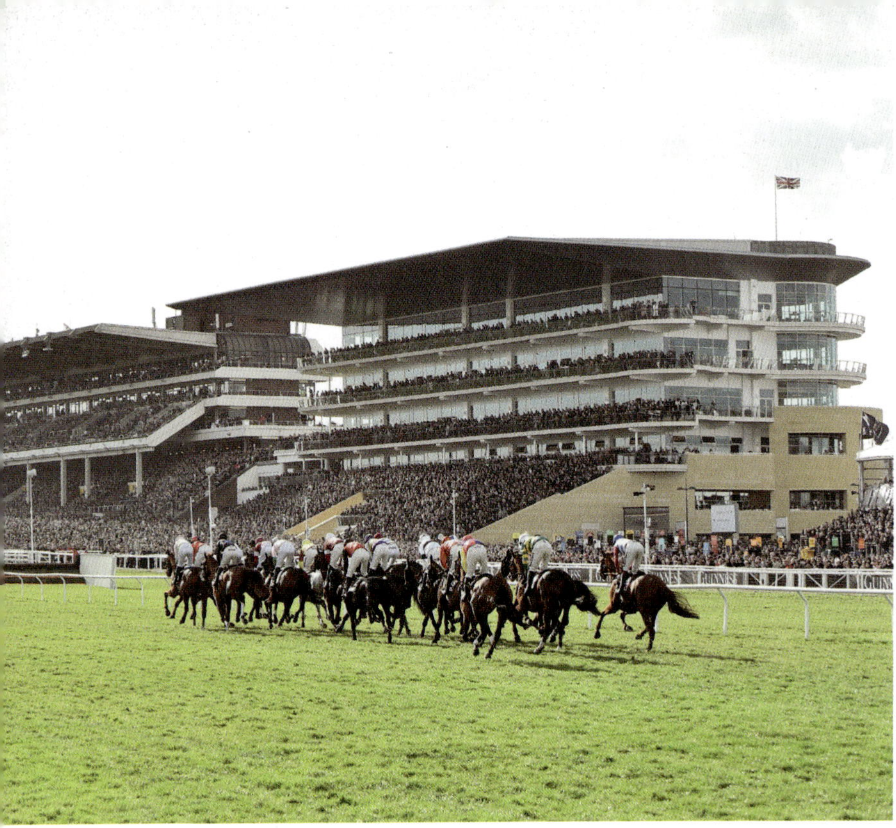

12 March 2020. Cheltenham Festival. Races take place in front of packed crowds. Many succumbed to the first COVID hurdle.

13 March 2020. Melbourne Grand Prix. Race abandoned and Ferrari team pack up equipment and leave for the airport.

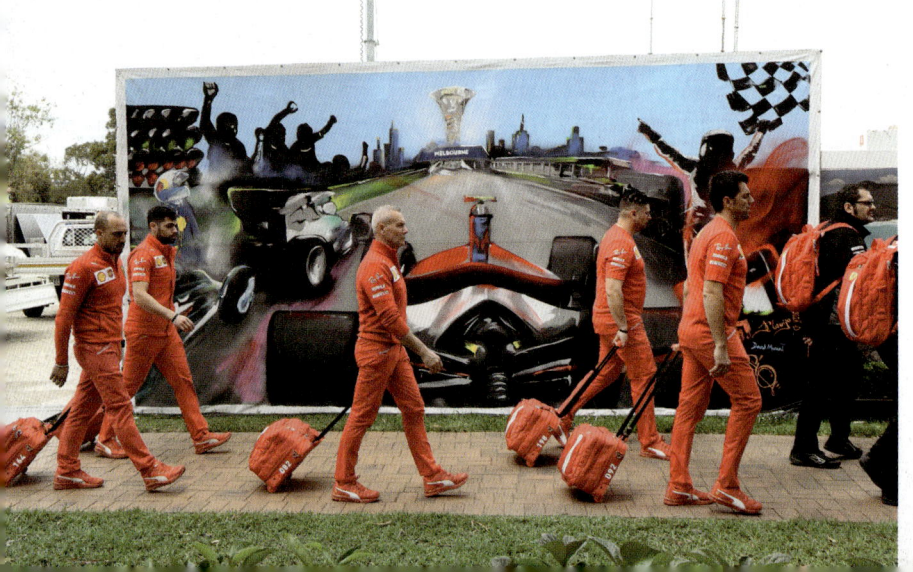

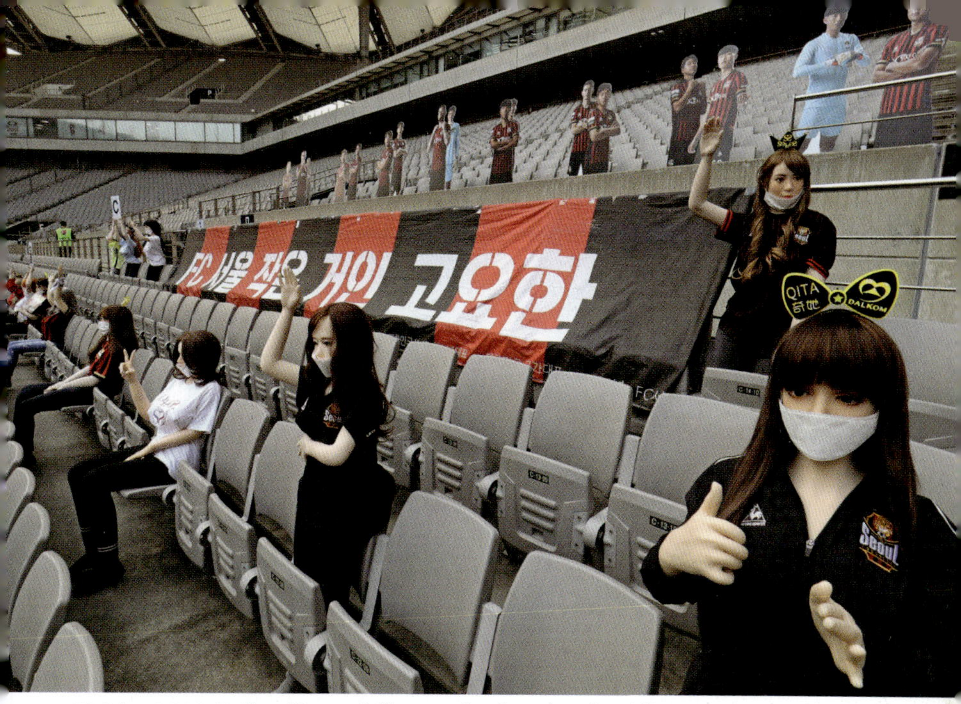

17 May 2020. Inflatable sex dolls mistakenly ordered to fill empty stands at FC Seoul.

1 July 2020. Northamptonshire cricketers return to training. 'One skin, one ball' mantra.

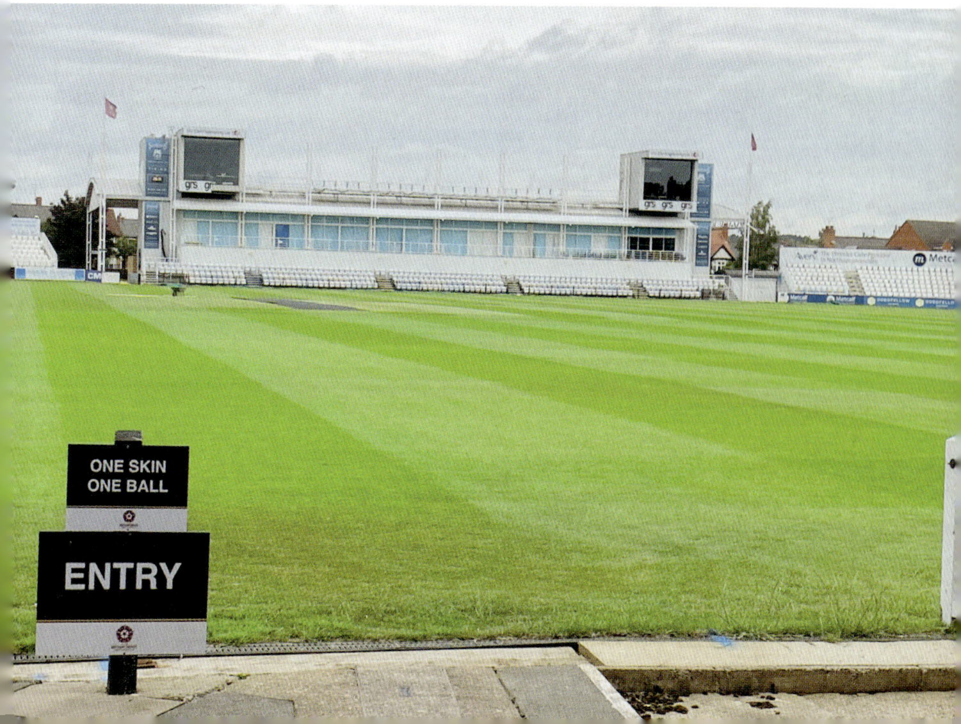

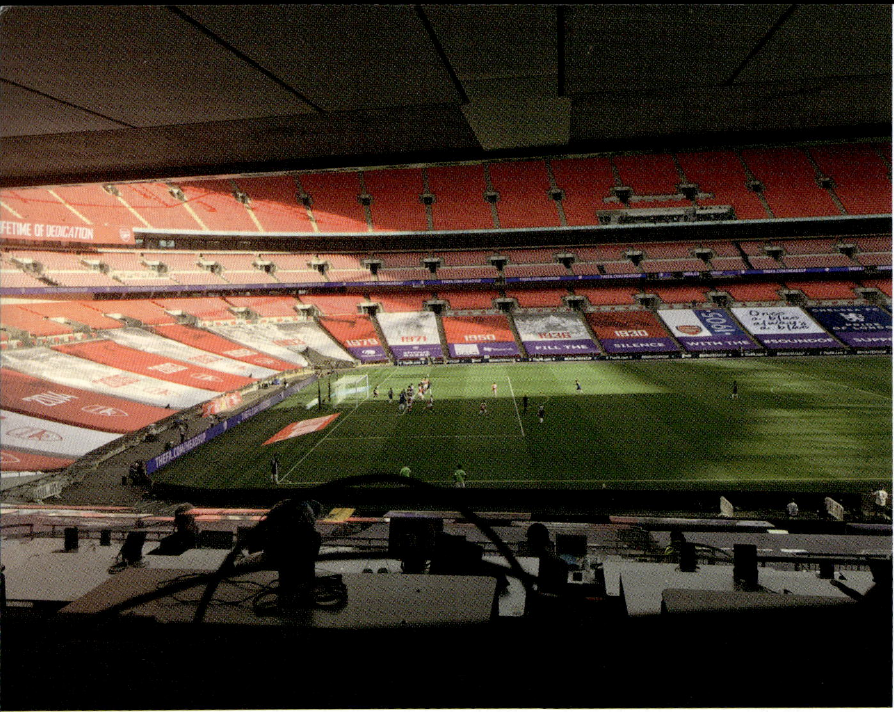

1 August 2020. FA Cup Final. Arsenal v Chelsea. View from the isolated commentary box at Wembley Stadium. 'Talking heads' but no specatotors.

23 August 2020. Storm clouds gather over the Ageas Bowl, Southampton. England v Pakistan third Test match.

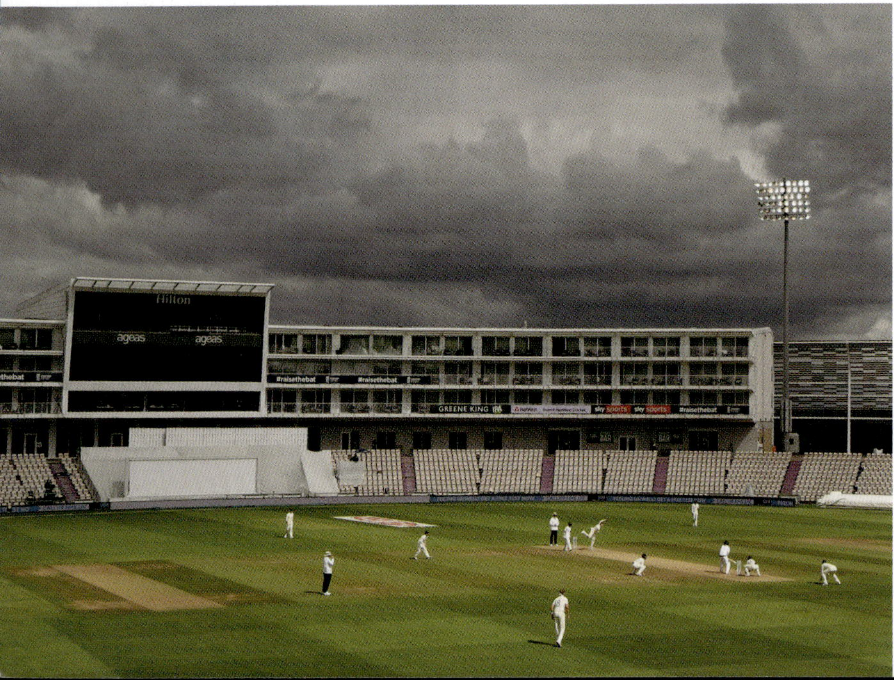

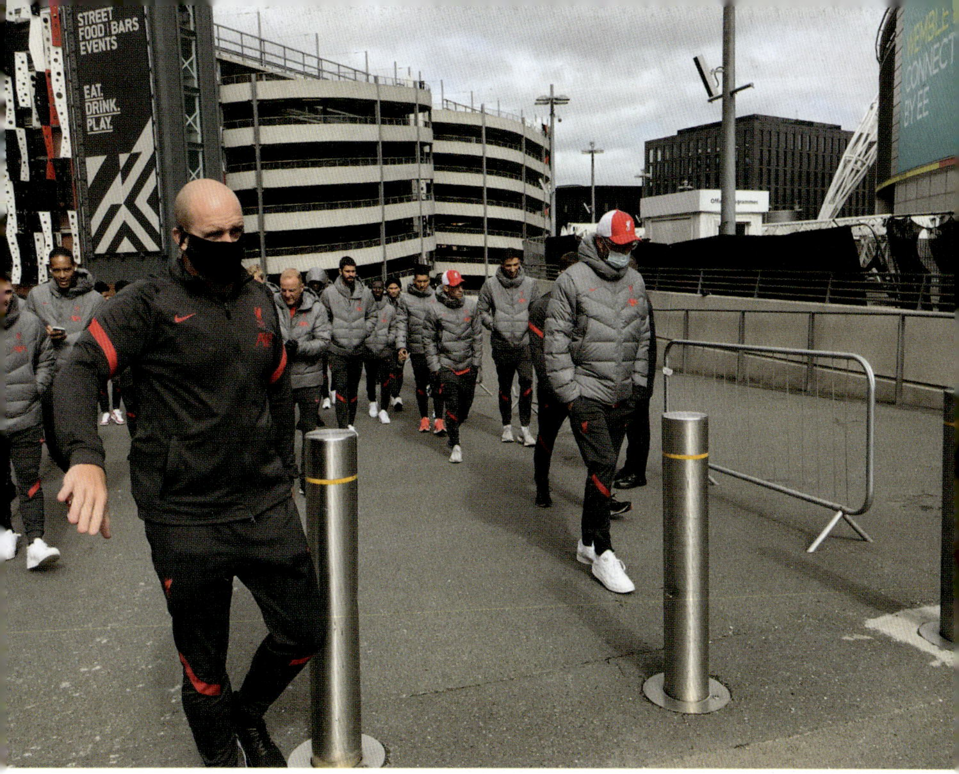

29 August 2020. FA Community Shield. Arsenal v Liverpool at Wembley. Liverpool players take a leisurely stroll around the complex. Jurgen Klopp in mask. Players without.

11 October 2020. LeBron James of Los Angeles Lakers takes a shot in the NBA play-offs in front of a cardboard cut-out crowd at Disney World, Florida. Not a Mickey Mouse in sight.

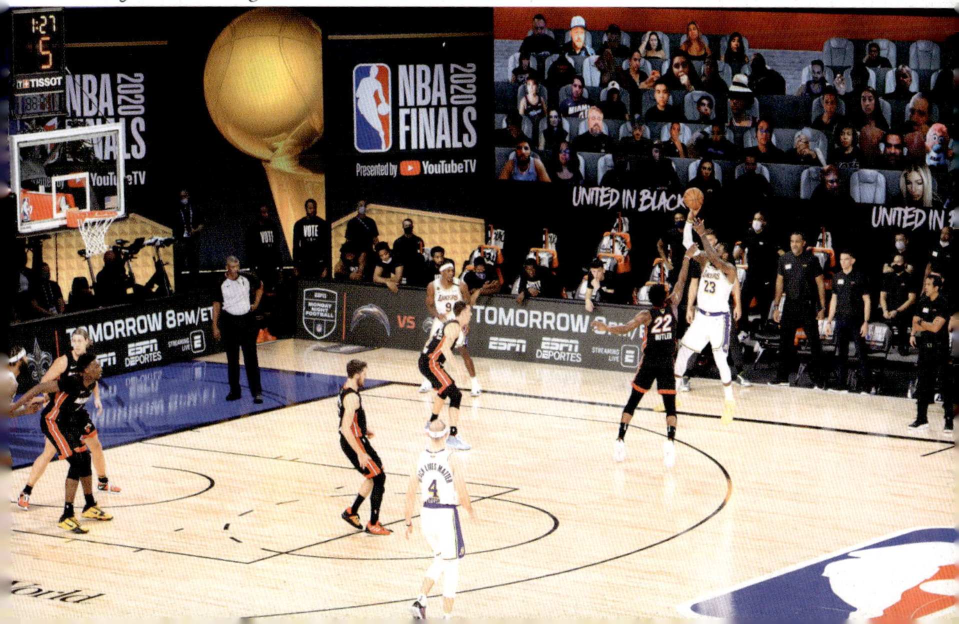

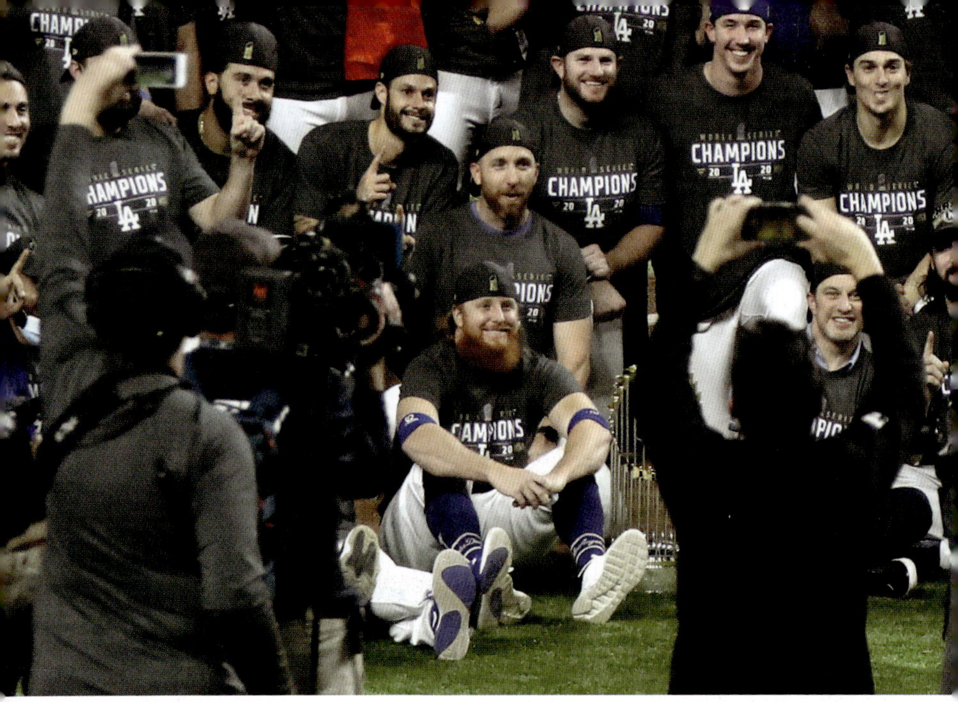

27 October 2020. Los Angeles Dodgers win the World Baseball Series at Globe Life Field, Arlington, Texas. An embarrassing strike out as Justin Turner (centre with red beard) poses with team-mates despite instructions to isolate with COVID-19.

12 July 2021. 'You did us proud.' The day after England lose the Euro 2020 final to Italy. Fans had rioted and charged the turnstiles, leaving English football in a terrible mess.

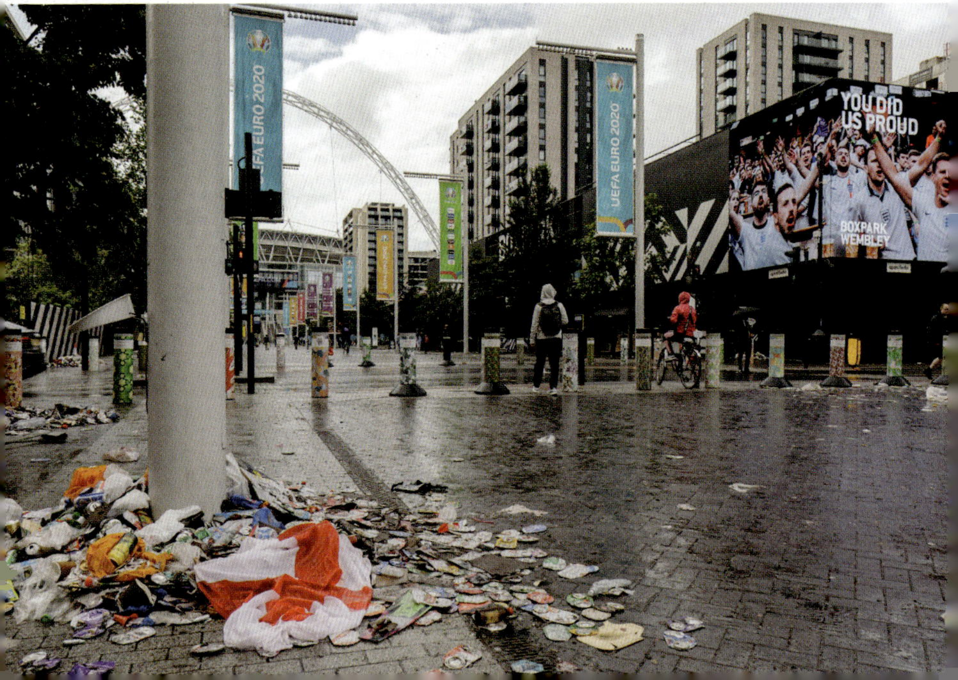

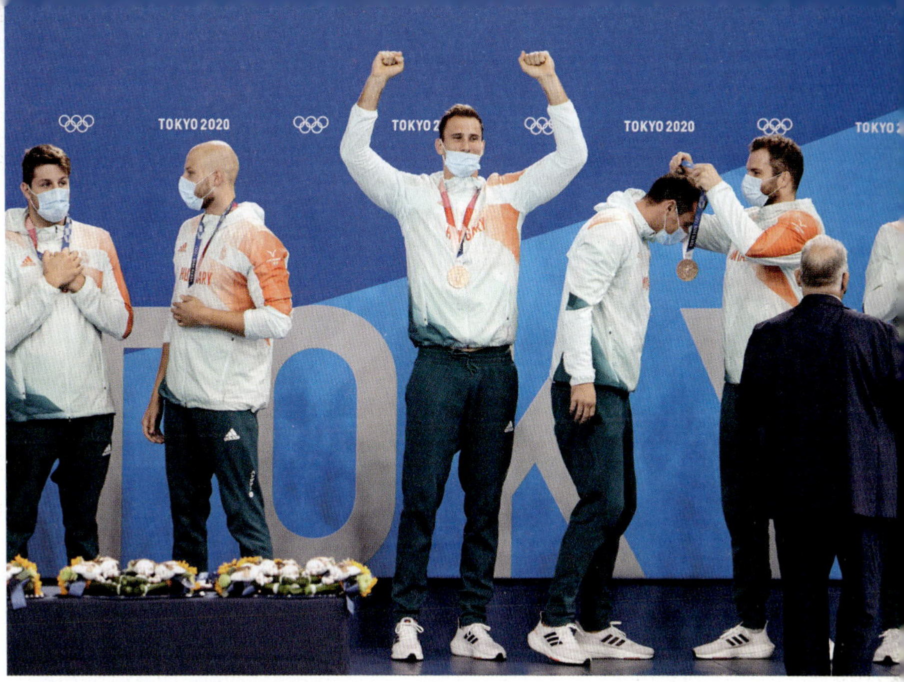

8 August 2021. Tokyo Olympics. Hungarian water polo bronze medallists in masks have to hang their medals around themselves or team-mates.

13 August 2021. Tokyo Olympics. Biting off more than he can chew. The Nagoya mayor nibbles the Olympic gold medal of bemused softball player, Miu Goto. The action caused outrage. The IOC issued a new medal to the athlete on the grounds of hygiene.

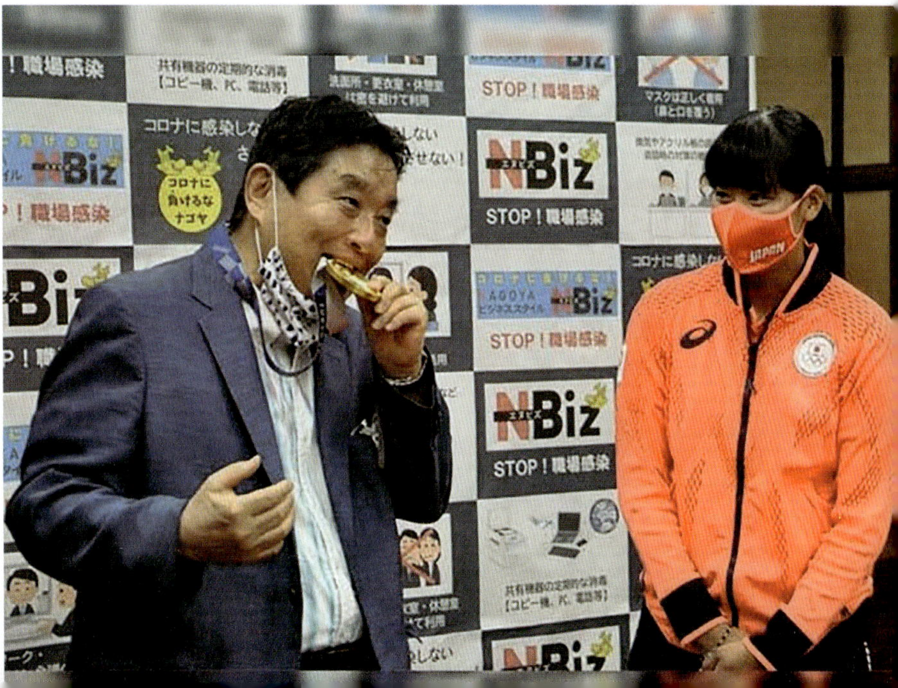

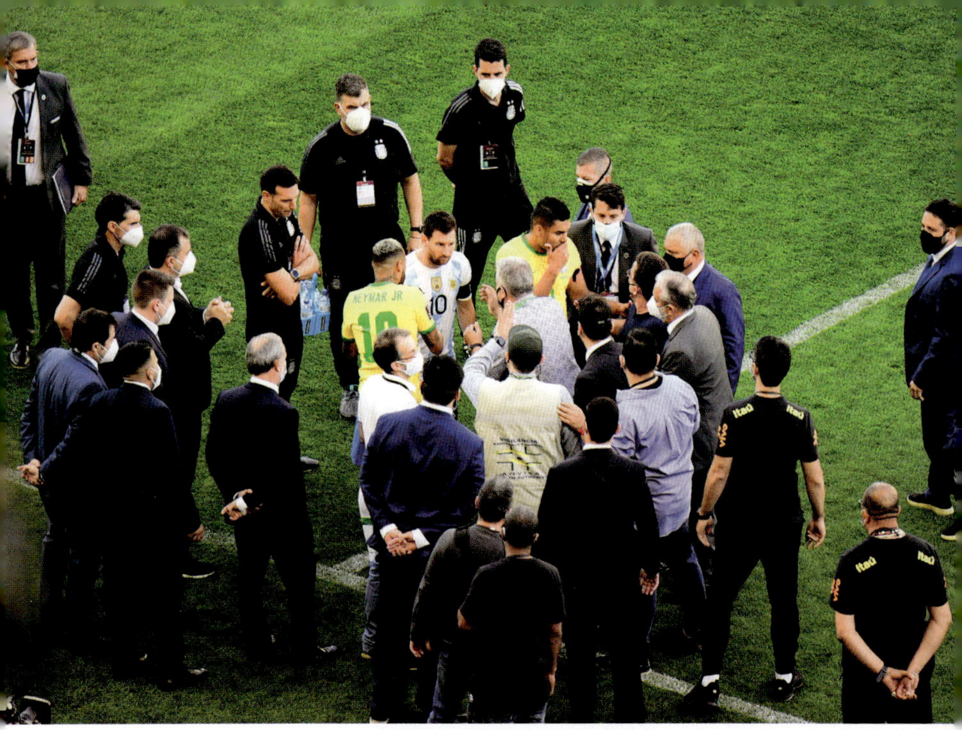

5 September 2021. Sao Paulo. World Cup football qualifier. Brazil v Argentina. It all gets Messi for the visitors. Match abandoned as health officials detain four Argentinian Premier League-based players for not following quarantine regulations.

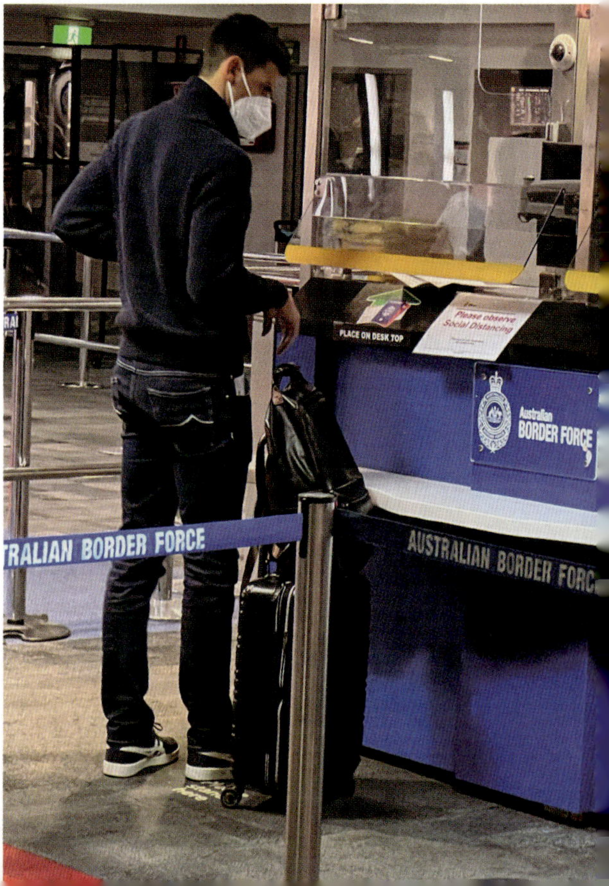

6 January 2022. Double-faulted in another court. Novak Djokovic at passport control in Melbourne airport ahead of the Australian Open tennis tournament. He was eventually deported.

Chapter 23

They Think it's All Over ...

Kenneth Wolstenholme's commentary on the closing moments of the
1966 World Cup Final

'I Have a Dream'

Song by ABBA. 1979

In 2012, Michel Platini, the later disgraced UEFA president, decided that his organisation should arrange a 'romantic' 2020 European football championship (aka Euro 2020). It would celebrate the 60th anniversary of its first competition. His quixotic dream was for cities spread across Europe to act as hosts. From the outset, thousands of fans, teams and media crisscrossing the continent was not UEFA's most eco-friendly gift to the planet. In the presence of a subsequent viral pandemic, the dream threatened to turn into a nightmare.

On 17 March 2020, faced with the first onslaught of COVID-19, UEFA took the only sensible decision. It postponed the competition for one year. The new dates would be 11 June to 11 July 2021. In a crowded international calendar, that would have knock-on effects. FIFA's inaugural 2021 World Club Championship was postponed.

The original 12 selected venues would host as planned. As the UK headed into its third national lockdown in early 2021, UEFA's president, Aleksander Čeferin, confidently stated, 'Vaccination has started, and I think we will be able to have full stands in the summer.' However, contingency plans were hatched. Hosts were given until Easter to confirm their capacity plans. Games behind closed doors were not an option. Dublin withdrew in late April. It had not received assurances from city authorities or its government that crowds would be admitted. Meanwhile, Boris Johnson, with his country still in lockdown, had earlier offered to host any games going spare.

To accommodate for COVID-19 infections, player fatigue and injuries (consequent upon the compacted schedule), new regulations were introduced. Squad numbers were increased from 23 to 26 players and five substitutes would be allowed during matches.

With games from Azerbaijan to Scotland, competing sides had to decide where to base themselves. Croatia and the Czech Republic had to abandon plans for Scottish bases because of quarantine restrictions. Scottish First Minister Nicola Sturgeon threatened to put entire squads into purdah if one player tested positive. Even Scotland chose their base south of Hadrian's Wall in Middlesbrough. Sweden, Slovakia and Poland were due to reside in the Emerald Isle until the host demitted from the party.

The championship build-up had the inevitable COVID-19 scares. Many teams posted positive player tests. Eight days before Spain's opener against Sweden on 14 June, their captain, Sergio Busquets, tested positive. Busquets and contacts were isolated. He missed Spain's two openers. Spain's final warm-up game against Lithuania was re-allocated to their under-21 squad. Three days later, the Spanish news got worse. Leeds United's Diego Llorente also tested positive. Manager Luis Enrique's potential headaches had been increased by his earlier decision to pick just 24 players rather than the permitted 26. Following the positive results, a 'shadow squad' (of under-21s and originally unpicked senior players) was selected. They trained separately to the main squad in case of further mishaps. Inadvertently, Sweden levelled things off. They reported that two of their players had tested positive and would not face Spain.

The eventual game finished fittingly in a draw but not before further twists and turns. Llorente's test turned out to be a false positive and he returned to training. Three days before the Swedish game, Spain decided to vaccinate its squad. It had been lobbying its government for preference ahead of other priority groups. The late decision to jab the team provoked an outcry at home. 'A group of 11 men kicking a ball have skipped the queue ahead of professionals who have saved lives,' said politician Aina Vidal. Luis Enrique was unhappy in case of adverse vaccine reactions. None were reported.

It'll Be Alright on the Night
British TV programme featuring 'bloopers'. From 1977

On 11 June, the opening game at the Stadio Olimpico in Rome kicked off in front of 17,000 fans. 'Nessun Dorma' was sung by Andrea Bocelli. Italy beat Turkey 3-0. All was well with the world again! The 36 group games would be played in front of depleted crowds. Only the Puskás Aréna in Budapest would seem close to full – 55,000 spectators.

Both Wembley and Hampden Park would be at one-quarter capacity. The three Wembley group games would trial COVID-19 passports for entry – full vaccination proof or a clear test. It was the first time such measures had been used for entry to a UK sporting event. Glaswegians did not have to show proof but were kept 1.5m apart. Long arms were required for passing a dram. Both venues gave fans ground entry time slots, required masks to be worn, and banned high fives, hugging and moving around at half-time.

The political games continued even after the matches started. Čeferin told the UK government that their COVID-19 restrictions were too severe. He threatened to move Wembley's semi-final and final games to Budapest. The UK's Freedom Day would not come until eight days after the final. Yet UEFA wanted 2,500 designated VIPs to attend Wembley matches and circumvent quarantine regulations. At the time, ten days' quarantine was required from amber-listed countries. The British government were caught on the horns of a dilemma. They were denying double-vaccinated nationals to travel abroad on holiday without restrictions but didn't want to upset UEFA when currying their support for Britain's 2030 World Cup bid.

The Auld Enemy

The group game that all Brits were looking forward to was the 18 June Wembley clash between England and Scotland. The visitors were only allocated 2,600 tickets. Over 20,000 Scots travelled south to London to watch the game in pubs and open spaces. Sturgeon asked fans to behave. Trains were packed with no opportunity for social distancing. The Met Police were issued with dispersal orders to assist with crowd control. After the 0-0 draw, the Scottish fans celebrated ecstatically in London and Glasgow. The Met Police arrested 29 men. In George Square, Glasgow large enthusiastic crowds congregated in defiance of their government's prohibition of unauthorised large gatherings. Swept along by all the emotion, Sturgeon appeared to have changed her tune. She tweeted, 'Yes, sir, you all boogied.'

The problems did not stop with the fans. An ill-fated end-of-game meeting in the Wembley tunnel violated PHE guidance. Players on both sides were put into confinement. Scotland's man of the match, Billy Gilmour, tested positive three days after the game. He was out of his country's crucial final game against Croatia in Glasgow the next day. No other Scottish players needed to self-isolate as potential contacts despite being within Gilmour's 'bubble'. However, later that day, two of England's players, Gilmour's Chelsea colleagues Mason Mount and Ben Chilwell, were put into isolation and forced to miss their country's final group match. They were seen as close contacts of Gilmour at the end of the game. Proximity during match play was not considered close contact. Earlier in the year, it had been reported that no cases of viral transmission during games had been identified in a range of sports.

England manager Gareth Southgate felt that standing down two of his players was illogical: 'It is a bizarre situation. They have spent 120 seconds too long in a fairly open space. It is full of contradictions. I don't understand it because there are teams travelling around by plane, coach and by bus in enclosed spaces for hours and our two boys have been pinged. I really don't get it.' All members of both squads continued to test negative except Gilmour. Southgate claimed the decisions were 'beyond comprehension'.

Twelve days later, Scottish authorities linked nearly 2,000 cases to the Euro 2020 championships. Two-thirds of the cases had travelled to London for the England game. Fifteen per cent of Scottish fans attending Wembley tested positive subsequently. Conversely, both of Scotland's two Glasgow games were linked to only 0.3 per cent of the crowd testing positive. Overall, six per cent of Scotland's national 32,000 cases since the tournament began were linked to football.

The revelation of cases associated to Euro 2020 led WHO to brand UEFA 'utterly irresponsible'. WHO believed the tournament had contributed to the reversal of the ten-week fall in cases across Europe, not only in the UK but elsewhere. The health officials said UEFA needed to look beyond the protocols at stadiums, to travel and hostelries before and after games. UEFA lamely replied that it was fully aligned with local health authorities' guidelines.

'Trains and Boats and Planes'

Song by Dionne Warwick. 1966

Meanwhile, some countries were racking up impressive Air Miles to fulfil their three group matches. Wales, playing in Azerbaijan and Italy, would accumulate 4,500 miles. Having travelled to the edge of Asia for their base, they could not paddle in the Caspian Sea, which beckoned from their hotel balconies. They stayed in separate rooms and travelled in several coaches amidst tight security to avoid multiple isolations following a positive case.

The 'round of 16' saw Wembley's fan allowance grow to half-capacity. England would take on historical rivals, Germany. A senior German doctor advised fans not to travel to Wembley for fear of contracting the Delta variant. The day before the game, German player Robin Gosens felt the decision to increase Wembley's attendance was 'far from optimal'. Germany departed the tournament after a 0-2 defeat. So did Portugal, Sweden and Croatia – who had all been disrupted with positive cases. After the game, Angela Merkel, the German Chancellor, expressed 'grave concerns' about fan numbers at Wembley and compared it unfavourably to the smaller number permitted to watch in Munich.

Next up for England would be a Rome quarter-final match-up with Ukraine. Few could travel from England because of the five days' quarantine requirement. Some had gambled and travelled early. Most English fans in the stadium were EU residents and numbered 2,500 out of a total attendance of 11,880. One fan was intercepted at the stadium and fined 450 euros for quarantine breaches and another 20 were told to stay in their hotel rooms and isolate. England beat Ukraine 4-0. Next up, Denmark in the semi-finals at an even more expanded Wembley – 65,000 fans.

Authorities warned Danish fans not to travel because of quarantine rules. Nevertheless, 6,000 tickets were allocated for the visitors. With 30,000 Danes living in the UK, it was expected the team would have good support inside the stadium. Danish fans attending the game would be sent flags and shirts by the Danish FA. Fans back in Denmark offered to teach their compatriots the best songs to sing at the game. An extra-time winner gave England a 2-1 win. It booked them into a major final for the first time since 1966. It would be Italy on 11 July.

'Do me a favour, open the door and let 'em in'

Lyrics from 'Let 'Em In' by Wings. 1976

The decision to allow attendances at Wembley-based semi-finals and finals to exceed 60,000 would witness the largest crowds at a UK sporting event since March 2020. The extra capacity was allocated as part of the ERP. The news had not gone down well in Italy. Premier Mario Draghi wanted the final moved from London because of rising UK cases. One thousand Italian-based fans could attend the game without quarantining – as long as they formed a 'fan bubble' with entry straight to the game and back to the airport afterwards.

The government had solved its 'horns dilemma'. It gave in to UEFA's demands for 2,500 VIPs – delegates, sponsors, TV company executives – to attend the final two games. They would be allowed to stay in designated hotels. There would, however, be no plus-ones. The media minister, John Whittingdale, had defended the decision by explaining that quarantine rules did not apply to 'important people', creating ill feeling amongst many people not allowed to go abroad on holiday.

Some Cabinet ministers were anxious that the crowds at Wembley, on public transport and in pubs were pushing up COVID-19 case numbers. A consideration to allow a full 90,000 crowd for the final was dismissed on medical advice and concerns over straining public transport. London Mayor Sadiq Khan asked fans to get themselves tested if they had been involved in wild post-match celebrations.

Sixty-seven thousand fans watched Italy win 3-2 on penalties after the game had finished 1-1 after extra time. The build-up to the game was marred by over 2,000 fans breaching security, forcing their way through turnstiles and gaining entry without tickets. It led to fighting inside the stadium. Another 6,000 were waiting outside for similar opportunities. Apart from the increased risk of spreading COVID-19, the incident reflected appallingly on the organisers' arrangements. The next day, the media reflected on how such scenes would be interpreted more widely as the country prepared (with Ireland) for its 2030 World Cup bid – which the PM had tried to improve by controversially waiving quarantine rules for UEFA VIPs and inviting Čeferin to Downing Street.

Commentators compared the flaccid security checks at Wembley with the four separate checkpoints at Rome a week earlier. Questions were being asked as to how such opportunity for overcrowding and violence could be allowed to happen at Wembley during the worst health crisis in anybody's memory. An independent review was announced by the FA to be undertaken by Baroness Casey. Three months later, UEFA ordered England to play their next two games (one suspended) behind closed doors and fined the FA £85,000 for disorderly behaviour.

The problems were not confined to England. Italian health officials claimed that celebrations at home after Italy's victory had sent COVID-19 cases soaring. A regional health official blamed Italy's football federation head, Gabriele Gravina, who backed the open-top bus parade: 'We are paying for the so-called "Gravina effect".'

Two weeks after the final, England's COVID-19 case numbers began to drop. The trend of falling cases started earlier in Scotland and was partially credited to the Tartan Army exiting Euro 2020 at the group stages.

Six weeks after the tournament finished, the UK government released figures on the effect of Euro 2020 on case numbers. For the final game, 2,295 people at or near Wembley were already infected and another 3,405 people attending the match potentially acquired the virus Wembley hosted eight games in total during the tournament – 3,036 positive cases attended and a further 6,376 became infected as a result.

Euro 2020. A perfect storm fanned by thugs

The initial concept of Euro 2020 had seemed hare-brained from the beginning. UEFA seemed tone deaf to the environmental and logistical problems they were creating. Cynics felt that this jamboree was becoming increasingly too expensive for one country to host. France had spent 2.8 billion euros on Euro 2016.

UEFA's decision not to refine the multinational extravaganza in the light of the pandemic was crass. German interior minister Horst Seehofer said UEFA's position was 'utterly irresponsible'. 'I cannot explain why UEFA is not being sensible ... I suspect it is due to commercialism.' UEFA's feeling of entitlement in requesting special privileges for its VIPs was matched by the UK government's passive acquiescence and appetite for political trading for its 2030 FIFA World Cup bid – an ambition abandoned seven months later.

The event's timing created a 'perfect storm'. People were tiring of lockdowns and restrictions. Britain had still not reached its date for the lifting of all regulations. Strict PHE guidelines relating to isolation and close contacts remained. The UK vaccination programme had only reached the under-25s during the tournament and enthusiasm for being jabbed had been waning since spring. The tournament contributed to a surge in cases across Europe and, undoubtedly, unnecessary deaths ensued.

Following Wembley scenes reminiscent of the worst excesses of the 1970s, the very real prospect of the country not being selected to host another men's football tournament again in our lifetimes was real. It was as though the previous 16 months of social restrictions and limitations from attending 'live sport' had deconditioned yobs from remembering what normal behaviour resembled. It is typical of football and its short-term memory that UEFA awarded Euro 2028 to the UK and Ireland only two years later. With the final allocated again to Wembley, will the authorities have learned any lessons?

Perhaps the last word should be those of Baroness Casey from her report: 'The Euro 2020 final was a potentially glorious national occasion that turned into a day of national shame. Our team of role models were in our first major final for 55 years. However, they were let down by a horde of ticketless, drunken, and drugged-up thugs who chose to abuse innocent, vulnerable, and disabled people, as well as police officers, volunteers, and Wembley staff, creating an appalling scene of disorder and coming perilously close to putting lives at risk.'

Chapter 24

Talk(ing)SPORT

Recollections from a broadcaster who has been around for a while

talkSPORT was launched in 1995 as Talk Radio UK. By 2012, it had dropped all its non-sport content. Broadcasting 24 hours daily, it featured discussions and commentaries on sport. It maintained its audience of three million listeners throughout the height of the pandemic – even in the absence of live sport to broadcast and analyse. To achieve this, it required a change of tack and lateral thinking by the radio station.

Mark Saggers joined the radio station in 2009 and hosted various shows and live commentaries. These included the evening weekday programme *Kick Off* along with the *Sunday Exclusive* and *Full Time Phone-In*. The broadcasts included topical debate from football commentators and ex-players as well as listener input. Throughout his broadcasting career, Mark had maintained assiduous notes on events. These are some of his recollections.

'Like a bolt out of the blue, fate steps in, and sees you through'
Lyrics from Walt Disney's 'When You Wish Upon a Star' from *Pinocchio*. 1940

'Not this time, not for the Pompey Chimes. Monday, 2 March 2020. It was unusual for me to drive to a football match with an uneasy feeling. The FA Cup fifth-round at

Fratton Park had all the makings of an exciting evening of commentary and reaction on talkSPORT. Portsmouth against Mikel Arteta's Arsenal. The game was a good one with the Gunners winning 0-2.

'We had heard whispers of possible coronavirus infection amongst one or two of a star-studded Arsenal squad earlier in the day. There was nothing to confirm this, but it didn't help that the press room would only allow four reporters in at any one time instead of the normal scrum.

'Our commentary team included ex-Portsmouth striker and Republic of Ireland international David Connolly. He was distressed. His father had been rushed to hospital with breathing difficulties. With no flights to Ireland, he decided to stay and kept in touch with family by phone. His father remained stable. Arsenal's win felt less important.'

'You'll Never Walk Alone'

Song from the musical *Carousel*. 1945

'Not for another three weeks at least.

'Ten days later, Mikel Arteta tested positive. Followed by four Portsmouth players. So much for fist bumps instead of shaking hands. Arteta's result and one from Chelsea winger, Callum Hudson-Odoi, prompted the shutdown of Premier League and EFL football. It changed broadcasting life for ever.

'It would be 21 days post-Fratton before Boris Johnson announced lockdown. Somehow sport was allowed to run its course at the four-day Cheltenham National Hunt Festival in front of over a quarter of a million fans from all over the country and Europe.'

Keeping the Sabbath

'My Sunday broadcast from London's South Bank continued. My routine of train to King's Cross and a walk to work became a different prospect. Suddenly, with lonely steps and separate spaces, it changed. Communication ceased as capital citizens stopped talking. Lockdown fear crept round every corner. Those walks reminded me of how important communication would be via television and radio mediums during lockdown.

'I was never comfortable being called a key worker, but interviewing and understanding the sporting needs of fans, followers, and those reliant on clubs for their own wages during this crisis became so very important.

'The word was out that football was fighting to carry on regardless. Sky's television deal relied on games being played and leagues completed. Clubs were already borrowing money against season ticket finance and future TV revenues to pay historic transfer fee instalments. It would easily precipitate a cash crisis if revenue stopped. The Premier League's deep pockets would help – but only their own. Everything looked on hold. It could soon lead to crisis and a costly mess.

'Lower down the leagues, desperation set in. Many clubs were mortgaged up to the hilt in the Championship. Chasing Premier League gold at the end of a rainbow was now being replaced by a threat from COVID-19 storm clouds. There was little time to balance the books. Football had always played fast and loose with revenue and debt and was now running out of time. With no prospect of matchday revenues and television fees, there was genuine panic.

'In early March, football convinced itself that it could just carry on. The game's governing bodies, government and broadcasters met on 9 March. Free football on TV was a major discussion. So was continuing matches – but behind closed doors.

'The Liverpool v Atlético Madrid Champions League second-leg match two days later went ahead with fans from both sides packed into Anfield. A decision that seemed to go against common- and possibly life-changing-sense for some fans. Even after the Liverpool game, UK football still thought it was a special case rather than a problem. The Bahrain Grand Prix would ban fans (and later be delayed for eight months), the Chinese Grand Prix was postponed, the World Snooker Championship at the Crucible gone, and there were calls for the Olympics in Japan to be delayed.

'By late March, we were in full lockdown. Even football. I presented the Sunday show from my study at home. The makeshift studio worked well enough. I wanted to make sure that we kept our listeners fully informed on how sport was coping with COVID-19. It became an opportunity for anyone to phone in. They didn't have to feel alone.

'Oxford United manager Karl Robinson gave us a weekly insight into how the club was coping. Players training alone, difficulties for furloughed staff, and strategies for staying in touch. Dale Vince, Forest Green Rovers' owner, outlined the struggles for clubs lower down the pyramid. Chris Munroe, Northern Premier League Basford United's chairman, debated the unfairness of finishing their season with ten games to go.

'None of it would have been possible without my fellow contributors, ex-international footballers Ray Houghton and Danny Mills. They described how footballers would be feeling and behaving. Football was in financial trouble. The situation laid bare, and they were turning against each other. The voices of fans, players, chairmen and owners all played a part in maintaining balance and communication.

'On that critical first May weekend, I invited Bill Ribbans to join Ray Houghton and Danny Mills on the programme. We reviewed the challenges and options for Project Restart after the first official government meeting with major sports. We discussed the changed role of the sports doctor working with elite teams over the previous six weeks. The challenges of advising and maintaining contact with players remotely and the mental and physical worries that we had for them. Views were exchanged on creating safe "bio-secure" environments for elite athletes, what resources and protocols would be required, and how different sports would be differentially affected. The ethical and financial challenges of testing in sport were examined. Looking forward, the physical pressures on the players from squeezing the fixtures lists were dissected

SPORT*

and how much time elite athletes required to regain optimal fitness and skill levels. It was a lively discussion with robust views expressed by the retired "pros". At the end of May and with games imminent, the same "crew" reassembled, assessing progress, debated testing regimes, specific risks for ethnic minorities, stadia preparation and implications for the next season.

'These were topics not seen on the *Sunday Exclusive* menu before.'

The gravy train restarts

'Sports broadcasting is huge business. With government backing, the Premier League's return was inevitable. I would soon be back on the road with the commentary team.

'Premier League CEO, Richard Masters, called the deal "a positive solution after all safety requirements have been met". Contact training with strict protocols in place at training grounds. It all sounded promising. It also showed how the Premier League was detaching itself from the football pyramid.

'The Premier League restarted a month after the Bundesliga and one week after La Liga on 17 June. One hundred days after the suspension. Aston Villa v Sheffield United and Manchester City v Arsenal needed to complete a round of games. That left every club with nine matches to finish. All 92 games were to be broadcast across Sky, BT, BBC, and Amazon Prime. No fans at matches. Just officials and restricted media.

'Liverpool won the Premier League with seven games to go. Thousands of fans descended on Anfield celebrating outside the ground and in the streets. Afterwards the police described the scenes as disgraceful.

'Protocols were different between club and later international matches for the rest of the pandemic. For domestic games, COVID-19 testing for accredited media was taken within 24 hours of kick-off. Self-administered, results notified via an app, and confirmation texted to the authorities. A system that was completely flawed. The individual took and then confirmed the result themself. Nobody seemed concerned about the illogicality. Wembley went a little further. Additional oxygen estimations and a temperature check.'

'There's a Kind of Hush All Over the World'
Song by Herman's Hermits. 1967

'Fan-free games changed the whole feel of live broadcasting. It affected the minds of some footballers. No longer under pressure from the "terraces". The squeals from footballers during physical challenges and instructions from managers and coaches audible. The eerie silence following a goal, or a result, produced a very different feel. If ever football needed to remind itself that fans make such a positive and atmospheric difference, this was it.

'The 2020 FA Cup Final was played behind closed doors. Chelsea v Arsenal. One of the strangest moments of my broadcasting career. The distance between commentators, the wearing of masks unless speaking, and a ghostly walk to and from the commentary box. I have always felt a sense of past glories, game-changing stars, and defining moments when visiting empty sporting arenas. This was different. No sound, no tension, no Bovril, no crowd. I felt privileged to be there – but with a sense of regret. For the fans denied access. For those that hadn't made it through COVID-19. Afterwards, as I walked back down a soulless Wembley Way in the early evening haze, I realised that this strangest of seasons was over. However, with COVID-19 still in charge, I felt neither contentment nor closure.

'I was back at Wembley faster than I expected. Just a month on from Arsenal's triumph, Liverpool would be their Community Shield opponents. The first match of the 2020/21 season. COVID-19 hadn't moved much. Neither had the football rules on fans. We were back behind closed doors. More empty chairs at empty hospitality tables. Social distancing still in force. Not long after breakfast on the morning of the match, I watched Liverpool led by Jürgen Klopp walk down Wembley Way and around the stadium. Not a fan in sight.

'How long would all of this be going on? Thanks to the brilliance of Oxford scientists, vaccinations rather than a winter vacation (unless you were a footballer in Dubai) would dominate the news by the new year. The long wait for capacity crowds would go on. A false dawn of restricted fans in December followed by a third lockdown. Unfettered turnstiles would have to wait until August 2021.'

'It's coming home'. The violence … if not the cup

'I never thought that UEFA's original idea for the Euro 2020 competition was a good one. Different countries for different group stages. It risked losing the essence of a coming together of fans with different identities and purpose. Instead, some long journeys. In and out in a heartbeat. Little feel for the country or their commitment to the match. At many stages it looked as if everything would be cancelled and not just rearranged for the summer of 2021.

'Eventually, an opening ceremony took place at the Stadio Olimpico, in Rome, before the first game. Group stages with vastly curtailed crowds and reporters. Many commentary teams had to work from studios back home in front of screens. Wembley would host the semi-finals and the final, which was good news for our talkSPORT team. I was presenting alongside commentator Jim Proudfoot, and experts Stuart Pearce, Sol Campbell and Jose Mourinho.

'England's subsequent quarter-final against Ukraine took place in Rome. The charade of consecutive COVID tests over six days began at pop-up centres in London. The feeling at the time was one of money-making schemes. Tests at outrageous prices paid for by TV companies. Those were the rules that continued in Rome. The centres seemed to disappear as quickly as they appeared. A lovely little earner for some all-round.

'Not all roads led to Rome in the summer of 2021. A walk past many iconic landmarks with so few tourists about was a pre-match afternoon never to forget. England's victory against Ukraine was comfortable. I had been at many World and European Cup tournaments over the last 40-odd years. This one should have been one to savour at home after all the COVID problems. Our country, England, still very much involved. Sadly, it felt so very different.

'Capacity at Wembley would still be restricted but the ground would be over half-full. Would the stewarding be able to cope? We had already noticed that social distancing had disappeared around the ground. There didn't seem enough staffing for the England–Denmark semi-final. Certain areas had little cover. Easy ways into the ground, without a ticket, felt possible. We needn't have worried. The semi-final went to the drama of extra time before England's captain, Harry Kane, won it. The excitement fizzed down Wembley Way. The country, closed like so many others for so long, had something to open up about.

'I always arrive very early for any live presentation from a football ground. It gives me time to feel the atmosphere. Assess the mood of the supporters. Savour the joy, or otherwise, of the occasion. A European final between two giant footballing nations is one of the greatest match-ups in the sport.

'At 10am on 11 July 2021, I arrived at Wembley for the Euro 2020 Final between England and Italy. The aroma of drugs and trouble in the air was overpowering even ten hours before kick-off. Many fans were already the worse for wear. The atmosphere had a jingoistic air to it. There was nothing new about cocaine, weed, and booze-fuelled posturing by England fans. There was only going to be one possible outcome. Trouble. I didn't hang around. I moved to the stadium to complete my COVID credentialling. My results were all clear. Relief. With COVID-19 restrictions in place, our commentary box was on a different side of the ground to normal.

'Earlier in the tournament, I had been taken by surprise more than once. As a veteran of so many of these occasions, it is the small details, or absence of them, that you notice. Sadly, I automatically scan the scene after seeing the senseless damage to people and property around the world perpetrated by football hooligans. What did I witness in the hours before kick-off? An apparent lack of connectiveness between stewards and police. A lack of attention to detail at flimsy so-called entrances to turnstile gates. The alarming naivety of young men and women employed for much-needed work as stewards for the day. I noted some real problem areas. From public walkways into ticketed fans' areas. These could be rushed by those looking to gain entry for nothing. The police had arrived and, like on so many previous occasions, I just hoped it would calm down.

'Eight days earlier, in Rome, I had been impressed by the Italians' attention to safety. Multiple "rings of security steel" had been established. The 12,000 fans and accredited media had to show their tickets and passes multiple times and at a distance from the ground. No whiff of a spliff or ticketless spectator could have got near the stadium.

'Back in London, nothing had seemingly changed with security for the final. It was going to be a long day. I understood the feeling of freedom. The excitement of being let out after months of lockdowns and anxieties. But hardcore troublemakers were there. Enticing others into their ways. If they were ticketless, there would be an assault somewhere at some point.

'The charge was something that the authorities didn't seem to contemplate could happen. In many ways it's no different from the looting of shops seen on social media posts – with little punishment following. It could have ended in a tragedy at any stage during the final. Police and stewards were overwhelmed. I can't say I was surprised. I was just relieved that there hadn't been serious injury.

'Wembley was the nadir of all the anti-social behaviour witnessed at grounds after elite sport opened to spectators again in 2021. England contrived to lose a final against Italy that they should have won.

'Dame Louise Casey's subsequent review found that it was a "perfect storm" of lawlessness which put fans' lives at risk; 2,000 ticketless fans entered the stadium, mass breaches of disabled access gates and emergency fire doors "jeopardised the lives of legitimate supporters and staff". She also found a "collective failure" by organisations in the preparations for a match of this stature. Alcohol and drugs were a key factor.

'I have seen and heard it all before. It was a thoroughly depressing day that should have been a celebration. COVID-19 finished the football season and the major European tournament in the way it started everything. Used as an excuse for others' failings and behaviour. It was a shameful episode that reflected dreadfully on Wembley and the FA. I drove home reflective and saddened by everything I had witnessed.'

Reflections

'What did I really learn? The Premier League and international football promises much to our football pyramid but delivers the bare minimum. Broadcasters need the experience and confidence to ask the questions that still need to be asked. Fans remain the most important part of professional sport and the delivery of a football regulator should be a government priority.

'I hoped it might encourage a new way forward. A more equal share of revenue. Realistic wages and transfer fees. Clubs helping each other and supporters having more input. I believe many clubs in the lower divisions have learnt and engaged with their communities in a much more open and inclusive way. The Premier League hasn't. Profligacy has never been greater.'

Chapter 25

A Pride of Lions

'We're going on a Lion hunt. We're not scared'

Children's nursery rhyme

The British Lions are rugby royalty. Since 1888, the cream of our four nations' players have sallied forth to take on the best of southern hemisphere rugby in their own backyards. Modern air transport and the congested rugby calendar had seen a dramatic contraction of modern tours from that 35-week opening sojourn. In the last half a century that same ease of travel has allowed a huge band of supporters to trail in their wake. In 2009, 30,000 British fans travelled to South Africa, boosting the Springbok economy. Five thousand more were expected in 2021.

A crowded playing field

The shortest tour in the Lions' history did not dampen the supporters' enthusiasm when the 2021 Springbok tour schedule was announced in December 2019 – ironically, as coronavirus was starting its own travels out of China.

Eight matches in seven locations would be played over five weeks throughout July and early August. Mid-2021 would allow the tour to take star billing on the global sporting stage and be the first where profits were split between hosts and visitors. Gate money, match-day spending, television and sponsorship meant that this was a £100m-plus tour. With full hotels and restaurants, the total injection was an estimated £350m into the local economy. There was genuine concern that the South African Rugby Union (SARFU) would go bust without the tour.

COVID-19 would take the stuffing out of these aspirations. When the pandemic struck in 2020, the world's sporting diary was torn up. Football's Euro 2020 and the Tokyo Olympics would be pushed back 12 months and a returning Wimbledon would all land in the Lions '22'. The summer of 2021 promised a feast for 'pandemic-ed out' armchair supporters, but rugby would struggle to get on to the televisual medals podium. In spring 2020, there were even discussions about moving the tour to autumn 2021 to accommodate a promised rescheduled global rugby calendar.

Will they, won't they?

However, the worst challenge would arrive in the shape of the second COVID-19 wave in early 2021 spearheaded by two variants – Alpha (arising from Kent) and Beta (arising from South Africa). At New Year, the prospect of any tour seemed bleak. Stephen Jones in the *Sunday Times* described the Lions and their fans as a 'Holy Union' that should not be cast asunder and threaten the trip's economic viability and SARFU's bank balance. A delay of 12 months might benefit the welfare of battered bodies that had had precious little rest since the COVID-19 restart in summer 2020.

The first quarter of 2021 saw various solutions trailed. A British Isles-hosted tour was one answer. However, the UK government was unwilling to underwrite any tour losses sustained. Australia offered themselves as hosts – even if fans of either side could not travel. Minimal financial guarantees supported by the Australian government were dangled like carrots.

On 23 March, the Lions announced that the tour would go ahead in South Africa – only 14 weeks before the first game. It was reported that the Lions had given their hosts an ultimatum to go ahead or wait four years. The final tour itinerary and the decision to play behind closed doors was announced in mid-May.

Major hurdles remained. The third spike of COVID-19 would begin in South Africa in May and peak around the time of the tour, caused by the India-originated Delta variant. No UK–South Africa direct flights were scheduled until the autumn. The Lions would be uninsured if the tour were to be pulled before or abandoned mid-tour with major financial repercussions for all. South African medics believed the tour represented a public health hazard. At the start of the tour, only one per cent of South Africans were double-vaccinated.

In mid-June, the Lions started ten days of training on Jersey before travelling to Edinburgh for a pre-departure game against Japan. Players were confined to their hotel, bussed to training and regularly screened for COVID-19. Some were absent because of club end-of-season commitments. There would be no room-sharing on tour – a tradition for bonding the four nationalities. Non-playing squad members would be banned from grounds. However, players felt that the stringent protocols would bring them closer together.

Injury would strike in Scotland. Lions captain Alun Wyn Jones injured a shoulder and did not travel to South Africa the next day. Successful treatment allowed him to be fit for the first Test on 24 July. A replacement was needed to travel at less than 24 hours' notice – who was tested and COVID-free. Jones was joined on the injury list by fellow Welshman Justin Tipuric.

Touchdown

As the Lions departed, South Africa's president Cyril Ramaphosa placed his country into lockdown. The medical situation in Gauteng province was parlous. Switching the two Johannesburg Tests to Cape Town seemed likely. The whole tour appeared to be in jeopardy.

The Springboks reported three positive tests. The whole group would isolate in Johannesburg. One case was rescinded a day later – another 'false positive'. Infection-free players were allowed 'out' to train. South African rugby was feeling the effects of COVID-19 elsewhere. The Bulls and Cheetahs game was cancelled because of cases in the latter's camp.

Case(s) history

The Lions played their first warm-up game in Johannesburg amidst continuing critical media coverage on 3 July. Four days later, their second Johannesburg game was overshadowed by the Lions' first COVID-19 problems. It involved a staff member and a player – causing eight players and four other staff to self-isolate. The need for quarantine was determined by factors such as team bus seating arrangements and a card game that had overrun the maximum 15 minutes. Card schools would be based outside in future.

The game was given the 'green light' only two hours before scheduled kick-off and held up for one hour while protocols were completed, only just before the nationally imposed curfew time. Eight Lions players were removed from the original 23. Some players were being overplayed while others were not getting enough game time. TV portrayed an empty stadium and a game lacking atmosphere if not intensity. Stephen Jones in *The Times* described the historic Ellis Park Stadium as resembling 'a mausoleum'. Stuart Barnes, in the same newspaper, called it 'the Lewis Carroll tour' and wrote that 'off-stage imperatives [economic drivers] seem to have driven us to take leave of our senses'. Beleaguered Lions chief executive Ben Calveley and coach Warren Gatland insisted that the tour would continue. Two days later, the single Lions player to have tested positive returned subsequent negative tests – yet another 'false positive'. His eight team-mates in quarantine were released.

Trouble was already brewing for their third warm-up game on 10 July. Four days before, the Pretoria-based Bulls announced five positive cases and the match was postponed. A rearranged game or alternative opponents were touted. The uncertainty was affecting the Lions' plans for trying out players and combinations ahead of the first Test on 24 July. Two days before the game, the Lions had no idea whether they would be playing or against who. It was announced that they would play against their Wednesday opponents, C Cell Sharks, on Saturday. But first, the Lions squad had to return negative tests. Their opponents were the only team who had been in mandatory isolation and returned negative tests. The decision brought criticism from many quarters. Former WRU player and ex-chairman Gareth Davies stated 'in a way the credibility of the tour is in question'. It 'makes a farce of things'. The Bulls' chief executive spelt out the economic realities. 'There is commercial value on the tour, and it is not about us but about the whole industry.' Sport was not sport anymore but an industry.

Ten of the Sharks squad were already away preparing with the national team. More of the team thrashed by the Lions three days before were rested. Effectively, the Lions would be taking part in a training exercise against a combined second/third XV of a provincial team. The one-sided Lions victory was described as an 'entertaining basketball match' and 'meaningless circus' by Barnes in the *Sunday Times*.

Starved of any games since their November 2019 World Cup victory in Japan, the Springboks had arranged two warm-up matches against Georgia. The first game was played on 2 July. Four days later, the hosts announced 12 cases in their camp and their opponents had six. The second game, for 9 July, was cancelled. Most of the Georgia team flew home but six had to remain for days in South Africa with their team doctor. The Georgian head coach Levan Maisashvili's situation deteriorated. On 17 July, he needed ventilating in a Johannesburg hospital with serious lung damage. He was in a coma for a month but miraculously survived.

The next week, the Springboks camp confirmed 26 positive cases – including their captain, Siya Kolisi. The entire squad were confined to hotel rooms with three doctors looking after them. The SARFU chief executive 'read the riot act' to the squad, reminding them of the financial implications of a tour cancellation. President Mandela's ex-bodyguard and the SARFU chief medical officer were brought into the camp to ensure adherence to COVID-19 protocols. Head coach Jacques Nienaber was in isolation and ex-coach Rassie Erasmus was brought in to lead the preparations.

The disruption to both teams was enormous. The Lions' stand-in captain, Conor Murray, had still not played a game because of self-isolation. It was announced that all three Tests would be played in Cape Town where both sides were ensconced, a decision made easier by a lack of crowds and not having tens of thousands of British supporters' travel itineraries to worry about. The nominated Television Match Official for the entire series, New Zealander Brendon Pickerill, was stranded at home because of COVID-19 protocols and a controversial South African brought in as substitute.

On 23 July, the Lions won the first Test. Seven of the home squad in that game had contracted COVID-19 recently. The Springboks fought back to win the second and last Tests to take the series over the next two weekends.

Aftermath of the tour

Afterwards, the Lions travelled back via Dublin where the Irish contingent were 'dropped off'. Half the squad went on to Jersey – even though local health advisers had warned against them arriving on the island. South Africa was on Jersey's red list – meaning ten days' isolation. The squad were offered special dispensation with release after a negative test if fully vaccinated or five days' isolation if not fully jabbed. The local consultant microbiologist advised of a dangerous travel precedent and its Scientific and Technical

Advisory Committee warned that Jersey would be viewed as a 'back door' to the UK. Two tourists departed directly for holidays abroad – Nigeria and Monaco – while coach, New Zealander Warren Gatland, spent two weeks quarantining in an Auckland airport hotel. Meanwhile, the Springboks moved en bloc to another bio-secure bubble in Port Elizabeth ahead of two games against Argentina.

There was relief that the tour was completed without further calamity. It was estimated that SARFU only earned £250,000. The games were played in empty stadia to service TV audiences. The local economies could not prosper from the expected huge influx of Lions supporters.

The Springboks were undercooked in terms of international exposure and likely weakened initially by COVID-19. The Lions players came off two incredibly compressed seasons (as did some of the Boks) with minimal time for preparation. For the most part, they had to endure warm-up games against inferior opposition that did not allow a comprehensive assessment of their own strengths. The itinerary resembled flotsam being tossed about on an angry sea. Both teams achieved miracles in the circumstances.

In the 133 years of proud Lions tours, this South African odyssey must be regarded as the most depressing and, in certain aspects, futile from a sporting perspective.

Chapter 26

Let the Games Begin?

The Games of the rising sun

In 2013, the IOC awarded the 2020 Summer Olympic Games to Tokyo. It was only the fourth time the event had been held in Asia and would be their second visit to Japan.

Importantly, for Japan it offered an opportunity to demonstrate recovery from the 2011 tsunami and Fukushima nuclear disaster, which claimed nearly 20,000 lives. Japan's economy had been stagnating; 2020 would allow the country to put all this behind it.

The dates were set for 24 July to 9 August 2020. The Paralympics would follow from 24 August to 5 September. Tokyo swelters in the summer. The 1964 Olympiad was held in October. The July start was at US television's behest to avoid clashing with later sporting events. The marathons were moved 600 miles away to cooler Sapporo.

The costs of hosting the planet's greatest multi-sport event increases with each celebration. The estimated bill for Tokyo 2020 rose from $7.5 billion in 2013 to $27 billion in 2019. The escalation drew sharp national criticism. Plans were clipped, including removing the main stadium's retractable roof.

The Tokyo Organising Committee for the Olympic Games (TOCOG) confidently announced in early March 2020 that the Games would proceed. The Olympics had faced microbial threats before – noticeably swine flu (H1N1) concerns at the 2010 Vancouver Winter Olympics and, more worryingly, Zika virus at the Rio de Janeiro 2016 Summer Games. Surely it would see off COVID-19? On 17 March, the IOC calmed nerves, 'No need for any drastic actions at this stage.'

Their bravado was torpedoed when growing international unease culminated on 23 March with Australia and Canada withdrawing. The Japanese PM, Shinzo Abe, supported a delay. The Games were up. The next day, it was announced that the Olympics would be delayed one year. The Games would remain 'Tokyo 2020' – preserving the millions of yen spent on branding. The knock-on effect of its delay on other sporting events has been described elsewhere. However, any further delays and 'Tokyo' would be abandoned.

The Olympic torch had been lit at Olympia in Greece on 12 March in a spectator-less ceremony. Following its arrival in Japan, its national relay was halted. The flame remained in Fukushima.

Isolation, improvisation and insecurity

The knock-on effect for Olympic competitors, delegations, overseas visitors, media, sponsors and the hosts was huge.

For many sports, the quadrennial event is their shining beacon for global coverage. Many competitors only get 'one shot' to call themselves Olympians. Some athletes may have been contemplating competitive retirement post-Games. Did they have enough in the physical and mental 'tank' to wait another year? There was no guarantee that form and health would hold for another 12 months. However, for others, with injuries or inexperience in 2020, the delay brought an unexpected bonus. Many athletes would contract COVID-19, causing disruption in their training schedules and potential long-term effects on cardiovascular fitness. The year 2021 would likely witness a host of different medallists compared to a 2020 celebration. The effect on future celebrity status and guaranteed post-career earnings could be scuppered.

The psychological impact of getting so close to their sporting ambition only to have it removed and the bearing on many sports experiencing a prolonged period of competitive suspension would be difficult to predict. Pre-Games, the British Olympic Association (BOA) announced that it was scrapping its medal targets predictions because of the lack of international competition in the previous year. A complete cancellation would have been even worse to contemplate. It would mean the end of the road for such Olympic icons as Mo Farah.

British athletes had to be inventive during the various lockdowns – 2016 Rio gold medallists Adam Peaty and Max Whitlock respectively imported a swimming tank and pommel horse into their back gardens. Pole vaulter Holly Bradshaw rigged up a homemade bar stretched across some rubbish bins. Paralympic gold medal swimmer Jessica-Jane Applegate trained in a Jacuzzi in her frozen garden. Oarsmen used indoor ergo machines in their lounges. The differential release of restrictions and the need for social distancing meant that individual scullers could get back in their boats before crews. Road cyclists were back on country lanes while the Manchester Velodrome for indoor cyclists was closed for seven weeks.

Medical staff and coaches tend to work in four-year cycles. Would the next job have to be shelved? Central funding for UK sports is based on Olympic cycles with budgets set depending upon previous Games' successes. New financial calculations were required.

Olympic competition is about more than the two weeks of the actual central celebration. Thousands of wannabe competitors start out in a raft of qualifying events across many sports in the years before. Qualifiers are spread out across the globe. Many sports would be affected, including archery, baseball, boxing, cycling, football, handball, judo, rowing, sailing, volleyball and water polo. Some teams just gave up. GB rowers had no international competition between September 2019 and April 2021.

For others, long periods of inactivity threatened to blunt their competitive sharpness. Travel restrictions became tiresome. Yachtswoman and Rio gold medallist Hannah Mills and her sailing partner were separated from their 470-class boat by 2,000 miles when the crisis began. Their boat was holed up in Lanzarote and required special dispensation from the Spanish government to allow them to travel in early 2021.

The bottom line

The global commercial insurance market, including Lloyd's of London, braced itself for huge claims from all directions in the event of complete cancellation. One observer noted that such an eventuality would trigger the biggest insurance payout ever of its kind.

The final decision to proceed with the Games rested with the IOC. Not TOCOG or the Japanese government. The IOC 'own' the Games. If the hosts had unilaterally pulled out, they would have been saddled with the liabilities. The *Nikkei Asia* publication assessed that the Japanese government would owe the IOC £1 billion for lost sponsorship and broadcast income. However, a joint decision would trigger compensation. Knowledge of the contractual entanglement its government found itself in increased anger towards the Games for many Japanese.

The delay added nearly an estimated quarter to the staging costs; £2.81 billion had to be spent on COVID-secure measures alone. TOCOG had bargained on $800m in ticket sales, which it would have to ask its government to make up in the event of empty seats. Three-quarters of the cost of the Games would be met by the Japanese taxpayer. They paid for a party to which they were uninvited.

At the beginning of 2021, the Japanese government, and its PM, Yoshihide Suga, were between a rock and a hard place. Three-quarters of Japanese people were against staging the Games. Opposition would remain at similar levels until its opening. The population received support from leading sports people, medical associations and companies – including Games sponsors. A viral surge related to the Games would likely spell the end of Suga's premiership. But the country had spent billions in readiness for the event.

Suga would eventually pay with his career. Two days before the Paralympics finished in early September, he resigned. His national popularity was at an all-time low. Infection rates remained high, the country was still under a state of emergency, vaccine rollout was slow, and the decision to proceed with the Olympics and Paralympics remained highly unpopular.

Having faced down the real prospect of abandonment in January, the same criticisms returned in mid-April as cases surged again. By late May, one of Japan's leading newspapers, *Asahi Shimbun*, called for the Games to be cancelled: 'We are far from a situation in which everybody can be confident they will be safe and secure.' The paper was one of the Games' official partners.

A petition against the Games reached 450,000 signatures. Ten thousand Games volunteers quit. Hospitals displayed posters on their windows with 'Stop Olympics' on them. Senior medics took to television requesting a cancellation. One observer stated, 'The Olympics has become a cult of commercialised sporting event and their arrogance is surprising.'

In late June, Tokyo's governor was admitted to hospital with 'exhaustion'.

Before the Games started, the IOC president, Thomas Bach, committed a major political blunder by referring to the hosts as Chinese. Leading sports figures from the UK had their say. Sebastian Coe felt the Games should go ahead without spectators. Matthew Pinsent felt it was 'ludicrous' to proceed.

Fuelling the 'fatted calf'

An abandonment of 'Tokyo' would have been the first ever in peacetime and an enormous loss of face and income for the IOC, whose financial streams are dependent upon staging major Games. It helps fund future celebrations and the work of agencies such as the World Anti-Doping Agency (WADA).

Most of its income is derived from media contracts and marketing. As only five per cent comes from ticketing sales for its events, a fan-free Games beamed worldwide would represent a relative 'win' for the IOC and keep 'on side' its major sponsors like Coca-Cola.

However, even after expenditure on projects, millions remain to keep the 'fatted calf' on the road. The IOC is not noted for its frugality. An IOC visitation resembles a royal state visit. Its demands on host cities are legendary for transport and hospitality requirements. Its IOC members are used to being cocooned away from the public in a hermetically sealed environment long before COVID-19 made it de rigueur for the rest of mankind. Cancellation risked a reduction in future hotel minibar sales and exclusive transport lanes for its entourages. One estimate in July 2021 claimed an abandonment would lose the IOC between £2.1 and £2.9 billion.

Three days before the Games began, Bach admitted to sleepless nights. He said that IOC doubts had to be kept to themselves to avoid them becoming a self-fulfilling prophecy and the Games falling to pieces.

Pill-poppers' licence to overdose?

An important part of any major sports occasion and its build-up is trying to keep one stride ahead of the drug cheats. WADA's purpose is to promote, coordinate and monitor the fight against illegal drug-taking in sport. To do this effectively, its agents need to be able to get out and test athletes. In the middle of a pandemic, with limitations on travel and social distancing in force, this proved difficult and potentially hazardous.

China temporarily halted testing in early February 2020. Before the official postponement of the Games, European agencies were scaling back on testing. Russia suspended all testing for three months. The UK undertook only five per cent of its normal tests at the same time.

The problems continued right up to the arrival of athletes in the Olympic Village in July 2021. Forty per cent of the Nigerian athletics squad were deemed ineligible for competition due to inadequate pre-Games testing.

Sampling the facilities

With the construction of facilities well advanced, the next mission was to stage test and qualifying events. Fifty-six such competitions were scheduled from 2018 but put into abeyance from March 2020. In 2021, they were restarted but with predominantly Japanese-only athletes. The international swimming authority (FINA) moved the marathon swim Olympic qualifier from Japan to Portugal in late May. FINA did not pull their punches: 'FINA sincerely believes that the Japanese government did not take all necessary measures to ensure a successful and fair organisation of the competition' and 'did not properly ensure health and protection guarantees to participants'.

The torch relay is reignited – but not the Japanese people

In late March 2021, the Olympic torch relay started a year late. No spectators were allowed at the lighting ceremony in Fukushima. It would wend its way for 121 days across Japan. Spectators lining the route had to wear masks. Cheering was banned. Half of the stages were cancelled. Some celebrities pulled out over COVID-19 fears. The officially recognised oldest person in the world, 118-year-old Kane Tanaka, withdrew from the relay in Fukoaka as she did not want to bring the virus back to her nursing home. A protester tried to extinguish the flame with a water pistol.

The relay bypassed the Tokyo streets and, instead, the capital's flame was lit in front of television cameras. The whole event had turned from a journey of pride, renewal and hope to one of unconcealed embarrassment.

Japan's early and swift response in 2020 had kept viral cases and deaths relatively low. Strict early border control helped. Its people's normal behaviour patterns made it easier to adopt social distancing measures and face-masking requests.

So where were the problems?

The central issues included the roller-coaster ride Japan was experiencing with COVID-19 in 2021, the slowness of vaccine rollout and the population's desire not to import the virus from abroad. At the beginning of 2021, TOCOG was trusting that the jabbing programmes in Europe and the USA would have a more positive effect upon the Games' viability than Japan's own internal programme.

Seven weeks before the Olympics began, Japan was in the middle of its fourth viral wave, its hospital facilities overwhelmed, and the host city remained in a state of emergency. Doctors and nurses reacted angrily to requests to divert personnel from front-line work to look after Olympians.

The problem was due to a combination of factors. Surprisingly, Japan (like France) had failed to develop its own vaccine early. It had to rely on buying foreign vaccines and joined a long global queue. Vaccine mistrust amongst the populace was high after historical issues with MMR and human papillomavirus (HPV) inoculations. The relative ease with which Japan had negotiated the 2020 waves had left its population less demanding of the jabs. A shortage of cold storage and refusal to give spare vaccines to those not on priority lists led to a lot of wastage.

By early June, only nine per cent of Japan's adult population had received its first vaccine dose – compared to the UK's 59 per cent. It seemed barely believable that an advanced country about to welcome the world to its shores had been so slow getting out of the starting blocks.

Annie Sparrow, an Australian public health professor, had advised the Games. She said that the organisers had not followed advice on areas like ventilation and improved testing. She described the IOC as 'the drunk guy in the bar who is determined to get behind the wheel of his car. All that we have been trying to do is to get him home without killing anybody.'

The moral maze. To jab or not to jab?

In late January 2021, the IOC and International Paralympic Committee (IPC) insisted athletes should not jump the vaccination queue at the expense of priority groups but hoped that athletes would be immunised pre-Games as part of their 'COVID-19 toolbox'.

However, over the following months, countries began to 'break ranks' on prioritising Olympians. New Zealand redesignated their athletes as people of 'national significance' to hasten their jabs. Australia announced that its 2,000-strong Tokyo-bound party would be jabbed pre-departure – six months ahead of their country's schedule. In early May, Pfizer offered to send vaccines to competitors pre-departure in their own countries. Japan offered vaccines to Olympic and Paralympic athletes, an offer not universally welcomed by a general population struggling to get vaccines to the elderly and vulnerable.

In late May, the BOA confirmed that all athletes and staff would be fully vaccinated ahead of the Olympics and Paralympics. The decision was justified by the UK government 'based on the unique position of having to travel to Japan to go about their work'.

A total of 93,000 athletes and officials would be entering Japan for the Olympics and Paralympics and separated from the general population. However, 300,000 local officials and volunteers would need to enter and exit the bubbles daily. The potential recipe for disaster was clear. By mid-June, TOCOG began vaccinating 18,000 key local officials.

Pre-Games it was estimated that 85 per cent of delegates would be vaccinated. Out of GB's 376 athletes only a handful refused because of worries that it would compromise their performance.

With or without you?

After much vacillation, the IOC announced, in late March 2021, that no international spectators would attend. It would have a substantial financial impact on TOCOG, the general Japanese tourism economy and beyond. Tens of thousands of ticket holders needed reimbursing.

In late June, TOCOG announced that up to 10,000 fans could attend venues – against the advice of national medical authorities. Two weeks later, the Japanese government revealed that Tokyo's state of emergency would be extended until 22 August – after the Olympics had finished. Although national cases were only seven per cent of contemporaneous UK numbers, it was too much for the Japanese people.

Two weeks before the start, TOCOG confirmed that no spectators would be allowed to attend Tokyo events. Katherine Grainger, UK Sport's chairwoman, felt a 'deep sense of loss' for athletes competing in empty stadia. It was felt that this decision would defuse the pressure on the government to cancel the Games. Half-capacity crowds of up to 10,000 would be allowed in venues away from Tokyo for football and cycling.

Athletes' rules, ok?

From the end of 2020, TOCOG started to provide advice to athletes and spectators on how to behave. The playbooks would be repeatedly updated until the Olympics started.

Athletes would be subject to strict social distancing, mask wearing and daily testing regimes. Pre-departure, all persons required two negative tests. GB's Amber Hill, one of the favourites for gold in the skeet shooting, tested positive only days before departure. A further LFT was required on arrival to get through airport customs. Although not quarantined, athletes were asked to eat alone, and not talk in lifts or official cars. Athletes would arrive at the Olympic Village no more than five days before their event and exit 'pronto' afterwards within two days.

They would be GPS-tracked for retroactive analysis for contact tracing. Officials were told not to shout or cheer at events. Two competitors were investigated for drinking in the Olympic Village park. Athletes were only allowed to imbibe alcohol in their rooms. Two Georgian athletes (both silver medallists) were expelled after taking a sightseeing trip into Tokyo.

In essence, it was more realistically a 'not playbook'. Olympic medal ceremonies would be socially distanced. Recipients would pick up their medals and hang them round their own necks.

It all sounded rather joyless and received this angry rebuke from the World Players Association, who represent 85,000 professional athletes: 'The playbook fails to deliver that trust and confidence.' The restrictions must have come as a blow to the swimming fraternity who traditionally spend the whole second Olympiad week boogying 'til dawn. Miscreants could have medals removed.

Into the midst of all this bad news was thrown the 'condom controversy'. Contraceptives are a staple diet of all Olympic Village welcome packs. Rio 2016 issued 42 per competitor. Japanese Sagami Rubber Industries had developed pre-Games the thinnest, but safest, contraceptive on the market. It had been tested to 'withstand 100,000 thrusts'. TOCOG had installed eco-friendly cardboard beds capable of withstanding post-competition celebrations for up to two persons. All of this would be redundant. It was later clarified that athletes would be presented with condoms as souvenirs on leaving the Olympics. Whatever happened to a sake set or kimono? Was it an upgrade on the London 1948 Olympics, when male GB competitors were presented with a pair of white Y-fronts to wear on return to their loved ones?

The compounded problems led to many leading competitors withdrawing from the Games, some with COVID-19 but most without. This was particularly noticeable in sports where the Olympics were not the only pinnacle of their seasons. Like tennis. Aussie player Nick Kyrgios said, 'The thought of playing in front of empty stadiums just doesn't sit right with me.' Australian protocols meant he had played minimal tennis in the previous year.

Training camps

Some cities withdrew their invitation to host training camps for foreign teams. One Japanese governor reported that he had rejected requests to secure hospital beds if required for competitors. As the teams arrived in Japan, they were subjected to tight hotel quarantine measures. Even before reaching Tokyo, athletes had COVID-19 scares to surmount. The Australian team had their pre-departure camp in Cairns, Queensland. At one stage, the entire team were quarantined in their rooms following a COVID-19 scare – which turned out to be negative.

The BOA confirmed that its distance runners were training on a Yokohama golf course when members were not playing. This was after they were banned from using public running trails. Both pre-departure and in Japan, the amount of meaningful warm-up competitions for athletes was extremely variable – dependent on local case numbers and travel restrictions. It all made for a very uneven preparation period for teams.

Fiji, the eventual winners of the men's Rugby Sevens competition, had their preparation hampered by COVID-19. The team went into training camp for a week in early April but never managed to return to their family homes because of the deteriorating COVID-19 situation in Fiji. Instead, they isolated together. They arrived in Tokyo on a cargo plane carrying frozen fish as passenger flights to and from the islands were grounded. Subsequently, they would face two weeks' isolation on return to Fiji in accordance with quarantine rules.

Jet jeopardy and Olympic positives

TOCOG had set up a 'Fever Clinic' in the Olympic Village for suspected cases. Confirmed patients would be transferred to an 'isolation hotel'. It would not be long before the system was tested.

After South Africa's Rugby Sevens squad arrived, 18 of their 21-strong party were taken to an isolation centre. They had sat close to a passenger who had tested positive on their Tokyo flight. Seventeen were subsequently released after review and allowed to play.

After their flight to Tokyo, six British athletes and two staff members were identified as close contacts of a fellow traveller who had subsequently tested positive. Athletes complained that there had been no segregation of athletes from other passengers on the flights and that they were travelling in economy class. They underwent 14 days of isolation despite returning twice-daily negative tests, and could train – but only if distanced from their coaches. It was for this reason that the BOA had flown in extra mental-health experts, to support such athletes. The isolation impacted upon performance; 400m hurdler, Jessie Knight, hit the first hurdle in the heats and fell. She had given up her schoolteacher job to pursue her Olympic dream.

The Czech team investigated their own outbreak of six cases, which put four athletes out of the Games despite the fact that they had chartered their own plane. After reports that masks had been removed on the aircraft, attention turned to the anti-vaxxer team doctor who had tested positive. The Czech prime minister described the episode as a 'scandal'.

All three members of the BBC Scotland team sent to Tokyo spent 14 days looking at the walls of their hotel rooms after being close contacts of an infected fellow passenger. The rules for non-athletes were different. Isolating athletes were still allowed to train.

Such examples confirmed organisers' fears that travel to the Games represented one of the most hazardous sections of the entire 'Games journey'.

Several other athletes made it to Japan but not much further. The entire Greek artistic swimming team were withdrawn en bloc after five team members tested positive and seven others required to self-isolate.

Let the Games begin

Confusingly, the Tokyo Games action began 48 hours before the opening ceremony. And not in Tokyo. Japan women beat Australia 8-1 at softball in Fukushima. The venue was chosen as it had been the epicentre of the tsunami and nuclear disaster ten years previously. The game was supposed to be an indication of recovery and celebration. Instead, the match took place in an empty Azuma Baseball Stadium and faced widespread opposition to the Games across the country.

On 23 July, a slightly muted opening ceremony took place in front of 1,000 invited guests, including sponsors, France's President Macron and America's First Lady, Jill Biden. GB was only allowed 30 of its 376 squad to attend to reduce COVID-19 transmission risk.

Boiled, bitten and blown off-course

The day after the opening ceremony, typhoons were forecast for Tokyo. Although later downgraded to a tropical storm, two days of rowing had to be rescheduled. Tennis players, golfers and footballers complained of the searing heat. Some events had start times delayed.

A Japanese female softball player had to be issued with a new gold medal after her city mayor had bitten her trophy.

'Germ medal' trended on social media and the politician had to apologise for his breach of protocols and lack of respect for the athlete's performance.

The closing ceremony of the Games on 8 August was a pared-down affair; 62 competing nations were not represented.

The athletes departed but for some it would not be an immediate heroes' hometown welcome. Returning Australian Olympians had to quarantine for two weeks. Those returning to Adelaide, South Australia were told to isolate for 28 days. The state government were concerned about the high risk of the Delta variant. The AOC's application for exemptions was refused.

Paralympics

Sixteen days after the Olympics finished, the 2020 Paralympics began. Over 4,400 athletes from 162 nations competed. COVID-19 cases in Tokyo had doubled since the closure of the Olympics. Paralympians were regarded as far more vulnerable than able-bodied competitors and bio-security protocols were expanded even further. Tokyo was experiencing a deteriorating hospital capacity. However, the hard work paid off and on the penultimate day of competition the Olympic Village had recorded no new cases for four consecutive days.

Was it all worthwhile?

The COVID-19 Games were stressful for all concerned with increased security, rules and testing. It held fears that the passenger two rows behind you on your inward flight might be carrying the virus, with the nagging worry that you might be pinged and removed to an isolation unit for two weeks, ruining five years of training and planning. Media at the Games commented on how Tokyo, despite its restrictions, seemed to be carrying on largely as usual, which made the sight of vast empty stadia even more incongruous.

The Games had effectively been reduced to a TV spectacular especially targeted at the American audience.

For the month around the Games, Tokyo daily case numbers increased fivefold. Organisers claimed that the Olympics were not directly responsible. Critics cited relaxed behaviours and reduced compliance of the local population during the Games. Despite requests to stay away, crowds had gathered at vantage points to watch outdoor sports, such as road cycling, triathlon and BMX. Surges in criticism of the Games by the hosts seemed greatest at times of mounting populace worry associated with increasing case numbers and medical capacity demands. It paralleled similar experiences of frayed patience and criticism of sport staged within the UK. The 1968 Mexico Olympics took place to the backdrop of riots and protests. However, never has an Olympiad been 'celebrated' when much of the host nation did not want it in its country.

By the time of the closing ceremony, there had been 438 positive cases from all the tens of thousands of people associated with the Games. Although some athletes had been prevented from competing, there had not been major uncontrolled outbreak within the Village.

The endeavours and accomplishments of GB's athletes and those from around the world proved inspiring. As for other major sporting events during the summer of 2021, like the football Euros, it provided an enormous tonic to sports' spectators.

GB equalled their medal haul of 2012 and were only two behind 2016. The team had defied all predictions. This was testament to the combined efforts, discipline, resilience and skills of the athletes, coaches, medical staff and sports organisations.

Despite the host of problems and heated debates, the athletes had performed to a remarkable standard – equivalent to most previous Games. Twenty-two world records had been beaten across all sports – only five less than the total achieved in Rio in 2016.

Chapter 27

Jabbing and Djoking

July 2021–January 2022

Getting the needle?

The UK COVID-19 vaccination programme began on 8 December 2020. Priority groups were published, starting with the over-80s and care home residents. Front-line workers came next. In March 2021, Boris Johnson was injected along with other over-50s. Priority group 9 had been reached and 26 million people had received their first dose. The UK's programme had been rapid and greeted with less scepticism than many countries, such as France.

Vaccination numbers peaked in spring 2021. On 17 May, it was announced that Tokyo-bound Olympians and South African-bound British Lions rugby players could jump priority groups for early vaccination. However, Euro 2020-bound footballers were denied access to early jabs. By mid-June, appointments were offered to anybody over 18. It was recognised that vaccine hesitancy was greatest in the young and some ethnic minorities.

When the Euro 2020 Final took place on 11 July, only half of 20-somethings had received their first jabs compared to 80 per cent-plus in the over-50s. Vaccinations numbers fell steadily from May and would not pick up again until a third 'booster' dose was offered in late September. By August, young people were being incentivised by the government to get vaccinated – including discounts on takeaway food, holidays, clothing and taxi journeys.

Euro 2020 hangover

As explained in chapter 23, the delayed Euro 2020 tournament contributed to a COVID-19 surge. Historically, summer is a time when viral cases dip. England's group games at Wembley had been the first UK sports events to require vaccination proof or negative LFTs.

The day after the final on 12 July, Johnson announced that England's 'Freedom Day' would arrive in one week. All restrictions would be lifted. However, he warned that the crisis was not over. Scotland would announce similar timings with Wales, delaying until 7 August. It was reported that young adults in hospital with COVID-19 were mostly unvaccinated and as likely to be as severely affected as the over-50s. In the five weeks between the start of Euro 2020 and one week afterwards, young adults' hospital admissions increased five-fold. Professor Neil Ferguson feared Britain faced difficulties with rising cases, hospital admissions and potential winter restrictions.

England manager Gareth Southgate urged young people to get vaccinated with his 'get your freedom back' message. He received more abuse for his stance than any aspect of his football activities. He supported vaccinated players worried about being 'nailed' for their public pronouncements. Later, Jürgen Klopp felt that people should be openly challenged on their vaccination status akin to 'drink-driving'. Mason Mount, the Chelsea midfielder, announced he had been jabbed, after missing two England Euro 2020 matches because of quarantine as a close contact. The Newcastle manager, Steve Bruce, made an impassioned plea for youngsters to get vaccinated. Bruce had witnessed first-hand the effects of COVID-19 on some of his players. His goalkeeper, Karl Darlow, spent a week in hospital and lost two stone in weight.

On 16 August more incentive to be jabbed arose. The doubly vaccinated need not self-isolate following 'close contact'.

Four days later, some sunshine broke through for sport spectators. The review of 37 'trial COVID-19 events' conducted via the ERP was released. The consensus was that infection numbers were 'largely in line with or below' community rates during the four-month programme. The testing period occurred after the Alpha COVID-19 peak in early 2021 with many people doubly vaccinated. It was deemed safe for big crowds to return while acknowledging that Euro 2020 had contributed to a spike in cases. Numbers infected at 'fan zones' or in pubs watching the matches was unknown. The many ticketless fans gaining entry to the final 'likely contributed to the increased infections data'. The same month, 350,000 people attended the Silverstone Grand Prix with 585 cases recorded. At Wimbledon, 300,000 fans returned 881 cases.

Who just went 'ping'?

The NHS COVID-19 app had really kicked into action. A record 700,000 people were contacted and told to self-isolate in the last week of July. It became known as the 'pingdemic'. Some industries, such as hospitality and supermarkets, were brought to their knees with staff shortages.

The football pre-season had been rocky with games cancelled because of cases. Arsenal (Florida) and Chelsea (Ireland) abandoned matches abroad. Domestic games were called off at short notice. The media speculated that a third consecutive season could descend into chaos. Manchester United goalie Dean Henderson contracted COVID-19 in early July and suffered extreme fatigue, which prevented him from playing for over five weeks. Arsenal boss Mikel Arteta was encouraging players to be vaccinated but admitted, 'At the end, it's a personal decision.' Premier League vaccination rates were difficult to establish as only three clubs revealed data. Others cited 'medical confidentiality' – something they ride roughshod over at other times of their choosing.

The new football season started during the middle of the pingdemic at the end of July with the EFL Cup. Newspapers reported that clubs and managers were encouraging players to switch off their NHS app to prevent isolation of players and teams becoming unable to field competitive sides. One club had three cases, requiring ten further players to quarantine. Newcastle had three goalkeepers isolating ahead of one pre-season game.

Passports at turnstiles?

The government was considering introducing double-vaccination proof from late September for any sports events involving spectator numbers greater than 20,000. The final three Euro 2020 games had allowed crowds of over 60,000. As at Silverstone and Wimbledon, all attendees provided vaccination proof or a negative test. Conversely, in Scotland, Rangers were limited to 17,000 for their season's opener on 31 July. Wales hoped capacity crowds could return by the beginning of the football season.

The Premier League wanted trials of COVID-19 checks ahead of the probable government announcement of mandated 'passports' for crowds of over 20,000. Tottenham Hotspur and Chelsea announced plans for testing in pre-season friendlies. However, while supporting a passport system, clubs felt that compulsory vaccinations of players and spectators were 'unworkable'. They were comfortable promoting the immunisation message. Newcastle United installed a vaccination bus for fans outside the ground. The Football Supporters' Association believed that demonstrating vaccination proof for entering grounds could cause 'chaos'.

The EFL season started properly on 6 August. For the first time since March 2020, most EFL fans would return without restrictions. Forty-eight out of 72 clubs were unlikely to attract crowds of over 20,000. An EFL supporters' code of conduct was sent to clubs to implement as they saw fit. However, Sunderland, with 31,549, and Ipswich, with 21,000 fans, insisted on vaccination proof or negative LFTs.

In the background were the final weekends of the Tokyo Olympics and South African Lions rugby tour played out in front of empty stadia. Travelling abroad was subjected to bewilderingly rapid changes to the traffic light system affecting quarantine and testing protocols. Eight thousand vacationing Brits in Mexico were waiting for emergency flights home. Later in August, Cornwall pleaded for tourists to stay away from the holiday county.

The next weekend the Premier League season started with capacity crowds for the first time in 19 months. Brighton, Chelsea and Tottenham insisted on negative tests or vaccination proof. Some other clubs undertook 'spot checks'. Clubs advised spectators that masks would be required – especially inside. A government scientist called the decision by 17 of the clubs not to insist on mandatory passports 'irresponsible'.

On 12 September, the government announced a U-turn on compulsory fans' passports. Plans would be kept 'in reserve'. Health minister Sajid Javid credited the decision to high vaccine uptake, improved surveillance and new treatments. A surprised Premier League announced that they still intended to extend spot checks to all clubs.

Testing tweaks

The season's start witnessed a variance in testing protocols. The Premier League would keep on testing and publishing results albeit reverting to LFTs rather than PCR tests to save money and speed up results.

Testing for the 2020/21 EFL season had cost £5m and was not sustainable for many clubs. The EFL issued two sets of guidelines – 'green' and 'red' protocols. Most clubs would be green and rely on daily symptom screening. In cases of large local outbreaks, government-imposed restrictions or protocol flouting within clubs, teams would be moved into the red. It would lead to anomalies. On 31 July, an 'untested' Nottingham Forest played Huddersfield, who continued with LFTs. The latter were still receiving 'parachute' financial payments following relegation from the Premier League in 2019.

A travelling, we will go?

On 24 August, European elite football clubs fired the first shots over players appearing in the autumn international breaks. Clubs wanted to block players from leaving. The issues involved quarantine travel rules to COVID-19 hotspots. Around 60 Premier League players needed to travel to 26 red-listed countries. Only eight players from the German Bundesliga were similarly affected. Such was the reliance of English clubs on players from these continents. The schedule had been in the diary for years but the restrictions not. Overall, 140 players from 14 leagues and 70 clubs across Europe were involved.

With World Cup qualifying plans potentially laying in tatters, FIFA asked the British government for exemptions, using the example of UEFA VIPs being granted exemptions for UK-hosted Euro 2020 fixtures. At the time, the government was hoping to 'curry favour' with FIFA and UEFA to host future tournaments – a hope dented by the fans' behaviour. The government declined, fearing a public backlash. It could cite the recent example of British Lions quarantining on return – albeit in Jersey.

Clubs claimed that they had a 'duty of care' and argued that ten days' hotel quarantine would result in 'welfare' issues, fitness loss and missing up to four club games in September. The same would hold for the October international break. FIFA increased tensions by unilaterally extending the release period for South American players during September and October. The European Club Association accused FIFA of 'destabilising the global calendar'.

It appeared that Premier League clubs would lose the argument. Experience should have taught everybody differently.

The keenly anticipated Brazil–Argentina World Cup qualifier had already been postponed twice because of COVID-19. Brazil wanted players released for the rescheduled 5 September game or bans imposed on those not released. However, for clubs, a maximum five-day player ban after the international break would be shorter than ten days in a quarantine hotel.

Premier League unity was fractured when four Argentinian players from Aston Villa and Tottenham Hotspur travelled directly to Brazil shortly after a Premier League game. The nine Brazilian players remained in England.

The infamous four had transgressed Brazilian quarantine requirements. The Brazilian president, Jair Bolsonaro, wanted the game to proceed in Sao Paulo. His health ministry, ANVISA, had other ideas. ANVISA were aware of infractions on Friday and held meetings with the 'institutions'. Attempts by police to enforce a quarantine had been 'frustrated'. Accusing the players of providing 'false information' and having 'failed to comply', officials marched on to the pitch after only five minutes. The game was abandoned; the four players deported from Brazil. The Argentine FA replied that the team had complied with all protocols.

Meanwhile, Premier League clubs with 12 Brazilian, Chilean, Mexican and Paraguayan players who had not travelled waited to see if they would be banned from the next weekend's games. On the Friday, FIFA announced they were free to play. The Argentina four travelled back via Croatia to avoid UK quarantine. Some trained with Hajduk Split during their enforced absence. Tottenham Hotspur's desire to fine their two players for travelling without permission was reported to face legal challenge from the players' unions.

Eventually, five months later, FIFA fined both countries and banned the players for two games. The game would be rescheduled for September 2022 but cancelled by FIFA as both teams had long ago qualified for the Qatar World Cup.

For the two weeks after 'Sao Paulo', confusion reigned. The next international October window loomed. Brazil wanted their English-based players released. As matters stood, they would have to quarantine for 14 days in Brazil, play the games and then quarantine for ten days in the UK. Spurs boss Nuno Espirito Santo wanted quarantine regulations changed so players would not have to miss club games.

The government was reported to be considering reducing international footballers' quarantine period, granting exemptions if private jets were used and players lived in strict bubbles while away. One *Times* reader commented, is there 'no end to their privilege?' Meanwhile, fans attending the October England–Hungary match would have to prove vaccination status or a negative test, despite it not being mandatory.

By early October, fully vaccinated players were allowed to travel to red-list countries but follow strict codes of conduct on travel, bubbles and testing. They would have to quarantine for five days on return in 'bespoke facilities' (such as training ground accommodation) while being allowed 'out' to train and play. Following further easing of restrictions in their home countries, all the Premier League's South American internationals participated in the October qualifiers.

Closer to home another farcical situation arose. At the Republic of Ireland media conference pre-Azerbaijan qualifier in Baku, West Bromwich player Callum Robinson was only allowed to be interviewed by fully vaccinated journalists. Robinson had refused to be jabbed, had self-isolated as a close contact before contracting COVID-19 in November 2020 and again in August 2021, causing him to miss the September Portugal World Cup qualifier. He was not alone in the Irish camp.

The whole sorry episode reflected poorly on several parties. FIFA wanted sovereign state laws relaxed to keep its World Cup carnival on the road. They compounded matters by unilaterally increasing player release periods. It lacked either the foresight or willingness to liaise and coordinate travel arrangements. It cannot have been unaware of individual countries protocols and advised teams accordingly. Better liaison and compliance in Brazil would have spared the embarrassment of Sao Paulo.

Club–country conflicts have been an increasingly thorny issue as foreign player numbers have increased over the last 30 years. There were only 13 in the 1992 Premier League and 367 in 2020. Clubs and spectators thrill at the skills of these players and the success they bring. However, release, particularly for non-European international matches, has often been granted grudgingly. Once the spectre of travel quarantine was added, clubs were quick to fly the flag of convenience. Duty of care. It frequently goes missing when issues such as fixture congestion and concussion are raised. Finally, within the UK populace, there was a growing weariness with football clubs' and players' demands for special dispensations when their own vaccination levels were poor, and while spectators and journalists were required to provide vaccination proof to watch or speak to refuseniks.

Time for all of us to roll up our sleeves?

The international release controversy was played out against a background of increasing irritation with low vaccination levels amongst professional athletes. The debate would continue throughout the rest of 2021 and into early 2022 where the story would morph into the Djokovic–Australian Open saga.

The problem of unvaccinated players was brought into focus by the Arsenal player and Swiss captain Granit Xhaka in early September. Having refused to be immunised, he tested positive shortly before a national game.

At the start of the 2021/22 season, only 18 per cent of EFL players were fully vaccinated. However, the messaging seemed to be effective as numbers rose to 49 per cent by the end of September. The August figures were half of 18- to 24-year-old nationwide numbers but approached equivalent levels by the end of September.

In late September, the Premier League were considering incentivising clubs with high player vaccination rates. Only seven of the 20 clubs had more than 50 per cent of players fully vaccinated. One option was relaxing restrictions at clubs once 85 per cent of players were vaccinated. Saracens rugby applied the 85 per cent rule in October 2020 – but still had to close their training ground and cancel fixtures two months later.

It was reported players had been sharing anti-vaccination messages on WhatsApp groups, including ex-Southampton player Matt Le Tissier's assertion that 15,000 Europeans had died from vaccinations. The PFA stepped in. Its chief executive, Maheto Molango, warned players of 'myths and lies'. Jonathan Van-Tam joined the conversation with Premier League and EFL club captains. One Premier League club had a particularly low vaccination rate and was accused of being arrogant by others. Manchester United were apparently having problems convincing players.

Commentators questioned whether they were aware of their hypocrisy in enjoying special privileges denied to fans and NHS staff, described in *The Times* by Henry Winter as 'naivety and selfishness'. The unworldly elite 'dressing room culture' divorces its inhabitants from normal society. It allows beliefs to become entrenched and anoints anonymous social media 'influencers' with more medical knowledge than senior doctors whose long careers had been immersed in this work. Ex-footballer Gregor Robertson wrote, 'It's hard to escape the fact that there is a deep strain of stupidity and selfishness running through changing rooms up and down the country.'

By Christmas, 16 per cent of Premier League players were still refusing first jabs while Liverpool, Leeds and Wolves had close to 100 per cent rates. A reflection of general club culture and tolerance of the unhealthy influence of individuals in anti-vax changing rooms?

Aston Villa manager Steven Gerrard announced that vaccination status would be a factor considered when buying a player in the January 2022 transfer window. Despite the U-turn on mandatory player vaccinations, it was not 'off the table' and clubs were concerned that games might be postponed if they involved clubs with large numbers of anti-vax players quarantining. Their fears would be realised.

Vax view from abroad

The 'hands off syringes' approach towards anti-vax footballers worried about jabs affecting their performance in a game or in bed contrasted to approaches from other sports and countries. Frequently, decision-making was based upon sport having to kowtow to local health restrictions or an acknowledgement that their international fixture list required adherence to the strictest protection measures.

In Germany, Bayern Munich's Joshua Kimmich's anti-vax stance dismayed doctors worried about encouraging vaccine hesitancy. Germany's Chancellor, Angela Merkel, advised Kimmich to seek further medical advice. In November, Bayern announced no pay for unvaccinated players required to quarantine. This was in line with edicts from the city of Munich. At the time, they had six players self-isolating – including Kimmich. The latter developed lung problems from COVID-19. It kept him away from team-mates for seven weeks. Kimmich admitted he regretted his previous stance and that he intended to be vaccinated. Shortly after, his team-mate Alphonso Davies developed myocarditis from the virus. By the end of 2021, Germany, Italy and Spain's top football leagues all reported player full vaccination rates of greater than 90 per cent –

higher than their countries' average for their age group. America's NBA basketball stars had achieved that level by mid-October.

In the USA, the NBA tested unvaccinated players more frequently. Golden State Warriors' Andrew Wiggins could not play home games in San Francisco as local regulations would not allow fans or athletes to attend indoor events unvaccinated. His request for exemption on religious grounds was dismissed. A week later, he was jabbed, but revealed later his regrets despite having the best season of his career. His club went on to win the NBA championship for the seventh time in their history.

In mid-October, NBA team Brooklyn Nets stopped their unvaccinated player, Kyrie Irving, training or playing. He breached a New York City mandate requiring all athletes to be jabbed. He could have played in most away games, but his franchise chose not to select him until he could be a full squad participant. Irving missed 35 games and lost $14m in salary. The player was an admittedly 'big conspiracy theorist'. He had previously apologised for his 'flat Earth' beliefs and had shared Moderna vaccine microchip theories. His club relented in early 2022 for away games with other players out with COVID-19. It would be late March before he made his home debut once New York City lifted its ban. Ironically, he had been allowed to watch from the stands! Six months later, Irving revealed that his stance had cost him a $100m-plus contract extension with the team.

Washington State University American football coach Nick Rolovich and his four assistants were dismissed for refusing to be jabbed. He lost his £2.25m salary as all workers in the state of Washington had to be vaccinated. By the end of the year, 95 per cent of NFL players were vaccinated. The England men's cricket team were fully vaxxed. In January 2022, Formula 1 announced that all within the paddock – including pit-lane visitors – must be fully vaccinated. No room for manoeuvre there.

Pennies dropping and matches missing

The concerted cocktail of criticism, potential sanctions, quarantine as close contacts, knowledge of stricken fellow players and education began to reap dividends. By mid-October, 68 per cent of Premier League players were fully vaccinated and 81 per cent jabbed once. However, 25 per cent of EFL players refused to be vaccinated.

Football managers, administrators and government pleaded with players to reconsider. On 17 December, six of ten Premier League fixtures were postponed because of outbreaks at clubs. Unvaccinated players had to quarantine as close contacts and were increasing the jeopardy of fixtures proceeding. The vitriol reached its nadir on 15 December. Only hours before their game at Burnley, Watford cried off following a squad outbreak. Coaches of fans had arrived at Turf Moor before the announcement. Isolating unvaccinated players was reported to have added to the problems. The next day, *The Times'* Henry Winter took aim, 'All clubs should demand that their players are double-vaccinated and have the booster jab … Some may have ethical reasons for not getting the jab. If so, they have to stay at home.' Rod Liddle in the *Sunday Times* opined that 'entitled footballers … still deserve to get it in the neck for not getting it in the arm'. Jürgen Klopp felt players had a moral obligation to be vaccinated as over half the games in the top four tiers were lost on the pre-Christmas weekend. Leeds CEO Angus Kinnear talked of players' civic duty. NHS staff vented their spleens on the toll on ICUs and waiting lists caused by unvaccinated people.

By 1 February 2022, Premier League footballers' vaccination rates outstripped their contemporaries in the UK – 80 per cent against 74 per cent for 25- to 29-year-olds. It coincided with a fall in positive tests in the league for the fifth week in a row. Meanwhile, EFL figures from December continued to show less appetite for helping the national effort – only 69 per cent had one vaccination.

It had been a dispiriting second half of 2021 for sport – particularly football. Certain athletes and administrators had demonstrated staggering insensitivity to the general public. It was all in stark contrast to the contrite 2020 statements promising COVID-19 would push the reset button.

No vax

The vaccination debate washed up on the shores of 'planet tennis' as the 2021 US Open was due to start in New York on 30 August. Beforehand, Andy Murray said that players travelling the world had a public responsibility to be vaccinated.

New York required vaccination proof to access indoor dining, fitness spaces and entertainment facilities. Spectators at Flushing Meadows had to be jabbed. For players, vaccination was optional. Just over half of the male players were. Stefanos Tsitsipas, the Greek third seed, was criticised by his own government for his anti-vaccination stand. The *Sunday Times'* David Walsh wrote that it revealed 'the athletes who only think of themselves'.

Players avoided the designated accommodation of 2020 but were tested every four days. Vaccinated players avoided the need to isolate if identified as a close contact and wearing masks at the venue. Unvaccinated Frenchman Gilles Simon withdrew after his coach tested positive.

On 10 September, these controversies were quickly forgotten as a sporting miracle occurred. The unseeded Emma Raducanu lifted the women's singles title and became the first player to win a grand slam via qualifying in the open professional era. Novak Djokovic lost in the final and with it the chance to win a calendar grand slam.

Vaccination take-up by globe-trotting players remained slow. By late October, 40 per cent of women and 45 per cent of males remained unjabbed. The spectacle of compulsorily vaccinated fans watching unprotected competitors remained. Players continued to contract the virus – most notably

Raducanu, Rafael Nadal and Ons Jabeur at the Abu Dhabi tournament in December. Raducanu received BBC's the *Sports Personality of the Year* award in isolation in a Middle East hotel. The recovery blighted her build-up to the Australian Open and was partly blamed for her poor form later in 2022.

By that time, tennis was already on a collision course with Australian authorities.

Walking where the Association of Tennis Players (ATP) and Women's Tennis Association (WTA) dared to tread, unflinching Aussie politicians had declared in October that unvaccinated players would not be welcome for the January 2022 Open. Victoria's state prime minister Daniel Andrews declared, 'On behalf of every vaccinated Victorian who has done the right thing, my government will not be applying for an exemption for any unvaccinated player.' In August, the organisers had outlined plans for a 'hotel-tennis court bubble' to avoid the 2021 debacle of 72 players spending a fortnight cooped up in hotel rooms. The restrictions seemed to act as a spur. By the end of November, 85 per cent of the men were immunised.

Novak Djokovic would not commit himself to defend his 2021 title or reveal his vaccination status. His father claimed his son was unlikely to play 'under these blackmails and conditions'. The nine-times Aussie Open champion was respected in the country. He had earned 'brownie points' when organising a $500,000 players' donation for relief efforts during their 2020 bush fires.

In April 2020, Djokovic stated that he was 'opposed to vaccinations and wouldn't want to be forced by someone to take a vaccine'. However, early in 2020, he had donated over $6.6m to Serbian health authorities and more monies abroad.

In May 2020, Djokovic announced that he was organising an elite eight-player tour of the Balkans, the Adria tour. The official world tennis tour had been suspended until at least August. The first tournament was in Djokovic's hometown of

Belgrade on 13 June. The organiser said, 'I'll do everything in my power to be a good host.' The games were greeted with dismay abroad as full, unmasked crowds watched players who provided autographs, and exchanged hugs and high fives. One sports commentator described it as 'shocking'. Videos emerged of the players partying and dancing shirtless with fans. Eleven days later, it was cancelled. Four players, including Djokovic, tested positive. There was widespread criticism from the tennis world over the antics. There were calls for him to step down as president of the ATP Player Council. A sheepish Djokovic tweeted, 'I am so deeply sorry our tournament has caused harm … everything … we did with a pure heart and sincere intentions.'

'You must be Djoking'
Front-page headline from the Brisbane *Courier Mail*. 4 January 2022

Less than two weeks before the 2022 tournament, the Serbian ace announced that he had an Oz travel exemption relieving him of being jabbed. The Brisbane *Courier Mail* led with the headline 'You must be Djoking'. Seventy per cent of Aussies didn't want him in the country. Many Australians remained marooned abroad nearly two years after the pandemic started. Melbourne hosts were fed up with sanctions and the six lockdowns totalling 262 days, making it probably the most locked-down city in the world. Australia was experiencing a surge in Omicron cases – over 68,000 on 5 January compared to 4,762 on 5 December. Their very own tennis demigod, Rod Laver, said, 'I think it might get a bit ugly.'

Djokovic's anonymised application for a waiver had been vetted by two medical committees. Twenty-five other players had followed a similar path – only a few were successful. One reason for a waiver was proven evidence of COVID-19 in the previous six months. Djokovic declined to reveal the reasons for his exemption.

On 5 January, the tennis star was photographed standing at an Australian passport booth before being held for eight hours in an airport room with policemen standing guard. The Serb had apparently applied for the wrong visa – only discovered once he was airborne.

The player had landed into a political storm. Australia's prime minister, Scott Morrison, was seeking a fourth term of office in the May general election. Faced with surging COVID-19 cases, he did not want to antagonise voters. In the event, both Morrison and Djokovic would be the losers.

The sorry saga lasted until 16 January – the eve of the tournament. Australian federal authorities overrode the state and medical boards' decisions. Visitors needed medical grounds for not being vaccinated.

Pending the deportation appeal, Djokovic was placed in a detention hotel normally inhabited by asylum seekers. It was much removed from his usual accommodation standards and his request to be moved to a private rented apartment was denied. His mental state was speculated upon and his former coach Boris Becker felt that his stance risked his career.

The next day, female Czech player Renata Voracova joined him in the hotel after an application review. She had already played in a warm-up tournament and was willing to leave the country. Later, she revealed that she had been ordered to strip during a six-hour interrogation.

Crowds protested outside of the hotel and in Serbia. Police used pepper spray on fans gathered outside his lawyers' offices. His parents claimed he was a prisoner. The government riposte was that he could leave the country whenever he wanted.

Five days later, a judge found in Djokovic's favour and ordered his release. The authorities had not followed procedure by denying Djokovic time to consult with lawyers and Tennis Australia before having his visa revoked. Within hours of his release, Djokovic was on court at the Rod Laver Arena practising with his team.

His lawyers claimed that Djokovic had contracted COVID-19 on 16 December and, thus, fulfilled criteria for a vaccination waiver. It did not help. Photographs appeared of him presenting awards to Serbian youngsters one day after the positive test. Two days later, and knowing he was positive, he was interviewed by the French newspaper *L'Equipe*.

His travel declaration form specified no travel in the 14 days pre-embarkation for Australia – but he had visited Marbella at New Year. This potentially put him in hot water with Spanish authorities. He should have produced his vaccination status or exemption certificate on arrival. He was forced to admit his mistakes two days after the court decision.

Waters were muddied following detective work by the German paper *Der Spiegel*. They 'QR scanned' the PCR test result. Initially it read negative but, when rescanned an hour later, it changed to positive. They described anomalies in the test's time stamp indicating it may have been undertaken ten days later – on Boxing Day. The Serbs countered with explanations for the seeming conundrum. The test's validity was questioned for weeks afterwards.

As Rod predicted, this was getting uglier.

Players criticised the circus around Djokovic, which was detracting from the normal tournament build-up. The previously 'vac-sceptic' Stefanos Tsitsipas told Indian network WION News, 'He [Djokovic] has been playing by his own rules. No one would have thought, "I can come to Australia unvaccinated and not have to follow the protocols they gave me."'

On 13 January, the competition draw was made with the Serb in it. The next day, the government revoked his visa on 'health and good order grounds'. Djokovic appealed. The court sat on Sunday morning – 24 hours before the tournament began. The application for a review of the decision was denied. Djokovic had run out of road, ran up the white flag, and flew out of Australia. Potentially, the deportation order could keep the Serb out of Australia for three years. Serbian President Aleksandar Vucic claimed the hearing was 'a farce with a lot of lies'. By September, Djokovic claimed that he had no regrets and hoped to play in Australia in January 2023.

The tournament was played in front of 50 per cent crowds to mitigate COVID-19 spread. Tennis Australia deeply regretted the impact the saga had had on fellow players. The organisers acknowledged there were 'lessons to learn'. Tennis Australia announced an annual loss of £53m – largely due to COVID-19 protocol expenses for the 2021 tournament. This farce did not help replenish their coffers.

The aftermath of Oz

With other countries beefing up entry requirements, Djokovic's 2022 schedule risked being shredded. President Macron in France revealed his strategy towards unvaccinated people. 'I really want to piss them off, and we'll carry on doing this – to the end,' he told *Le Parisien*.

America was getting tougher on the non-jabbed entering the country compared to September 2021. Austria was introducing mandatory vaccinations for all over-14s from February and Germany was planning similar moves. It appeared that life was going to get difficult for unvaccinated athletes.

What was the fallout from this saga? Djokovic was now in a minority. While Djokovic was in Australia, the ATP confirmed only three of the top 100 tennis players remained unjabbed. Djokovic thanked all his Serbian supporters including the president. He was consulting lawyers about suing the Australian government for £3.2m for lost prize money and his quarantine conditions.

Later, Voracova suffered depression and dramatic weight loss and considered retirement. She was not an anti-vaxxer and had provided a genuine medical reason for exemption. She was exonerated subsequently by an Australian inquiry. Without Djokovic, she claimed she would have been allowed to stay.

Djokovic's 2022 started belatedly on 21 February at the Dubai Open. It had no vaccination requirements. The rusty defending champion lost his world number one ranking after defeat in the quarters. He was excluded from two early American tournaments.

Only in the middle of May did Djokovic take his first title – the Italian Open. He lost in the French quarter-finals to Rafael Nadal before triumphing at Wimbledon in early July against Nick Kyrgios in the final. It was Kyrgios that had called Djokovic a 'tool' over the latter's COVID-19 demands in the build-up to the 2021 Australian Open. After his win, an emotional Serb spoke about his mental state after Australia and his need to 'weather the storm' that ensued.

No sooner had the SW19 triumph been completed than Djokovic had to consider the September US Open. His world ranking had slipped to number seven. US regulations required all visitors to be vaccinated. Djokovic stuck to his principles and did not appear stateside. Another opportunity to add to his 21 grand slam singles titles had gone begging.

Redemption would come for the Serbian in the shape of the new Australian government. In November, the Labor administration quashed his three-year entry ban to Oz. The maestro expressed his relief. It would not all be plain sailing. In early 2023, the US authorities extended their ban on unvaccinated visitors to their country. Djokovic would not be able to play in the prestigious Indian Wells and Miami Open in March. However, the player arrived in Australia in good spirits.

Despite some heckling from a spectator, his dodgy hamstring and his father posing with supporters of Vladimir Putin, he was in imperious form. He breezed through seven rounds with the loss of only one set. With his tenth Australian title in the bag, he equalled Rafael Nadal's record 22 grand slams and regained his world number one ranking. By September 2023, the Serb was allowed to reappear in New York. Having won the French Open in June, Djokovic took the US Open, taking his grand slam singles titles to 24.

Chapter 28

COVID Chaos from Cape Town to Cardiff

Rugby reality 2021–22

Rugby union hoped that late 2021 would signal a semblance of normality returning to its sport. The British Lions had returned finally to their homes and teams. The English Premiership, French Top 14 and United Rugby Championship (URC) would start in September, with the northern hemisphere autumn internationals scheduled for November, and the European Champions Cup commencing in December.

Teams could begin crisscrossing countries and continents. Coffers could be refilled. What could possibly go wrong? Someone testing positive for COVID-19 in New Zealand for a start.

South of the equator

The 2021 Rugby Championship involving the four southern hemisphere powerhouses took several twists and turns. The Springboks had been prevented from participating in 2020 by government regulations.

On 14 August, Australia were thrashed in New Zealand in the opening fixture. Six days later, the All Blacks announced that they would not fulfil the return fixture in Western Australia and, additionally, cancelled their two South African games. They cited the reimposed New Zealand lockdown regulations (after the country's first case in six months) and Australia's quarantine requirements. South Africans could not be admitted to New Zealand. Australian coach Dave Rennie said he was 'bloody angry' and cited Aussie willingness in 2020 to isolate for two weeks in Wellington in order to play. Sixty thousand advance tickets had been sold for the Perth game.

Rescheduling the entire series in Europe or South Africa was mooted. Eventually, Australia was chosen as host. The Perth game was played two weeks late. Queensland was chosen for the rest of the tournament, having been less affected by the Delta variant. Teams were allowed 'managed isolation'. All went swimmingly … until the final match.

Six Argentina players and two staff crossed the state border into New South Wales to visit a tourist haunt. On their return, the border police refused to let them back into Queensland to play against Australia on 2 October. The miscreants were only allowed to join up with their mates for the flight back to Buenos Aires. New Zealand won the tournament. Argentina lost all six of their matches.

'Mutual confidence will sustain us to the end!'
Quote from Wilkins Micawber from *David Copperfield* by
Charles Dickens. 1850

The 2021 autumn rugby union internationals began with all the optimism of Mr Micawber.

In general, crowds would be allowed to return in large numbers to five of the Six Nations' grounds. Italy remained with significant restrictions. Twickenham and Cardiff saw the return of full crowds for the first time since the pandemic started. Wales played New Zealand at the end of October on a date outside of the agreed 'international window'. Both sides were under-strength due to injuries and clubs' refusal to release players. It helped the bank balances of the respective unions, which was probably the game's main mission. The

74,000 crowd had to show their NHS COVID-19 passes and arrived at times specified on their tickets to avoid congestion.

With England's squad reaching the prescribed 85 per cent vaccination rates, rules could be downregulated. Players could travel on the same bus and stand next to each other for national anthems. They could leave camp for coffee – so long as they sat outside. Everybody would have to PCR test three times per week.

Inevitably, sides would suffer COVID-19 withdrawals. England's game against Tonga was in doubt until hours before kick-off. Positive tests in the camp led to scrambled extra tests and the withdrawal of their captain, Owen Farrell. Cancellation would have been a financial disaster. One player recounted the stress of not knowing if the game would go ahead. The next day, Farrell's test was found to be a 'false positive'. It would not be the only sport to suffer from spurious results. The RFU had sought to eradicate such problems in the spring when dumping testing company Randox after Bath had returned 19 'false positives' in January – all but one was incorrect. Further 'true positives' would dog England's November schedule. One involved prop Joe Marler. The player would test positive again two months later as England prepared for the 2022 Six Nations.

Again, the worst problems would be reserved for the 'last knockings'. The Barbarians would take on Samoa at Twickenham at the end of November. They would try to do better than the 2020 shambles. They didn't succeed. Ninety minutes before kick-off, the Baa-Baas camp discovered six positive cases. The Samoan side were in the changing room and 41,000 people were arriving at 'Billy Williams' Cabbage Patch'. A Baa-Baas game was cancelled for the second time in 12 months. Chairman John Spencer threatened legal action after ex-players accused the 'club' of being shambolic. The next day, the Barbarians were on the back foot as rumours spread that players had visited the Hyde Park Winter Wonderland in the game's build-up. Sinoti Sinoti, the Samoan amateur player, was 'frustrated', having travelled 21,000 miles to play at considerable personal expense. It was to have been his final game before retirement.

United Rugby Championship

In 2021, the former Celtic League had been rebranded the URC. It comprised 16 teams with an ambitious 191-game schedule played across both hemispheres involving Welsh, Scottish, Irish, Italian and South African sides. The latter would be competing for the first time to qualify for places in 2022/23 European cup competitions. This was a brave new start for a post-COVID-19 era. Or so the organisers hoped.

The competition had reached round six on the last weekend in November. On Thursday, 25 November, England placed South Africa on the travel red list. Cases in the latter had increased twenty-fold in a month. Anybody arriving in the UK after Friday from South Africa needed to home-isolate for ten days. Even worse, passengers arriving home later than Sunday morning, 28 November, had to quarantine in a hotel.

Cardiff Blues, Llanelli Scarlets and Munster were already in South Africa preparing for weekend fixtures against the Sharks, Lions and Bulls respectively. They were the first Welsh and Irish sides to play in South Africa in the revamped competition and due to stay for games the next weekend also. The two Welsh teams had over 100 personnel. The deteriorating health situation for their hosts and the prospect of isolation on return meant that the sides had to abandon ship and seek an aeroplane home. Plans for a quick escape evaporated. Cardiff and Munster had cases and were held in Cape Town hotels.

The Scarlets escaped to Dublin on the Monday (29 November) and onward to a Belfast hotel to begin ten days' isolation. Despite no cases, they forfeited their 11 December game against Bristol Bears in the European Champions

Cup (ECC) citing concerns over player welfare and fixture preparedness. Despite having only 14 fit players in training, their request to move the fixture or borrow players had been turned down by the organisers. Bristol revealed that the cancellation had cost them £300,000.

Meanwhile, back in Cape Town, cases in the Cardiff and Munster camps were stacking up. Not only had the teams' two URC games been lost but the chaos threatened their opening games in the ECC scheduled to begin on the second weekend of December.

Bug-free Irishmen flew out on 30 November to isolate in the Emerald Isle, but nine cases remained behind. Amazingly, Munster won 35-14 at Wasps in the ECC on 12 December. The visitors were without 34 players and additional staff and played a young team with 12 of the 23 making their debuts. Wasps had eight players test positive the day before the game but had four reprieved with repeat negative tests and allowed to play.

Cardiff's 42 players and staff tried three times to leave. On one occasion their chartered plane's landing slot was removed. The Welsh government claimed there were no suitable quarantine hotels in Wales. It would have to be an English isolation hotel. Chartering a plane and quarantine would cost £250,000. Six positive cases had to stay put when they finally flew out on 3 December. The club wanted to fulfil their home European fixture against champions Toulouse, on 11 December. Profits from the game would be £200,000. Those players quarantining would miss the Harlequins European game on 18 December. Concerns were raised about players not training for three weeks and deconditioning, increasing injury risk when facing sides not similarly restricted. With players isolating across two continents, Cardiff lost to Toulouse 7-39. Their Harlequins game proceeded with 32 players unavailable because of COVID-19 and injury. A player came out of retirement to play out of position and Cardiff lost 43-17. The Blues stated that they would need persuading to return to South Africa after their experiences. Many players and staff had spent nearly four weeks in quarantine. Eventually, they did return to complete the fixtures (along with Scarlets and Munster) in March 2022.

The Premiership and European Champions Cup

The English Premiership had escaped lightly up to mid-December when Saracens had to close their training ground until Christmas Eve because of COVID-19. By forfeiting their away game at Pau in the ECC, they became the first English side to call off a game that season. Across the British Isles, new COVID-19 cases were forcing cancellations of league matches. Harlequins jettisoned their Christmas party to minimise the risk of their lucrative Northampton Saints game at Twickenham in front of 70,000 fans being lost on 27 December.

The WRU estimated each cancelled game cost clubs £100,000. All scheduled URC games on Boxing Day were cancelled because of COVID-19. The Welsh government decreed that all sport over the Christmas period must be played without fans. This prompted the Llanelli chairman, Simon Muderack, to claim that Welsh clubs were financially affected more from the pandemic than English clubs with less government support, large income reductions from the WRU, playing behind closed doors and reduced ability to attract sponsors. In England, Wasps coach Lee Blackett supported a 'circuit breaker' and rescheduling matches rather than play behind closed doors.

European games became more complicated on 16 December when the French government announced onerous restrictions to visitors including two days of isolation on arrival. If one person tested positive, the whole squad would have to quarantine for ten days. All seven games between French and British clubs were postponed the next weekend. The tournament organisers, EPCR (European Professional

Club Rugby), having stated previously that games could not be postponed, announced that they were reconsidering their options to preserve the competition's integrity. Eventually, the games were not replayed but declared 'draws'. Bristol had paid £35,000 for a charter plane to France for their cancelled game.

The French made things more awkward after Christmas. President Macron announced that all professional athletes needed to be fully vaccinated by 15 January. This posed issues for later ECC matches, the Six Nations Rugby game between France and England on 19 March and Chelsea's football match in Lille on 16 March. Visiting teams could not field non-vaccinated players. In France, 98 per cent of rugby players and 95 per cent of footballers were vaccinated.

Two days before the next round of ECC games, restrictions were eased. Vaccinated visitors no longer had to quarantine. Henry Slade, the Exeter player, announced he had now been vaccinated, allowing him to play for club and country in France. More European club cancellations continued during the group section of the competition before the tournament limped into hibernation and re-emerged in April for the less eventful knockout stages.

The 2022 Six Nations ran from early February until the middle of March without postponements. The tournament was played in front of full crowds. France took the championship and grand slam for the first time in 12 years. This was despite their coach, Fabien Galthié, contracting the virus before their opening game against Italy and having to communicate by phone with his coaching staff.

Rolling with the punches

The 2021/22 season had not turned out as planned. Clubs and national unions haemorrhaged money. Some sides had players and staff spread out thousands of miles apart. The integrity of competition was imperilled, and teams could not be sure only hours before kick-off that games would be played. It was not meant to be this way approaching two years since the pandemic reached these shores.

Chapter 29

Living with Omicron

To Plan B or not to Plan B? That was the question

England had been living under 'Plan A' throughout autumn 2021. However, poised like the 'sword of Damocles', 'Plan B' had been announced in mid-September – just 'in case'.

Vaccination was the first line of defence supported by free LFTs, Test and Trace facilities, and a legal obligation to isolate if infected or an unvaccinated contact. Hopefully that would suffice through the winter. If the Plan B button was pushed, measures like compulsory vaccination, face masks and 'work from home' advice could be back on the menu. In such a scenario, sport would be affected.

Problems created by positive cases during the autumn rugby internationals have already been described. In football, new Newcastle United boss Eddie Howe caught the virus and missed his first match in charge.

On 1 November, the last seven countries on the UK's red list were removed. Incoming passengers need not quarantine. One week later, 'ordinary' Brits were welcomed back to the USA after 20 months. However, foreigners remained wary of travelling into the UK. In early November, Liverpool played Atlético Madrid in the Champions League – a repeat of the much-criticised pre-lockdown fixture. Only 200 Spaniards came to Anfield compared to 3,000 in 2020.

A third booster jab was made available to all from December. Fortunately, it came just in time. By spring 2022, the vulnerable would be offered a fourth shot.

The Omicron variant was identified first in South Africa on 9 November. It would reach these shores 18 days later. Its easier transmissibility was not matched by the same lethality as its predecessors. Improved immunity levels gained naturally, or by vaccination, proved vital in protecting against the worst ravages of this new invader.

Despite some reluctance from younger age groups, UK vaccine hesitancy had been amongst the world's lowest. Vaccinations saved an estimated 20 million lives globally by summer 2022, including half a million people in the UK.

The prime minister warned of 'storm clouds that are gathering over parts of the continent' in mid-November. Tighter controls and even lockdown reintroductions were occurring in Europe. Holland placed all sport behind closed doors, including their World Cup qualifier against Norway. Austria's unvaccinated were told to stay indoors.

Wary of criticism of its own tardy response in 2021 to the Delta variant, originating from India, the government reimposed a red list for Omicron-affected southern African countries – only 25 days after changing its traffic light to green. With only a quarter of South Africans fully vaccinated, UK-bound flights were suspended. The effect on rugby teams marooned in Cape Town has already been described. Other arrivals would have to isolate until receiving a negative PCR result. The public went back to face masks in indoor spaces and had to isolate for ten days following contact with an Omicron case.

England would welcome in New Year 2022 under the watchful eye of Plan B – announced by Boris Johnson on 8 December. Pre-Christmas, 'work from home if you can' would be the mantra.

Plan B had implications for sport in terms of the NHS COVID pass requirement. Any English sports events with crowds greater than 10,000 would have to comply. Additionally, a pass would be needed for any unseated indoor venue over 500 people and any unseated outdoor venue with over 4,000 people attending.

In truth, England was following what had been the norm in the rest of the UK. Indeed, other home nations were more draconian.

At that time of the year, it would be professional football and rugby union most affected. It was the last thing sporting organisations needed as they looked to replenish coffers from turnstile activity over the festive period. The logistics of checking passes looked horrendous.

Which side of Offa's Dyke do you stand?

One feature of the pandemic had been the different stances invoked by each of the four home countries. In general, England had been slightly laxer and earlier to raise restrictions than Wales, Scotland and Northern Ireland. Scotland had limited outdoor sporting events to 500 spectators and indoor to 200 before Christmas 2021 – having opened their doors to all in August.

Welsh difficulties were highlighted by Chester Football Club playing in football's sixth tier. The Deva Stadium straddled the Anglo–Welsh border. The pitch was in Wales but the ground entrance was in England. Over Christmas, regulations relating to crowd attendances at sporting events differed in the two countries. The club had played two festive games with over 2,000 spectators present and were duly investigated by North Wales police. It would be February before they were allowed to play at home again.

Learning to live with it?

By early summer 2022, the UK was being told to learn to live with COVID-19. The government appeared set on removing all restrictions and getting the nation's economy going – or at least trying to stave off a recession.

On 14 March, the government announced that all COVID-19 requirements would cease that week. No more testing of the unvaccinated or passenger locator forms for people entering the country. SAGE members were stood down after two years of advising the government. As their relegation coincided with a weekly 50 per cent rise in cases, they did not all 'go quietly'.

The announcement coincided with 'Cheltenham week'. Crowds returned for the first time since March 2020 – an event seen as one of the 'powder kegs' at the start of the pandemic. The sea of humanity that arrived was described by Rick Broadbent in *The Times* as 'the gates opened, and a mothballed *Peaky Blinders* convention gushed in'.

Indicating that the population should confine the pandemic to the recesses of our minds (in the section marked 'my worst nightmares'), the plug was pulled on free LFTs for all but the vulnerable on 1 April. People with COVID-19 symptoms were simply advised to stay at home until they felt better. Following government advice, regular twice-weekly LFTs in many elite sports was phased out. Bill wrote to all Northants cricketers advising them accordingly during pre-season training. Only symptomatic athletes needed testing. Downing Street's plan was to change the mindset from one of a pandemic to an endemic virus that we had to learn to live with.

COVID-19 case numbers, freshened up by Omicron, peaked just after Christmas and, again, in higher numbers at Easter. Before Lent was out, cases in Scotland reached record levels with an estimated 1:11 infected. It was the highest anywhere in the UK since the beginning of the crisis. After that, numbers appeared to decline rapidly until the end of May. Abandoning free LFTs, weariness of becoming 'a slave' to the illness and outrage at the 'party' antics within Downing Street combined to make people less likely to test when symptomatic. Statistics were derived from weekly random testing of thousands of people by the Office for

National Statistics (ONS) rather than daily case numbers. COVID-19 death rates were less than a quarter of the early 2021 Delta-driven hump.

England's deputy CMO, Jonathan Van-Tam, had become popular during Downing Street COVID-19 briefings. He was fond of using football analogies to help messaging. Favourites included comparing the first few months of the pandemic as 'in the first half, the away team gave us an absolute battering' and likening the 2020 vaccine trials as 'to scoring in a penalty shoot-out'. He missed his knighthood investiture at Windsor Castle in mid-May after catching COVID-19 himself. More importantly, he missed two of his beloved Boston United's football matches, which he described as 'dreadful'.

In early June, the ONS reported that COVID-19 might be making a comeback with new Omicron subvariants. The population celebrated the Queen's Platinum Jubilee with thousands of street parties. The next week cases rose by 43 per cent with 1:45 of the populace infected. Certain restrictions remained into the summer. Compulsory face masks on aeroplanes remained on some European flights until May and in clinical settings until June.

However, the February Russian invasion of Ukraine, the induced cost-of-living crisis, and the Sue Gray inquiry into Downing Street 'Party Gate' allegations began to drive COVID-19 from the front pages.

Ice-olation

The Beijing Winter Olympics ran for 16 days in February 2022. Security was suffocating. Arriving unvaccinated athletes would need to isolate for 21 days. America insisted that all their team was vaccinated. Despite daily testing and compulsory use of the My2022 app to maintain health records, athletes were required to remain within the 'closed-loop management system'. For the second successive Olympics, the paying public would be excluded.

Cases still occurred. Like the Tokyo Olympics, some potential medallists didn't make it to China, after positive tests. Others were left weakened and underperformed after recovering from the virus. Anxious athletes felt that they were playing COVID 'Russian roulette' while travelling to China on scheduled flights.

Issues over host facilities, catering and the accuracy of testing pervaded the competition. The Australian curlers were packing for a flight home after conflicting multiple tests before being reprieved 15 minutes before a match. A Finnish ice hockey player isolated for 18 days – despite his team doctor claiming that he was no longer infectious. A Polish short-track speed skater tested positive and was later released but tested positive again, until finally a negative test allowed her to compete. The Canadian and Russian women's hockey teams took to the ice wearing masks until negative test results were released during their game. After 45 PCR tests in three weeks, a missed event and lost luggage, American speed skater Casey Dawson finally realised his Olympic dream – on borrowed skates.

It was not the joyous celebration of global youth planned.

Gaming and games, protocols and postponements

The 2021/22 football season would be even more disrupted than the year before. Perhaps it was inevitable. Encouraged by government, society was trying to return to normal and the highly contagious Omicron variant was at large. Hugging would be allowed again. It came as a surprise to most. Players appeared to have been cuddling throughout most of the previous season in defiance of protocols.

From pre-season games onwards, cases mounted. The opening Premier League fixture of August saw Arsenal thumped 0-4 at newly promoted Brentford. The Gunners had four out with COVID-19 despite Mikel Arteta's pleas for them to be jabbed. As previously described, players' vaccination status became one of the talking points of autumn.

The day after Plan B was announced, football acted. The Premier League reverted to emergency COVID-19 measures – masks, social distancing, minimal physiotherapy treatments and medical staff in full PPE. The EFL moved from 'green' to 'red' protocols. It was probably all too late. By mid-December, the frequency of player testing was increased.

Team doctors were expecting the season to be halted. Several managers supported them. Brentford's Thomas Frank and Brighton's Graham Potter wanted a temporary suspension. Norwich's Dean Smith said that carrying on was 'bordering on negligent'. Henry Winter in *The Times* said, 'Fans are suffering – players need to get vaccinated or stay away.'

Clubs expressed concerns for player welfare resulting directly from viral complications, fixture congestion and restricted training opportunities. They had a point. Injuries for the first half of the season were up ten per cent on historical figures. Leicester's manager Brendan Rodgers believed players' careers were being jeopardised by a combination of fatigue and infection. Matters had been aggravated when the Premier League reverted to three substitutes for the 2021/22 season despite FIFA allowing five. 'Smaller clubs' felt that larger matchday squads favoured richer clubs.

Just before Christmas, the authorities decided to continue the season. Games would proceed if clubs had 14 fit players, including a goalkeeper. AFC Wimbledon wanted clubs calling off games to be held to account. The Dons had few cases and claimed that this was due to good practices and investing in resources compared to other, better-financed clubs.

Premier League positive tests topped out at Christmas with a record 103 weekly cases. January would see an improvement, but lopsided league tables appeared. Chelsea had played six games more than Burnley by the end of the month. The Clarets only managed eight games in 14 weeks. Liverpool postponed their early January Carabao Cup semi-final against Arsenal. Wanting quick test results, Liverpool used a local firm (four-hour turnaround) rather than the normal Milton Keynes company (up to 24 hours). It resulted in 13 false positives and a game being deferred.

Across December 2021 and January 2022, 22 Premier League games were called off due to a combination of COVID-19, injuries and international duties.

Europe was not seeing the same problems. Germany's Bundesliga 1 and Spain's La Liga lost no games. The French Ligue 1 postponed three games and Italy's Serie A only five games after 22 rounds of action.

In Spain, 200 players in their top two divisions contracted the virus. Games carried on so long as a club had five fit senior outfielders and a goalie. At the end of November, Belenenses, in Portugal's Primeira Liga, played the mighty Benfica with only nine fit players after COVID-19 swept their camp. A goalkeeper played in midfield. The game was abandoned when Belenenses were reduced to six fit players and 0-7 down.

English football's postponement directive was not working. Arsenal cancelled their game at Spurs in mid-January after one positive test. They did have injuries and players away on Africa Cup of Nations duty, however, Granit Xhaka was suspended, and they had allowed two players to go out on loan knowing that they would be short-staffed. They were still smarting from not having their Brentford fixture postponed five months earlier.

There was a feeling that some clubs were continuing to game the system. Comparisons were drawn with teams happy to play their youngsters in cup competitions and 'dead' European games but not in the league. By the end of January, rules were changed again with no postponements allowed until at least four players had COVID-19. However, the crisis was abating. By the end of February, the Premier League lifted all emergency COVID-19 measures in line with the government's 'Living with COVID' mantra.

Football's English Premier League finished on 22 May. Six days later, in Paris, Liverpool lost to Real Madrid 0-1 in a Champions League Final marred by security issues outside of the ground. Liverpool fans were robbed, tear-gassed, pepper-sprayed and many denied entry to the ground. The end of the domestic season had witnessed worrying scenes of pitch invasions at many grounds.

After little rest, the clubs were back in pre-season for 2022/23. Traditionally, many teams venture abroad. However, some players did not have to locate their passports. America was still not welcoming unvaccinated travellers. Chelsea and Manchester City were among clubs forced to leave stars at home. Their managers were variably described as being disappointed and frustrated.

Summertime blues

On 27 June 2022, another staple of the English summer, Wimbledon tennis, arrived. The crowds were not entirely enthusiastic. Despite diehard fans being allowed to queue again overnight for the first time since 2019, spectators for the first three days were down 11 per cent compared to pre-pandemic. The players were not required to regularly test. After four days, three men from the singles draw contracted the illness and withdrew – including the 2017 and 2021 runners-up.

COVID-19 remained an issue abroad too. Cycling's Tour de Suisse endured 29 riders pulling out before the start of stage six, including the race leader. Four teams pulled out completely, leaving the organisers crossing their fingers as the race limped across the line 48 hours later. It was won by Welshman Geraint Thomas. July's Tour de France saw 176 riders embark on the Grand Départ. Seventeen were forced out after contracting the virus during the three weeks.

Sweaty scrums and southern series

Incredibly, rugby union's English Premiership regular season continued until 4 June with two weekends of play-offs to follow. It produced a 40-week campaign. Additional games were introduced to accommodate an extra 13th team caused by a moratorium (for a second season) on relegation. Outside of the two 'COVID seasons', fixtures had only ever been allowed to spill over into early June on two previous occasions.

Summer 2022 saw southern hemisphere tours of European rugby union teams re-established: England to Australia; France to Japan; Wales to South Africa; Scotland to Argentina; and Ireland to New Zealand. For the Argentina Pumas, it would be the first games in front of their fans since 2019. The All Blacks hosted a northern hemisphere team at home for the first time since June 2018 and Japan since their own World Cup in autumn 2019. France played in Australia only after undergoing strict entry quarantine.

After the 2021 British Lions tour was played in front of empty stadia, South African authorities only relaxed restrictions on crowd numbers in June 2022. Wales' game, in Pretoria, in front of 52,000 fans, was the first time the world champions had played to a home capacity crowd since being crowned in November 2019.

No sooner had England landed in Australia than winger Jonny May contracted the virus. He missed selection for the first two internationals and had to hotel-isolate for seven days.

In New Zealand, the All Blacks head coach, Ian Foster, along with his two assistants and three players tested positive before the first Test. They were joined by two infected Irishmen. Cue panic. Joe Schmidt had to be rushed into the All Blacks setup a month ahead of his official start as coach to take over duties.

The COVID-friendly Games

The Birmingham-hosted 2022 Commonwealth Games was awarded in 2017 and scheduled to run for 11 days from 27

July. It hoped to be one of the summer's central sporting events. COVID-19 changed that.

Birmingham would not have the summer to itself.

Events resembled 'a line of dominoes'. Euro 2020's delay meant its women's equivalent was also displaced 12 months to overlap with the Commonwealth Games. Similarly, the 2021 World Athletics Championship, in Eugene, Oregon was pushed back a year by the rescheduled Olympics and finished only days before the Games. The 2021 World Aquatics Championships were moved back one year in Japan to accommodate the Olympics. However, continuing Japanese Omicron cases caused the 'meet' to move to Budapest. It would now be held in late June rather than May. The European Athletics Championships would start one week after the Games. Tournaments competed for media attention and athlete participation. Brum pushed its own start date back a day to reduce clashes.

The pandemic put paid to the original Games Village. The intended Perry Barr development was abandoned due to delays from the 2020 lockdown. Instead, student residences and a hotel sufficed.

The previous October, India declared its hockey teams would not be competing due to 'biased' COVID-19 restrictions. Ten days' quarantine on arrival was required for subcontinent arrivals. Indian vaccines were not recognised by the British government. It seemed a precipitous decision. No one knew what the situation would be like nine months later. India reversed its decision in December and won medals in both men's and women's competitions.

The organisers wanted a COVID-friendly Games with cases treated on an individual basis. Overall, three per cent of athletes and officials tested positive on arrival at the Games compared to four per cent of the UK population at the time. Australia thought the protocols lax and planned to impose stricter monitoring of their squad. Despite this, an Aussie women's cricketer tested positive on the morning of the gold medal match. She played and won a gold medal. Attitudes were changing towards the disease. However, if the player had been home in Oz, she would have had to isolate for one week.

Lionesses roar

The standout summer sporting extravaganza was the Women's Euro 2022. Delayed a year, it was played out across August to large, enthusiastic and well-behaved crowds across the country. The England Lionesses overcame all opponents, and COVID-19 to players and manager Sarina Wiegman, to beat Germany after extra time in the Wembley final.

After over two long years, it appeared that sport was beginning to come home.

Misshapen and spit-free balls

Some COVID-19 regulations were jettisoned for the 2022 domestic cricket season. Umpires could hold bowlers' caps, sunglasses and sweaters again. Crowd numbers were uncapped from the season's start. However, some 'temporary' regulations remained. Banning saliva use to maintain a ball's shine was made a permanent law. COVID substitutes during play continued for early red-ball games but not for white-ball competitions. The first COVID substitute had been used in October 2020 in New Zealand and in England in May 2021.

Players underwent a proper pre-season conditioning programme for the first time since 2019. Overseas warm-weather spring tours were re-established. The COVID-contrived Bob Willis Trophy regionalised group format for red-ball cricket was discarded and the two-division County Championship was reintroduced. Promotion and relegation places from 2019 were dusted down. The red ball, made by Dukes, was soon criticised for poor quality, with balls becoming soft and misshapen. COVID-19 amongst skilled leather tanning workers during manufacturing was one potential cause espoused.

Echoing bad behaviour at end-of-season football matches, T20 cricket supporters were criticised for drunken and boorish behaviour. Two years of sparse pickings for devotees of live sport continued to cause some to forget how to behave.

The summer's opening Test series was against world champions New Zealand. The second Test was bookended by Kiwi skipper Kane Williamson contracting COVID-19 on the eve of the game and two Kiwi players and two backroom staff testing positive within 48 hours of the game finishing. While preparing for the third and final Test, England's batting coach Marcus Trescothick went down with the virus. During the game, England's wicketkeeper Ben Foakes tested positive and England whistled up a COVID substitute in Sam Billings. He was allowed to bat and field behind the stumps for the game's last two days. Poor Foakes failed to shake off the virus and missed the delayed 2021 fifth Test against India at Edgbaston the next week.

T20 trouble spilt over into Test matches. Brawling broke out amongst the Barmy Army during the third New Zealand Test at Headingley.

Eventually, on 1 July, the final India–England Test match scheduled for September 2021 started. A review of the two sides selected reveals how quickly international sport moves on. Only half of the original 2021 selections were left standing. Both countries had new skippers – Ben Stokes for Joe Root and Rohit Sharma for Virat Kohli. However, Sharma succumbed to the virus and joined England's Foakes in isolation before the game. India's wicketkeeper Rishabh Pant made an explosive 89-ball century in an eventful Indian first innings leading to the predictable media headlines 'Pant's on fire'. The game finished in carnival atmosphere as England cantered to a seven-wicket victory chasing a record total of 378 runs.

By the Australian summer of 2022/23, regulations meant that cricketers playing with the virus became more common – so long as they felt well and had separate dressing rooms.

Australia's T20 Big Bash League, Test matches and the T20 World Cup all featured actively infected players.

A pyrrhic victory?

By the end of 2022, COVID-19 and sport resembled two heavyweight boxers slugging each other to a standstill over 12 rounds. Mutation and immunisation had taken its toll in the red corner. Weariness and financial uncertainty had diminished the blue corner.

It was time for life and sport to try and recover. The year 2023 would see better days but the coronavirus tail occasionally wagged to remind us of its presence. Cycling's Giro d'Italia in May saw 13 riders, including first-placed Remco Evenepoel, forced out with the virus. Post-stage media interviews were conducted with masked cyclists.

The virus had indeed become endemic. It retained the capacity to randomly disrupt competition and the economic health of teams and organisations.

Chapter 30

COVID Conversations

THE TASK of getting sport up and running required the work and dedication of tens of thousands of people – politicians, clinicians, financial experts, administrators, coaches and athletes. Most made their contribution unseen by the sports people they facilitated.

The following are recollections of nine people from different sports and walks of life.

Brendan Rodgers. Leicester City manager (2019–23). FA Cup winner 2020/21

'I learned a lot about myself and my team during COVID-19 – particularly when I caught it early on. The virus took more out of me than when I climbed Kilimanjaro.

'Right from the start, with all our players, I decided upon an open-door policy. Communication was key. Many had concerns about whether they would be safe. Twice-weekly testing was vital. We followed all the measures put in place by the police and, of course, the Premier League.

'It was up to players to choose whether they felt right about returning. There was no pressure on players or their families if they had fears. In the end, it was important for us all to get back into a routine.

'Later in the pandemic, with an FA cup semi-final at Wembley looming against Southampton, I had to revert to

343

stricter discipline. I don't want to say too much since it was a private meeting between staff and the players. However, James Maddison, Ayoze Perez and Hamza Choudhury were all dropped for one Premier League match for breaching COVID-19 rules after a party. They apologised to their team-mates, which was accepted. We quickly moved on.

'Winning the final against Chelsea was a great moment. We deserved it. As I said at the time, Youri's [Tielemans] winning goal was old-school – but don't forget Kasper Schmeichel's save.'

Professor Kiran Patel. Sports cardiologist and the first doctor in the world to prescribe the COVID-19 vaccination, for Margaret Keenan in Coventry

'As the pandemic emerged, took grip, and influenced all of our lives, it did the same to elite athletes. Early on, athletes of a BAME ethnicity were rightly concerned for the risks to themselves and their families by being exposed to COVID-19 in a return to play and this required careful psychological support and communication of emerging evidence when it came to ethnicity. I certainly recall gathering evidence about the drivers of ethnicity-related risk and discussing it directly on Zoom calls with players and staff from sports teams.

'It was a pleasure to be part of the FA governance group supporting a return to play, and developing a consensus of opinion where evidence was absent. When it came to COVID-19 we learned rapidly that athletes, by virtue of being at lower risk of co-morbidity and having better physical health, would be at lower risk themselves. Of course, athletes needed to adhere to social distancing and all the behavioural interventions to mitigate transmission risk.

'From a cardiac perspective, the risk of complications was incredibly low. The dreaded risk of myocarditis was minimal, but we had to manage anxiety related to this. We took few chances. The use of ECG, troponin levels and inflammatory markers to guide a return to play after symptoms or infection quickly enabled a safe protocol to support pre-participation screening after infection. Within a few months of the pandemic starting, in football at least, we had a safe and systematic process to guide return to play.

'On 8 December 2020, I was privileged to prescribe the world's first COVID vaccine outside of a clinical trial. Serendipity had placed me in a position where we knew the vaccination protocols. Athletes had to wait their turn. We vaccinated the most vulnerable first. It was a challenge to ask athletes to wait their turn. However, when it came to their turn to be vaccinated, there were those who relished the opportunity to get vaccinated and got on with it. Others were influenced by social media – particularly the much-hyped-up risk of myocarditis secondary to vaccination. Subsequently, we found this to be an exceptionally rare complication, which UK regulatory agencies are still collecting data on.

'I recall arranging for an entire football squad to attend our vaccination centre one day and even despite attending the centre and having direct discussion with myself, only 50 per cent of the squad got vaccinated that day. The power of social media and myth was incredible to see. We did our best as medics to allow informed consent from our athletes when it came to vaccination, but it was not easy.

'Overall, COVID-19 itself and the vaccines posed little risk to athletes when it came to heart complications. There were a handful of cases where we saw myocardial [heart wall] scarring likely to be secondary to infection, but even these individuals are safely competing with reassurance and surveillance to this day. Being a cardiologist during the pandemic to elite athletes really did bring out all my skills of communication, persuasion and empathy.'

Nikki Woodward. Performance manager at Oxfordshire's Abingdon Gymnastics Club

'During lockdown periods, coaches maintained contact with gymnasts using Zoom. Providing support, advice, and strength and conditioning programmes. As an indoor activity, gymnastics suffered in similar ways to sports like netball. Outdoor classes were scheduled when weather permitted. Gymnasts returned in short bursts between lockdowns, but full uninterrupted training would resume only 14 months later in May 2021. The club noticed a small "drop off" in numbers over the next six months.'

Nikki felt there were two important factors: 'Gymnastics requires regular training sessions. Some youngsters had simply gotten out of their routines, moved on to other activities, or found it difficult to re-commit to the same level of dedication. Additionally, that vital 14 months had seen teenagers naturally grow. In normal times, continuous training allows the gymnast to adapt. Lockdown restrictions had removed that opportunity. Some athletes found that they could not "catch up" and undertake the exercises and routines that had been embedded in pre-pandemic times. Their comfort with various apparatus had been removed.'

Ben Smith. Ex-cricketer and professional coach

'During the pandemic, I was coaching with Cricket Ireland. We were embarking on a one-month tour of the UAE for the ICC T20 Cricket World Cup in late 2021.

'I had flown into Dubai separately and met the rest of the travelling party at Dubai airport, where we jumped on the tour bus to our hotel. All this travel had been under strict COVID-19 guidelines. Masks, sanitising, social-distancing and group herding. It was intended to keep us in the best possible place to avoid contracting the virus.

'Immediately, on arrival at the hotel, we went to our own rooms to carry out a six-day quarantine period. Three meals a day were delivered outside your door. Fortunately, we had rooms with a balcony and one piece of exercise equipment. Mine was a bike.

'We had our first COVID-19 test on the third evening. This test was the big one. If you got through this, you tested once more on day six. If clear, you'd be released for full duties at the World Cup. However, I tested positive. It was the worst possible news.

'UAE rules were a ten-day isolation following the result. I had to get my head around spending a total of 13 days in isolation. My initial feeling was of panic. I don't suffer normally from anxieties. However, I felt my chest tighten. I wondered how the hell I was going to do this. Three days had been long enough. One of my main concerns was that I had seen our team analyst go through this on a previous tour. He was carted away to a high-rise "Covid hotel" in the middle of Dubai. He had a room with no opening windows, 24 floors up, all air con and no fresh air. My worst nightmare. Fortunately, I was allowed to stay in my original room following a request from our science and medicine team (aka mental health department).

'The days ticked by slowly helped by plenty of Facetime, Zoom and remote contact with family and the outside world. The exercise bike became my best friend. No choice of food. The daily same old food options became pretty boring.

'I hadn't expected what was to come after release. Once out of isolation, the effects of being away from the group and "out of the loop" became apparent. I felt off pace with where the squad had got to for their game preparation. My connection with the players was slightly off the mark. Normally this wouldn't worry me, but the first group game was in a couple of days. I didn't have time to drag this back. On top of the mental strain, the isolation had inflicted other problems. I underestimated how drained I would be. How this would affect the physical demands of my job.

'I came away from the tournament with mixed emotions. I had been involved in a very prestigious competition. However, I would have liked to have been more myself. Given everything I had from day one. Something that was taken away from me by COVID -19.'

Professor James Calder. Consultant Orthopaedic Surgeon and government adviser

Calder is one of the country's leading orthopaedic sports surgeons. Having served eight years in the SAS, he was accustomed to situations requiring operational skills and a clear strategy.

'I was approached in early April 2020 by government officials regarding the feasibility of restarting sport amid the pandemic. I was appointed as the independent chairman of the group tasked with appraising the risks involved. Such independence from government and major sporting organisations was pivotal in developing effective and reasoned dialogue and developing trust between all parties.

'Throughout April, I consulted with senior doctors in all our major sports. Collectively, we resisted the Premier League's wishes to negotiate separately with government officials. I believed that allowing all sports to be party to protocol development was vital and beneficial to the common cause. Once the safest, incremental pathway had been established, it was up to individual sports to undertake their own risk assessments. The intrinsic nature of certain sports like the two rugby codes meant that they would have to delay return to training compared to activities such as football.

'I was impressed by the speed in decision-taking by senior government ministers and the support I received from senior PHE doctors. Before sport could return, amendments had to be made to the Coronavirus Restrictions Act, with changes to the law allowing elite athletes to train and then compete.

'Once sport had returned, my colleagues and I from Imperial College and Bristol University set about further risk assessments for virus transmission from sports equipment and being spread by exhaled lung aerosols and droplets. We opened the doors of our clinic's orthopaedic clean-air operating theatres to the London Philharmonic Orchestra and Royal Opera and measured the amounts of particles spread during singing and the playing of wind instruments.

The answer was no more than speaking at the same volume. We set elite rugby players off on static bikes until close to exhaustion to measure aerosol and droplet generation. Aerosol emission rates during vigorous exercise were no greater than conversational speaking. It left me with the impression that indoor gyms could safely reopen with suitable ventilation and social distancing. We also conducted live virus studies on sports equipment in the Category 3 laboratories of Liverpool Hospital for Tropical Medicine using sputum from patients with COVID-19. This showed that the virus died rapidly and rugby, soccer, cricket, tennis and golf balls, and sports shirts, were very unlikely to be a source of transmission of the disease. I am not aware of any cases of COVID-19 transmission proven to have occurred during outdoor sport.

'In February 2022, I disagreed publicly with Novak Djokovic's decision to refuse the COVID-19 vaccination. Personally, I think he was poorly advised and would have been better off having the vaccine because the risks of COVID-19 and the complications that can ensue in elite athletes are greater than the potential risks of having the vaccine.

'My experiences have shaped my views on facing future similar pandemics. The initial response would have to be similar while the nature and virulence of the organism was established. Science will still have to establish effective testing mechanisms and determine how quickly vaccines could be developed. Although the "at risk" groups would need protecting, the balance between house isolation and sensible outdoor exercise for the healthy would need re-evaluating. The negative impacts of restricted physical activity and social seclusion on physical and mental health and socio-economics must be acknowledged in future planning.'

Ray Payne. CEO of Northamptonshire cricket (NCCC) since 2015

'Northants is one of only eight non-international venues in English first-class cricket. It derives a high proportion of its income from ECB funding. In the five years pre-pandemic, the club had eradicated its debt and was financially resilient enough to withstand the 2020 economic crisis.

'The 18 counties have a five-year cycle of guaranteed funding from the central organisation. A new agreement of core funding started in 2020. The Infrastructure Fund guaranteed each club £300k per year to improve facilities and their operations. It would be crucial to retaining financial stability for the counties. Sky TV's agreement to extend their cricket package to 2028 with extended hours of coverage, including the women's game, had been important. Government schemes helped to support staff. NCCC withstood the loss of £1m annual income from non-cricketing activities and had rebuilt these revenue streams to pre-pandemic levels by 2023.

'Since the pandemic, spectators have become used to booking advance tickets online. What was once a thousand "walk-ups" has become a trickle on matchdays. Online streaming of games has become important to maintain contact with fans. The women's 2020 Hundred games were due to be played independently of the men's competition at separate grounds. Playing the men's and women's editions back-to-back in 2021 was easier from a bio-security viewpoint and proved an enormous success – even if some grounds, like Northampton, fell out of the calendar.

'All 18 clubs emerged intact from the pandemic, which is a good advertisement for the stability afforded by the central funding model within the game. Although it does demonstrate cricket's reliance on media deals and sustaining lucrative media contracts for international and domestic cricket.'

Scott Field. Director of communications, British Olympic Association (BOA)

'Within sport's administration, so much happens very slowly. Suddenly, decisions are needed. Matters move very quickly.

This was true of the pandemic. I was sitting in my garden with my children at home wondering whether there would be a Games at all when the IOC and Japan made their announcement.

'A quick decision for a year's postponement but with total confidence of making 2021 happen. The clarity allowed us to prepare properly. But how would we work within that environment and deal with collateral damage? Most Olympians understood their responsibilities. They were used to hygiene routines and mask-wearing. They like certainty and support. Some competitors had spent their whole adult life training for just two, five or ten minutes of action at a specific Games. Sadly, some retired knowing the delay would be too late for them.

'Having observed the 1,000mph decision-making within elite football, the opportunity to put our "foot on the ball" and work closely with the team allowed for rational assessments – helping swimmers install plunge pools in their back gardens, understanding the psychological impact when six athletes were forced to quarantine after close contact with an infected individual following their flight to Japan.

'Our considered planning paid dividends. The BOA was the only delegation to take full teams to both the Tokyo Summer and Beijing Winter Olympics and have no positive COVID-19 tests during either. The British media travelled with the team and understood their responsibilities. Every Olympic day is day one for someone within that team. Two medals in modern pentathlon on the final day proved how tight and together the team was.'

Ian Thomas. Director of members' services, Professional Cricketers' Association (PCA)

'The PCA support present and ex-professional cricketers. In the first month of the pandemic there was "radio silence" from our members. Like sport in general, our members were initially stunned.

'Afterwards, the PCA were active advising players about restrictions in place. They were desperate to stay fit and practise at local grounds. By the end of 2020, the PCA were very busy. There were more cries for help for mental health support from retired than present-day cricketers. Mostly anxiety and depression.

'During 2021, psychological support requests increased again. Of active players, one quarter was female as more professional contracts were issued in this sector of the game. By 2022 and 2023, the PCA were funding small but increased places in residential programmes for alcoholism. Other sports, like football, were experiencing similar trends and COVID-19 was often cited as an initiator.'

Kieran Maguire. Academic, author and broadcaster, specialising in football finances

'The pandemic exposed both the noble and dark facets of the football industry. Initial concerns about the survival of many clubs proved unfounded. Smaller clubs utilised the furlough scheme, received grants from the Premier League, benefited from large TV audiences (and broadcast revenues) despite empty stadiums, and witnessed fans graciously forgoing season ticket refunds. Consequently, only Macclesfield Town succumbed, primarily due to owner-related issues rather than the pandemic's direct impact.

'Numerous heartwarming instances emerged as clubs and their personnel engaged in acts that filled fans with pride. Players and managers reached out to isolated fans by phoning them at home, facilities were repurposed for community initiatives, and NHS staff received support through free accommodation and other initiatives, fostering a sense of unity often absent in the cut-throat quest for on-field success.

Surprisingly, transfer fees continued to flow, with Premier League clubs shelling out £1.7 billion in 2020/21, even amidst empty stadia, and even League Two clubs managed to spend £820,000. Premier League wages, defying expectations, rose by six per cent, despite fewer matchday staff due to empty stadiums and the unusual demands of then Health Secretary Matt Hancock to reduce them. Clubs contended that technical factors justified the wage increase.'

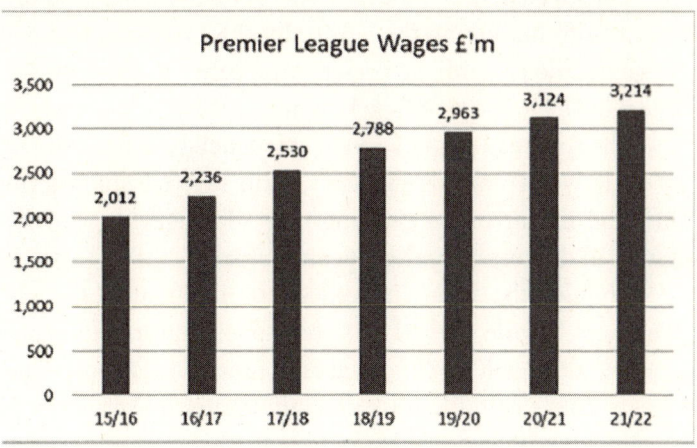

'However, the pandemic-induced decrease in revenue, stemming from the loss of matchday sales and broadcaster rebates, coupled with increased expenses related to players and COVID-related travel, accommodation and testing, resulted in significant financial losses for football clubs.

'Over the 2019/20 and 2020/21 Premier League seasons, operating losses totalled £2.3 billion, while the EFL Championship incurred £1.1 billion in losses. Owner support, borrowing and player sales were the primary avenues through which these losses were absorbed.

'The downside of the COVID-19 crisis also unveiled opportunistic endeavours in the form of Project Big Picture and the European Super League. The former aimed to consolidate power, decision-making and money within the hands of a self-appointed elite in the form of the "Big Six" clubs.

'Meanwhile, the latter venture saw the "Big Six" and their European allies attempt to concentrate power, decision-making and money. It's always money, isn't it? There were a dozen clubs, all averse to the idea of earning their European competition places through the merit of winning football matches in their domestic leagues.

'Those owners behind the two schemes were notably absent from marketing the new order that they sought from the game, too cowardly to present themselves to the fans and others in the game that they hold in contempt.

'The financial desperation of smaller clubs was exploited by their wealthier counterparts, who offered short-term financial incentives in exchange for a long-term, two-tier system in domestic and European football.

'Thankfully, fans, spurred on by influential figures like Gary Neville, united in fierce opposition to the Super League, ultimately forcing its abandonment ... for now. The owners cried crocodile tears and said they had learned their lessons, but will no doubt regroup for further attempts to take control of what was once the People's Game.'

Chapter 31

Damaging the Crown Jewels

Letting the 'air out of the tyres'

To the public, it is called 'being out of shape'. For athletes, it is an 'exercise deficit disorder'.

Worries expressed by managers and coaches over the brevity of preparation time in mid-2020 have been recounted earlier. There is a sweet spot for athletes. Being either undercooked in terms of groundwork or burnt to a crisp in the furnace of rapid overtraining are both recipes for injury. Each end of the spectrum would appear.

Detraining causes losses in bodily adaptations acquired by exercise. The wheels come off highly tuned athletic chassis quickly. By 12 days, an athlete's VO_2 max (a good fitness indicator) falls significantly. Less blood is pumped out of the heart each beat; by six to 12 weeks, muscles' ability to use oxygen changes. They risk swimming in lactic acid. There is even a tweak in athletes' muscle fibre types from low to high fatigability forms. Their VO_2 max falls further, increasing injury risk – probably influenced by quicker exhaustion.

Serious athletes have carefully designed schedules. COVID-19 ran a 'horse and cart' through this. The sporting calendar is so tightly packed that even short, unscheduled stoppages could cause competition chaos. Additionally, what would be the longer-term effects on bodies and minds of squeezing even more into an already overflowing sporting diary for the years ahead?

Keeping athletic engines turning over to maintain some semblance of fitness was going to cause headaches. Medicine and science have come to appreciate how these physiological wonders of the modern world respond best. Training periodisation is designed to progress fitness, strength and skill acquisition ahead of engaging in combat. It reduces the risk of these sporting icons (and even 'weekend warriors') spluttering to a halt halfway down the new season's runway. What happens when the emergency brakes have been applied and, subsequently, the programme 'jump started' again without adequate warning to all those bodies 'on board'? Exercising at home individually was never going to replicate the intensity and variety of work available at the training ground with team-mates.

Sport had some experience of the likely consequences on participant health. Sports scientists refer to alterations in the ratio of acute/chronic workload ratios (ACWR) when training frequency and intensity is ramped up. Research had demonstrated a 5-7x injury rate increase in Premier League footballers when ACWRs rapidly climb.

In the 2011 American NFL industrial dispute, 'locked out' players were denied access to doctors, physiotherapists, trainers and coaches. When the dust settled, players were 'granted' a 17-day training period before the first pre-season game instead of their normal 14-week programme of progressive conditioning. A four-fold increase in Achilles tendon ruptures occurred in the shortened pre-season. Historically, it's an injury from which one third of players never sufficiently recover to play professionally again.

Project Restart. 'You can pull your hamstring now?'

Sporting organisations were worried about finances. Government needed a sop to the increasingly impatient 'masses'. Televised sport could ease these worries. Set against these, what are a couple of torn hamstrings amongst team-mates?

Footballers sustain an average of two injuries in a normal season. English Premier League clubs paid out £177m in wages to injured players in 2016/17. Long pre-seasons and avoiding fixture congestion had been demonstrated to reduce injury risk. Playing twice per week multiplies the damage.

British sports tried to help. Football introduced five substitutes instead of three and introduced 'mid-half' drinks breaks. Rugby union confined players to no more than three hours' game time weekly. County cricket cancelled one competition, reduced the number of games, daily overs bowled overall and per player, and the length of innings. Rugby league jettisoned scrums.

Football's German Bundesliga was first up and running. The high early injury rate was described earlier. Was it maintained? Matches restarted 64 days after lockdown. Injury rates tripled – with particularly high rates in pre-season and the first game. In Italy, Serie A restart games were played over six weeks at double the normal frequency and paid the price. Matchday injuries were significantly higher post-lockdown. Injury rates during post-lockdown training tripled compared to 2019.

Comparatively, Norwegian and Japanese elite football start their seasons in spring. Both delayed the start. Each play fewer games with lower intensively than the Premier League and showed no difference in injury levels compared to 2019. Japan suspended relegation to reduce strain on players at the season's end. However, Japan still had a notable increase in muscle injuries in the two months after restart.

In American sports, baseball injury rates doubled during the delayed 2020 season compared to the two seasons before. This was despite the season being shortened from 162 to 60 games. Pitchers were almost three times more likely to require surgery to ruptured elbow ligaments. Pre-season had been shortened. It increased the ACWR and reduced sport-specific training. The increased numbers of double-header games contributed further.

However, it was not all doom and gloom. Step forward American basketball and English domestic cricket and rugby union as role models?

The NBA completed their season in the bio-secure bubble in an Orlando theme park. The eventual finalists spent three months incarcerated in this Florida playground. Inside Disney World, injury rates decreased, despite the increased density of games. Forced isolation bucked basketball's increasing injury trend over previous years. Historically, injuries were more common 'on the road'. Now all teams were 'at home'. Lack of sleep and recovery time and jet lag caused by long-distance travel across American time zones had been shown to dull players' reaction times. One welcome from Mickey Mouse and friends and all these factors were eliminated. Security effectiveness resulted in no players contracting COVID-19.

English domestic cricket started nearly four months late. In the County Championship and T20 Blast, only 37 per cent of the normal cricket days were played. Travel was reduced. Players came back into training for one month before. The 2020 cricket injury profile resembled previous years. Like other sports, the proportion of soft-tissue thigh injuries increased but was balanced by reduced hand and spine problems. No lumbar spine stress fractures were recorded in 2020 despite jettisoning an advised normal pre-season preparation time for fast bowlers of eight to 12 weeks. The control of workload had clearly been effective.

The concerns that English Premiership Rugby faced concerning specific infection risk and match congestion has already been described. For 12 weeks, players had no access to training facilities, coaching or routine medical help. This was followed by four weeks of non-contact and, subsequently, six weeks of contact training. Protecting playing time seemed to work. Injury rates in the post-suspension period were significantly lower than equivalent periods in the preceding three seasons and the 2019/20 pre-stoppage section.

Feeling the strain after COVID-19 infections

Any athlete catching COVID-19 was subjected to the prescribed isolation period and detraining effect. Combined with potential effects upon heart and lung function, such episodes clearly impacted upon fitness, increasing injury risk, fatiguability and sport-specific skills. Added to that were overarching psychological worries for many. Research indicated that the virus affected oxygen transport within muscles. Excessive lactate increases muscle fragility. Enhanced fatigue affects muscle power.

It is why return to full training post-infection needed careful monitoring.

Belgian professional footballers had a five-fold increase in muscle strains in the first month after COVID-19. Injured players had spent three days longer quarantining on average compared to infected players without damage. In Italy's Serie A, players with symptomatic COVID-19 had a 69 per cent increase and in Spanish football a double increased risk of muscle injury post-virus.

An American study including 72,000 high-school athletes found a nine times increased risk of concussion in those involved in collision, field or court-based sports within two months of COVID-19. Other simultaneously reported illnesses did not increase concussion rates. The authors speculated that as well as fatigue and deconditioning, the virus might cause nerve inflammation and affect mental processing and balance.

Getting COVID-19, even as a young fit athlete, was not a totally benign event.

Did the pandemic create hangovers?

What would be the effect of a shortened 2020/21 pre-season preparation, the impact of further societal lockdowns and fixture and player disruption as new COVID strains infected sport? Coping with rearranged events like Euro 2020 and the Tokyo Olympics and Paralympics?

The Premier League scrapped its 2021 planned winter break just when it needed it most. It was first introduced in 2020 after 25 years of debate. European clubs in leagues without such a 'holiday' historically lost players for an average of 303 days more per season. English football voted against continuing with five substitutes for 2021/22, choosing to revert to three.

In France, the 2019/20 season had been abandoned under government pressure. Players had rested; 2020/21 injuries, including muscle damage, were all reduced compared to 2018/19. The company Howden produced a report on the economic costs of injuries in the five main European football leagues for 2020/2021 – England, Italy, Germany, France and Spain. Despite France's frugality, there was an overall 14 per cent rise in injuries compared to 2019/20. The Bundesliga and Premier League led the way with crocked players.

With a short pre-season and compressed fixture list, it was not surprising that English clubs experienced a 67 per cent rise in recorded injuries. However, injuries appeared less severe judged by recovery times. The average injury cost, in terms of salaries to 'stricken strikers', was £140k per episode.

Surprisingly, the top half of the table experienced 37 per cent more injuries than the bottom half. It challenged the view that richer and more successful clubs benefit from larger squads. Arguably, increased progress in domestic and European competitions added to their burdens. Average times between games was two days shorter than 2018/19. Players were getting injured for the first time earlier in the season. In November alone, 100 Premier League players across the 20 clubs suffered soft-tissue injuries.

The pain did not finish in May 2021. Many top European clubs would lose players to Euro 2020. Increased injuries in the season following a continental or global football competition are well recognised and 2021/22 would be no different. The response of worried managers, like Brendan Rodgers, was outlined elsewhere.

Howden reported that in the first half of 2021/22, injuries had rocketed again. The Premier League had sustained, at the halfway point, 70 per cent of the total injuries of the previous season. In September 2021 alone, clubs paid out double (£20.4m) the amount in wages for unavailable players compared to the same period in the year before. December 2021 was the soft-tissue injury acme. It coincided with high COVID-19 cases and postponed fixtures. The 'five leagues' had 256 COVID-19 absences in December and another 140 in January. Healthy players were feeling the increased strain and deconditioned infected players were returning to busy schedules.

After successfully negotiating the shortened 2020 season, domestic cricket continued to fare well in 2021. Despite pre-season COVID-19 restrictions, injury rates remained at their lowest since 2016. Similarly, time loss from lower back injuries was at its lowest for many years. The figures were probably helped by continuing restrictions on red-ball matches.

The year 2022 saw the reintroduction of two-division red-ball cricket. Helped by a hot and dry summer, 20 per cent more overs were bowled in the country compared to 2021. Unsurprisingly, with the increased workload, injuries and low back problems rose again, approximating pre-COVID-19 levels. By May 2022, expressions of worry surfaced over England's injury crisis.

In less than two years, England had played 72 fixtures. – more than any other team. The side's reward would be a summer of 22 matches in 15 weeks. New Test captain Ben Stokes called the schedule 'ridiculous'. Seven potential fast bowlers were unavailable for the first New Zealand Test. Four had lumbar stress fractures.

In American NFL football, the 2019/20 season was over before lockdown. However, there were disruptions to the 2020/21 pre-season. The normal four pre-season games were cancelled. There was limited access to gyms and normal training equipment. The players would go into the new season seriously 'undercooked'. Compared to 2018/19, researchers found a 52 per cent increase in soft-tissue injuries during the season. The lack of a proper pre-season and the increased ACWR were blamed.

After the successes of the Disney bubble in reducing injuries, the 2020/21 basketball season was back to normal injury rates and more. There was considerable uncertainty for players and coaches as to when the season would start, with several false dawns. It started two months late and finished a month late with ten games shaved from each franchise's schedules. Many games were postponed. It still represented a higher density of games than in recent seasons. Teams had problems at times fielding full squads. The season saw a much higher number of individual injuries and games missed by players compared to the two seasons pre-COVID-19.

The news was no better for American baseball. The 2021 MLB's injury rates remained similar to the shortened 2020 season and 70 per cent higher than 2019. Researchers believed that the cumulative effect of lockdowns had created deconditioned players as the 2021 season started in the spring. Pandemic restrictions had affected players' pre-season build-up, affecting mood and sleep quality and increasing fatigue.

There was one encouraging note. Echoing the positive results from the 2020 NBA restart in an empty Disney World, the delayed Tokyo Olympics and Paralympics produced reassuring news for athletes in 2021. The largely spectator-free and hermetically sealed Olympic Village and venues ensured injury levels were similar to the previous three Olympiads. The Paralympics went further with fewer injuries than the previous two celebrations.

Mental health

Most sporting organisations employ psychologists to facilitate athletes working on the mental side of their performance. However, no counselling could have prepared them to develop resilience to the microbe. The early psychological challenges were outlined before.

Pre-pandemic it was recognised that elite athletes were at heightened risk of mental health disorders. Added to the generic triggers (for example life events) faced by all, athletes face sport-specific factors (for example injury and deteriorating performance). Symptoms may be present in between 15 per cent and 35 per cent of Olympians. Home confinement, fears for health, financial worries, concerns about body changes, athletic identity and an uncertain future fuelled the flames of anxiety and depression in sports people during the pandemic. Studies from around the world in numerous sports reported between doubling to quadrupling of mental health symptoms in elite athletes.

It was a truism that sports that successfully excluded the virus from the team environment through rigorously enforcing Fort Knox-level 'bubbles' risked storing up mental health problems going forward. By the end of 2020, players' tolerance of such isolation was appreciated to be short. By July 2021, England cricketing icon Ben Stokes announced that he was taking indefinite time out from the game 'to prioritise his mental well-being'. His exile lasted three months. That summer, tennis's Naomi Osaka and gymnastics' Simone Biles withdrew from major competitions to safeguard their mental health.

The FIFPRO football world players' union reported after the Qatar 2022 World Cup. Two months later, 43 per cent of involved players reported increased mental or emotional fatigue compared to normal at that stage in their domestic seasons. This was coupled with 44 per cent experiencing physical fatigue and 20 per cent with injuries at the same juncture. English-based players fared the worst; 63 per cent reported reduced mental well-being.

Are we any the wiser?

Sufficient information existed to understand how elite athletes would respond to the chaos and congestion occasioned by the pandemic. The voiced worries of those involved with their welfare and performance was based on sound science. The health crisis has provided the sporting and scientific world with additional information and experience about the limits of the athletic body and mind when faced with sudden and ongoing disruption.

From a participants' viewpoint, the safest way to minimise physical harm has been for sports administrators to 'cut their cloth' according to the calendar. Those sports that have finished on the credit side of this health crisis are those that adopted safety measures to reduce athletes' workloads. This has taken various forms. Abandoned seasons, reduced and spaced fixtures, sufficient preparation time, less travel, capped individual workload and adequate time to recover from COVID-19 infections. American basketball, English international cricket and the Tokyo Olympics have shown that basing athletes at one venue and adopting scrupulous bio-security measures can help minimise infection and injury levels. However, there is a psychological limit to how long athletes will tolerate bubble isolation.

Numerous studies have demonstrated that soft-tissue injuries, such as muscle damage, made up most of the increased workload for sports clinicians. Player availability will affect team performance and, ultimately, affect the integrity of the competition in which they are involved.

It is difficult at times to confidently detach the 'COVID-effect' from other contemporaneous factors risking athlete welfare. Unfortunately, the people charged with determining the fate of sport come predominantly from the business and financial sectors. There is little evidence that they have heeded the welfare messages. Indeed, some sports seem hell bent on increasing workload going forward. FIFPRO estimates that football's plans to expand the European Champions

League and introduce the FIFA World Club Championship could add 11 per cent workload to leading players. There is simply no hiding place for talented athletes – especially the young. David Beckham only played 829 minutes of elite football before he was 20. Jude Bellingham had played 14,445 minutes. Some would counter that, in some sports, players and agents, by demanding ever increasing Monopoly money in wages, have been a major contributor to the rocky business model of sporting organisations. They have crossed their own personal Rubicon and are consequently expected to lay their bodies and minds on the line to save the hand that feeds them.

Premier League football has set itself apart with its huge television contracts, salaries for its stars, and belief in its right to bulldoze aside any outside decision-makers. The sheer physicality of its game increases player risks. However, its determination to finish its 2019/20 season, start the next instalment uncomfortably soon and ditch safety valves – the winter break and extra substitutes – speaks of decision-makers who place athlete–employee welfare low on the priority list.

Was it too much to suggest that organisations like Premier League football might have taken a leaf out of Wimbledon and the Open golf's ledger books? To use part of their extraordinary wealth to insure their sport against such eventualities? It would have removed one of the principal drivers for a rushed return.

What will not be known for many years is the long-term toll that COVID-19 has extracted from our sports people. It seems logical from present knowledge that certain athletes' careers will be shortened by the excessive physical and mental loads imposed upon them during this period.

Doctors and sports scientists will continue to compile the data. It is important that everybody involved in decision-making in sport makes themselves aware of the outcomes.

Chapter 32

The Long-COVID View

WHEN POLITICS and economics decreed that elite sport should return for all the reasons previously discussed, the outstanding issue was safety. How to safeguard athletes and those around them.

Safety first

Early health concerns were outlined in chapter 6. In summer 2020, all that was available were thermometers, symptom self-reporting and common-sense risk management strategies like PPE, ventilation and distancing. Some elite sports had the finances to purchase hugely expensive tests. Others had to take their place in the queues at NHS testing centres. Team doctors, like Bill, had to complete weekly COVID-19 reports and upload them on to centralised sporting databases. Around the world, each sport had to develop protocols for return to training of proven cases. Some countries applied more exhaustive checks than others on infected players.

It was inevitable and wise to take a safety-first approach. An overwhelmed public health system did not need extra cases from the world of sport. Strictly imposed bio-bubbles could eliminate the virus. English-based international cricket had no infections throughout the summer of 2020. Sensible protocols and disciplined personal behaviour could minimise infection – even in elite sports where athletes returned home at night. Domestic English cricket only had three infections and eight players required to isolate as close contacts in the 18 first-class counties during the truncated 2020 season.

By 2021, vaccinations were available and cheaper investigations, such as LFTs, made testing more universal. Virus variants appeared. By 2023, the lethality of the virus appeared to be waning. Risk assessment reviews reflected the changing landscape. How robust was sport and its athletes? When faced with another such threat, what can sport and medicine learn from our handling of COVID-19?

Supermen and superwomen?

The personal response to the health crisis amongst sports people mirrored that of the general population. Many watching the news bulletins and rising death tolls were terrified. Others believed themselves to be 'bullet proof' and possessing superior physiques and physiology. As we know, some didn't think at all.

At the elite level, athletes are a rare breed. Varying combinations of genetics, opportunity, freedom from injury and psychological resilience separate them out as different from mere mortals. Adding in their relative youth, this cohort should be particularly equipped to deal with the vicissitudes of facing down the virus.

Were athletes more, or less, at risk than Joe Public of catching or developing complications from COVID-19? Would minor physical (or psychological) scarring from the illness affect athletic performance that the rest of us would not notice in our more sedentary lifestyles? Answers take time and the accumulation of significant chunks of data.

In 2022, a Brazilian team reviewed global research involving 11,518 infected elite athletes during the early waves of the virus. Were athletes more likely to carry the virus without symptoms? There was no evidence to suggest that these super-engineered bodies could suppress symptoms from the virus. Stratifying elite athletes' symptoms found that 25 per cent were asymptomatic; 68 per cent mild; six per cent moderate; and 1.3 per cent had severe acute responses. Comparatively, one third of the rest of us had no symptoms. However, engagement in regular sport reduced the risk of COVID-19 infection by 11 per cent. The acute symptoms experienced by elite athletes were not dissimilar to the rest of us. Half lost taste and smell. Headaches, fevers, coughs and fatigue featured prominently.

American data suggested athletes were only half as likely to have severe forms of the disease compared to a normal matched young population – 1.3 per cent and 2.7 per cent respectively. Regular exercisers were less likely to require hospital admission. It underscored the beneficial effects of exercise. It laid to rest some initial concerns. Early in the 2020 pandemic, experts suggested athletes might be more at risk of serious pulmonary involvement as strenuous exercise favours deep inhalation of the virus within lung tissue.

There were other factors likely to favour athletes. Obesity was recognised early as a risk factor for severe COVID-19 disease. The beneficial effects of exercise on weight control cannot be overemphasised. Athletes were more likely to have better nutrition and sleep quality. Both have been identified as enhancing our immune response to infections.

Whisper it quietly, but not training at almost maniacal levels imposed by lockdown might have been a good thing. Particularly when the disease was at its most virulent.

Regular exercise is beneficial in fighting disease. Thirty to 60 minutes' daily workouts at 60–80 per cent of maximum capacity three to five times weekly appear ideal. It increases our immune defences. However, heavy exercise periods can suppress the immune system and make athletes more prone to infection, including COVID-19. It takes a temporary hit in the hours after heavy exertion – anywhere between 15 and 70 per cent. Risks increase when there are repeated cycles of heavy exertion, for instance during competition. It has been calculated that two to 18 per cent of elite athletes experience illness episodes during international competition. Females and endurance athletes are particularly prone. Other illness risk factors for athletes include depression or anxiety, highly concentrated training periods with large intensity fluctuations, international travel, winter competition, sleep deprivation and low energy intake.

'The Air That I Breathe'

Song by the Hollies. 1974

A virus that affects primarily the lungs could have profound effects upon any athlete. The initial wave of COVID-19 caused some hospitalised patients to have severe lung involvement with viral pneumonia. Chest X-rays looked awful. This can lead to scarring of delicate lung tissue, compromising its ability to expand and exchange vital gases. Patients who had suffered badly from the virus were often left with breathlessness, abnormal lung function and a reduced capacity to exercise. All outcomes to avoid for an athlete.

Deep inhalations, high asthma rates and depressed immunity during intense exercise were signposted as potential additional risk factors for athletes.

Like many within our populations, most athletes' symptoms involved the upper respiratory tract – 'above the neck'. The presence of lower respiratory symptoms was associated with a week's longer symptoms and ten days' longer return to sport in UK's elite athletes. Chest symptoms tripled the likelihood of being off sport for over a month.

One small study found that COVID-19 affected athletes' cardiorespiratory fitness. Cross-country skiers reached aerobic threshold earlier, which has a detrimental effect upon training intensely without building up muscle lactic acid.

'Don't Go Breaking My Heart'

Song by Elton John and Kiki Dee. 1976

A common feature of many viruses is their ability to cause heart wall inflammation (myopericarditis) and had been implicated previously in the sudden death of young athletes. Exercise during the recovery phase, particularly when acute inflammation exists, is a particular risk factor.

A combination of a new virus causing heart damage in the severely ill, the known risk of myopericarditis causing catastrophic health problems in young athletes, and the nearness of sports people during activity were main considerations in suspending sport and wariness in reopening.

In America, some well-known athletes developed the heart condition in 2020, leading to media headlines and increased concerns. Boston baseball pitching star Eduardo Rodriguez was diagnosed shortly after rejoining the team following COVID-19. He was removed from the sport for the season. Nine days later, it was revealed that the same condition had been found in at least five leading players in college football. Cardiologists commented that the return of the sport in the autumn might be in doubt as a result. Early research using a battery of sophisticated testing suggested that 1:43 student athletes had evidence of heart inflammation. Three-quarters were asymptomatic. To avoid serious medical problems, some of the most influential universities (the 'Big Ten') decreed that all athletes post-COVID-19 (regardless of their level of symptoms) should undergo extensive investigations pre-sports return.

As more global research became available later in the pandemic, advice and management of athletes post-COVID-19 became more balanced. Overall, about one to four per cent of athletes (especially in those subjected to heart MRIs) showed cardiac inflammation. Heart MRI scans are expensive and need to be undertaken as early as possible to diagnose acute myocarditis. It was not clear if the detection of athletes without symptoms and normal other tests were at risk of a cardiac catastrophe. It was the classical problem found in all health screening programmes – cost against societal benefit. Reassuringly, there was no incontrovertible evidence of arrhythmias (irregular heartbeats), cardiac arrests or sudden deaths in athletes.

The expert consensus was that the tool should be reserved for selected individuals with persistent symptoms and other abnormal investigations rather than subject thousands of young athletes post-COVID-19 to expensive cardiac MRIs. The variation in diagnostic tests between sports and countries was very variable. Some simply used LFTs and retested until negative. Others resorted to more sophisticated tests like electrocardiograms and blood tests for detecting signs of heart wall damage, like troponin levels.

The long and winding COVID-19 road

George Garton caught COVID-19 as part of the England one-day cricket squad in June 2021. Many players were infected, but he had yet to make his international debut. After mild post-viral fatigue, he recovered. Roll forward seven months. He contracted COVID-19 again – probably on a plane trip from Australia. Initially, all appeared well. He made his T20 England cricket debut in Barbados in January 2022. A life's ambition achieved. However, on return home, he developed fatigue and breathlessness on exertion. Investigations revealed some myopericarditis. His heart rate was sky-high. He had 'to learn to breathe again'. Six months later, further tests revealed he had developed a lung blood clot. He had contemplated retirement but fortunately recovered and returned to first-class cricket.

The great footballer Lionel Messi became infected in January 2021. He missed two Argentinia games and three club matches. He described how he had difficulty running for six weeks because of lung involvement. He regretted trying to come back too quickly, which prolonged his recovery. In June 2023, as he prepared to leave Paris Saint-Germain and join Inter Miami, he reflected on how COVID-19 and, later, exhaustion after the World Cup had affected his integration with the French club.

In July 2021, Newcastle United goalie Karl Darlow travelled south to watch the Wembley Euro 2020 Final. He returned north with COVID-19, describing 'razor blades in my throat'. He spent three days in hospital. Afterwards, he felt 'awful fatigue' and lost five kilos in weight. He played only eight games in the 2021/22 season. It followed on from team-mates Jamaal Lascelles and Allan Saint-Maximin suffering badly from the virus at the end of 2020. Like Darlow, they experienced severe fatigue, meaning they couldn't train for weeks or play for two months. Club manager Steve Bruce criticised the anti-vaccination campaigners after their experiences.

Shrewsbury Town football manager Steve Cotterill missed the second half of his club's 2020/21 League One campaign. The 56-year-old spent 33 days in hospital, including ICU, after contracting the virus in January 2021. Two weeks later, he was in hospital again with COVID-pneumonia. He spent 69 days out of 80 in bed and admitted that sometimes 'I was frightened to go to sleep because I wasn't sure if I was going to wake up'.

Long COVID, according to the UK's National Institute for Health and Care Excellence (NICE), occurs when symptoms remain four weeks after an acute infection. If problems persist over 12 weeks, a state of post-COVID-19 syndrome is diagnosed. One year after the pandemic started, the English NHS had established 69 multi-disciplinary long COVID clinics. By mid-2022, two million UK residents had developed long COVID with 800,000 symptomatic for over 12 months.

By summer 2022, 15 per cent of American adults experienced long COVID after the initial infection. The numbers were even higher in the UK. Thirty-two per cent of healthcare workers experienced symptoms at three to four months. Oxford university studied over a quarter of a million infected people; 1:3 had symptoms between three and six months. The rates were significantly greater than with influenza. Long COVID rates were higher with worse initial infection in women and in the young. Lower vaccination rates in the young were one possible explanation for higher long COVID rates.

How common was it for athletes to suffer from symptoms suggestive of long COVID? The answer was surprisingly high. While most athletes returned to play within five to ten days after symptoms abated, research suggested that between four and 17 per cent experienced post-acute symptoms. As expected, taste and smell disturbances, cough, fatigue, chest pains and headaches were the most frequent symptoms. In 2021, UK Athletics reported that over a quarter of those infected were not back in full training at one month. The risk of prolonged symptoms in this group was three times longer than other respiratory illnesses.

'Will it hurt, Doctor?'

We know many athletes were reluctant to be vaccinated. The reasons were manifold including a conviction that as young adults their risks of serious complications were unlikely and that vaccinations were not without problems; a preference for the viewpoints of team-mates and social media than for senior medical advice; a concern that the after-effects of a jab might affect training and competition; and the knowledge that being vaccinated does not inure you from being infected.

The difference in vaccination hesitancy between football clubs was striking. It attests to the slightly unreal, cocooned life some athletes inhabit. The global vaccination programme aimed to reduce deaths and the more serious viral complications. Like all immunisation programmes, its intent was to reduce microbe transmission and protect the elderly and vulnerable. To create 'herd immunity' in a population, a huge proportion of its people need to be jabbed. The numbers depend upon microbe infectivity (the R number) and vaccine effectiveness. Ideally, everybody should roll up their sleeves for the 'common good'.

Research suggested that in its first year of use (2021), vaccinations saved the lives of 20 million people worldwide.

UK work indicated that adverse vaccination effects were 'moderate in frequency, mild in severity and short-lived'. Symptoms usually lasted only one to two days. In 2022, a publication appeared on vaccination safety in GB Olympians and Paralympians. Its findings mirrored those of the general population. Athletes were advised to reduce the intensity of training for a few days and expect that physiological measures would return to normal within four days.

The rate of heart muscle inflammation after vaccination was 1:20,000 – multiples less than post-infection itself. Long COVID problems were reduced in people triple-vaccinated in both the UK and USA.

With a quarter of UK athletes off full training for one month following infection, it was a matter of considering relative risk.

Giving the virus a 'sporting chance'?

Was playing team sports a significant risk factor for contracting COVID-19? Was Boris Johnson right to declare in June 2020 that cricket balls were a 'natural vector of disease'? The frenzy of sporting analysis by scientists was touched upon earlier. Footballers spent on average less than 90 seconds 1.5m or closer to another, potentially infected, player during a game.

UK researchers studied virus survival on sports equipment. COVID-19 was coated on to surfaces. Within one minute, less than one per cent of the virus could be detected on average. Absorbent surfaces like tennis and cricket balls were least transferrable. Non-absorbent material like rugby balls and horse saddles fared slightly less well. The conclusions were that 'it seems unlikely that sports equipment is a major cause for transmission'. It was human behaviour that needed to be worked on. It was sensible to stop players spitting and lathering saliva on cricket balls. Low compliance with protocols was reported to be behind the high incidence of COVID-19 in Brazilian footballers after their own Project Restart. At 12 per cent, their rates would not have been out of place in high-risk environments, like healthcare workers.

When BSL rugby league restarted, it was without scrums. An analysis of 36 games revealed eight participants testing positive soon after. PHE guidance was applied. Twenty-eight other players were deemed close contacts during the matches and isolated for two weeks. Subsequently, one tested positive. Five non-close contacts developed the infection during the fortnight. All six positive cases were thought more likely to have contracted the disease from social spread than while playing. Researchers could find no evidence that transmission from the rugby ball or tackling increased the risk of transmitting disease.

These works suggested that playing sport outside was safer than originally believed. Boris didn't get it right.

'When can I go out to play again?'

In 2020, advice to athletes on return to sport had to err on the side of caution, to provide simple and universally applicable parameters. The main fears of too early resumption were creating serious and/or long-term heart and lung complications. Sensible guidelines suggested ten days of abstinence after symptoms began followed by another seven days of graduated exercise – 17 days in total. Some sports added additional tests and required cardiology clearance in symptomatic athletes before giving the green light. It created a frenzy of activity surrounding such sports people's return to play.

Inevitably, as our knowledge grew, advice could become more nuanced and personalised. The worst fears for the widespread development of cardiac complications in athletes were not realised. The nature, site and number of symptoms became important predictors. Features, such as severe initial fatigue, were recognised as indicators of likely prolonged recoveries.

The addition of vaccination protection and waning potency of COVID variants further helped the athlete and sports doctor. There was never a time for relaxing the guard, but medics were entering the 'ring' more knowledgeable about the opponent in the opposite corner.

Are we any the wiser?

So, athletes are not superheroes when it comes to fighting microbes. They get infected like the rest of us – although engagement in sport gives anybody greater protection. Post-infection symptoms affect a not-insignificant minority of sports people, and they were not immune from long COVID. A careful, perhaps overcautious approach was necessary initially. Conventional warfare has historically mandated medicine to learn quickly. This battle was no different. Initial and specific concerns for athletes could be tempered as data was acquired. There is no evidence that vaccinations of athletes (compared to the general population) created extra complications and conferred benefits to themselves and their communities. Finally, sensible outside exercise, including throwing a cricket ball, has far more positives than negatives for our physical and mental well-being.

Chapter 33

W(h)ither Future Generations

HOW DID the general population respond to forced exile from their normal exercise routines? What did home working and study do for our physical and mental health? What did we learn about the nation's health and readiness to withstand the onslaught from this crisis?

After impositions were lifted, our arms repeatedly jabbed and the virus's lethal intent weakened, how did we respond? Were the length and depth of the restrictions enough to break exercise habits and develop new ones? What were the longer-term effects on our youth? Is it true that COVID-19 created a 'lost generation' of athletes?

'And you put the load right on me'
Lyrics from 'The Weight' by The Band. 1968

In early April 2020, the UK's prime minister had a near-death experience.

Boris Johnson developed COVID-19 lung complications and was placed into St Thomas' Hospital ITU. One week later, he was discharged, on the day that UK COVID-19 deaths breached 10,000. Deputy prime minister Dominic Raab described it as a 'sombre day'.

Johnson had a high BMI. It was reported that his personal experiences had made him passionate about tackling the country's obesity crisis. Costs to 'UK Ltd' in dealing with obesity gobbles up three per cent of our GDP and £58 billion annually. The causes are complex and multifactorial, including economic, environmental and social factors. While 40 per cent of Americans are obese, the UK cannot be complacent with a 'figure' of 27 per cent.

Weight was recognised as a major risk factor for developing COVID-19 complications within the pandemic's early months. By August 2020, it was reported that a BMI of over 30 increased hospital admission rates by 113 per cent and deaths by 46 per cent. Lockdowns led to greater overeating and reduced physical activity in the obese. Apart from the risks for a multitude of illnesses, research indicated that vaccine effectiveness could be impaired in people with high BMIs.

Just over two months after Johnson's hospital admission, the government published its 'obesity strategy'. Within six months of its launch, the Social Market Foundation reflected that the report's warnings had been 'largely ineffective'. It believed that government ministers placed too much emphasis on 'individual willpower and not enough on the environmental and economic aspects of obesity'.

By the end of 2020, only 28 per cent of obese individuals were trying to lose weight following the pandemic. Two years after its launch, the King's Fund reviewed the early effects of the strategy. In 2020, obesity rates rose across all sections of UK society. The gap between the most well off and deprived sectors widened. The percentage of obese primary school children in poorer areas was more than double the levels in more affluent neighbourhoods.

The Fund claimed that the government had not delivered on its promised policies and criticised the withdrawal after one year of grants of adult weight-management services, which were claimed to be delivering significant interventions.

For young children, obesity changes from the pandemic were pronounced. Kept out of school for prolonged periods, their routines were changed. They had reduced opportunities for sport and, for many, proper nutrition. Trying to resist rising childhood obesity levels was akin to the little Dutch boy planting his finger in the hole in the healthcare dam created by the virus, trying to hold back the weight of calories behind it. It was no contest. The dam burst across the world.

In 2018–19, ten per cent of UK Reception class children (aged five) and 20 per cent of Year 6 pupils (aged ten) were obese. In 2020–21, these levels rose to 14 per cent and 26 per cent respectively. There was evidence that levels were stabilising by 2022–23, or even beginning to fall, as activity levels and diet began to normalise. Nine per cent of Reception children and 23 per cent of students entering secondary school were officially obese.

Similar findings were reported in the US, where the trend in schoolchildren for increasing BMI doubled during the pandemic. The youngest students and those already at the 'wrong end' of the weight spectrum suffered most.

'She's my little nicotine gal'
Lyrics from 'Hev Yew Gotta Loight, Boy?' by
The Singing Postman. 1965

Sitting at home inactive had other effects upon our health.

We smoked more during lockdown. An estimated extra 625,000 young people took up the habit during lockdown.

With pubs closed, reduced car commuting and various sources of stress, many Brits drank too much at home. The number of people exceeding safe alcohol levels rose by 50 per cent during the first lockdown. Once again, the issues were greatest in poorer communities. Two years later, the Institute of Alcohol Studies conservatively predicted an extra 10,000 deaths from chronic alcohol disease in years to come if people's consumption did not ease.

Mind games

During the pandemic, forced domestic incarceration, financial and career worries, loss of educational opportunities, isolation from friends and families, and health fears for self and loved ones inevitably took their toll. Many were denied a key 'stress de-fuser' that is access to regular sport. It became a recipe for anxiety and depression for many.

The British-based charity Mind studied the pandemic effects on mental health. As in physical illness, the toll was felt greatest in areas of most deprivation. The young suffered significantly. Perhaps predictably, those with pre-existing mental welfare issues were most likely to experience the greatest deterioration. However, a quarter of adults and one sixth of youngsters developed some form of mental distress for the first time during the pandemic. American mental health issues appeared even worse than in the UK. A third of adults were suffering from anxiety or depression by June 2020, three times higher than in 2019. Young adults, especially those in higher education, would have double these rates.

The positive relationship between physical exercise and mental well-being is acknowledged. The benefits apply to all. An American study demonstrated a significant increase in depression in those who stopped exercising during the pandemic compared to those who continued. The authors believe that physical activity disruption was a major contributor to mental health issues.

The effect on elite athletes of lost opportunities for training and competition, economic uncertainty over funding, contracts and long-term income streams, and being deprived of the camaraderie of the 'changing room' have been underlined in other chapters. However, the mental strain was felt right through the 'sporting pyramid'. Physical activity is associated with better academic outcomes and sleep, with reduced substance abuse and risk-taking activities.

American studies revealed that up to 70 per cent of adolescent athletes suffered from anxiety and/or depression during the early pandemic months. Once again, children from low-income families and ethnic minorities were disproportionately affected. Team sport players suffered more than those engaged in individual pursuits.

There is some positive news. Once students had been allowed to return to normal sport in the spring of 2021, large-scale US studies showed that mental health and perceptions of quality of life improved although remained at lower levels compared to pre-pandemic.

As in other aspects of our recovery from COVID-19, the recovery of mental well-being in the youth ranks will remain an issue into the future. Sport England's post-pandemic report of 2022 showed that mental well-being was positively correlated with engagement in sport as society recovered from the restrictions.

'When the feeling's right I'm gonna run all night'
Lyrics from 'Run to You' by Bryan Adams. 1984

So, if sitting on the sofa eating burgers during lockdown was bad for us, what about the opposite? The lifelong health advantages of involvement in regular sport are well documented. Did physical fitness hold any additional rewards in coping with the pandemic?

Research emphasised repeatedly the effect of regular physical activity in protecting against the worst excesses of the virus. Maintaining the minimum WHO recommendation of 150 minutes of weekly moderate exercise seemed to be helpful. It wasn't necessary to embark on an Olympic training programme to derive positive benefits.

Data from millions of people around the world showed that regular exercise caused significant reductions in infection risk, severe illness, hospitalisation, ITU admissions and death. From Spain, regular exercise reduced mortality from COVID-19 six-fold. In the UK, it was found that 30 minutes of daily exercise reduced the risk of severe COVID-19 infection by 37 per cent in women and 16 per cent in men.

Physical activity improved our response to vaccination. Regular exercisers had a better antibody response to vaccines, which was maintained at six months. Immuno-compromised patients mounted better responses to jabs if they exercised.

Countries around the world embarked upon campaigns to encourage people to remain active during confinement. Over half of the UK population admitted that government guidelines had stimulated their interest in doing more exercise. However, it did not always translate into 'action'. The first lockdown appeared to drive a wedge between the sofa surfers and 'Energizer Bunnies'. Sport England found that 41 per cent of people did less exercise and 31 per cent did more during restrictions. As with health outcomes from the virus, the pandemic had a more profound effect in terms of reduced activity and obesity levels upon the poorer sections of society, ethnic minorities, the young and the chronically ill.

Exercise patterns in 2020 were forced to change. Walking, running and cycling saw large rises. However, it did not offset the large numbers lost to gym closures, indoor sports and outdoor team sports. Even when restrictions were lifted for a few months in the summer of 2020, activity levels remained subdued.

UK surveys, such as the Nuffield Health Healthier Nation Index, revealed the profound effect that the pandemic had on adults' exercise patterns in the year that followed. Three-quarters of adult Brits failed to reach the weekly target of 150 minutes of moderate exercise. Half of millennials (25–34 years old) admitted to having fallen out of love with exercise and lacked motivation to restart. Women's participation in sport dropped because of working from home and increased childcare demands. A quarter of over-55s took no exercise at all in the year after the pandemic started. An estimated 3.65 million people had not exercised due to long COVID effects.

It did not improve quickly. Half of women and a third of men did not exercise regularly in 2021–22. One in seven women reported that they had stopped exercising completely since the pandemic. They cited lack of motivation and embarrassment as important impediments.

By late 2022, the country's appetite for sport was returning but the recovery was uneven. For both adults and children, some sectors of society would remain under-exercised. Sport England recorded that over 60 per cent of adults achieved over 150 minutes of moderate exercise weekly – similar to pre-COVID levels. Worryingly, a quarter did less than 30 minutes. Women's activity levels recovered more slowly. The same applied in less affluent communities and ethnic minority groups. In the 16- to 34-year age bracket, half a million UK citizens were less active. By 2023, 400,000 more UK residents were registered as long-term sick three years after the pandemic finished compared to beforehand.

'Run Baby Run'

Song by the Newbeats. 1965

The effect on UK childhood activity paralleled that of obesity trends. Sport England reported that a third of children – over two million – were classed as inactive following lockdown restrictions. Despite less time spent in formal education and with parents freed from commuting, children struggled to amuse themselves exercise-wise. Never was there a better advert for organised youth sport. Even after the easing of the third lockdown in 2021, UK youngsters' activity levels did not return to pre-pandemic levels.

To be classed as active by Sport England, schoolchildren should participate daily in over one hour of exercise. Just under half met this threshold by 2022 but had, at least, returned to pre-pandemic levels. Like their adult counterparts, boys' sport rebounded better than girls'. The exceptions were for young, black male students and girls' football. The latter had 100,000 more players than five years earlier and would be greater after the inevitable boost from the Lionesses' Euro 2022 triumph and appearance in the 2023 World Cup Final.

'School's out for summer, school's out for ever'

Lyrics from 'School's Out' by Alice Cooper. 1972

The pandemic's global effect on children's academic and physical education was calamitous. A UNICEF report calculated that the average child around the world missed half of their classroom instruction in the year following March 2020. Inevitably, the burden was greatest in the world's poorest regions weighed down by restricted healthcare resources and less-developed educational systems. Latin America and the Caribbean were most affected. One hundred and sixty-eight million schoolchildren in 14 countries missed an entire year's schooling.

In the UK, the prolonged closure of school gates impacted not only on academic progress but on levels of obesity, paediatric mental health and child abuse. Many senior school students endured up to six months' absence from their classrooms in 2020 and a further period at the beginning of 2021 – precious time that could never be completely caught up.

Sports within the school environment perform many important functions. For many youngsters, it is their only exposure to physical activity. It provides relief from academic learning, a welcome opportunity to release stress and expend energy. It burns up calories in society's quest to reduce childhood obesity levels. It develops strength, endurance and proprioceptive skills for the growing body. It embeds motor skills that can be maintained for life. As importantly, it teaches 'softer skills'. It fosters teamwork, respect and camaraderie. It teaches correct ways to accept and respond to adversity.

All of this was put under threat by the 'stop–start' policies towards schools in 2020–21.

In many ways, the return of physical education was slower that the re-institution of academic teaching. Continuing restrictions on indoor sport, including the much reintroduced rule of six, affected staple school sports like gymnastics, netball and basketball. Team sports, like rugby union and rugby league, laboured under the emergency protocols to minimise 'close encounters of a viral kind'.

La crème de la crème

What about the next echelon of youth sport? The academies. It is where young athletes with precocious sport-specific skills assemble. Their ultimate ambition might be anything from proficiency and local success to potential Olympic champions.

Academies span the spectrum from local gymnastics clubs to multi-million-pound Premier League nurseries. Recently, some sports and academies have drawn criticism for their ruthless process of 'talent sifting' and associated safeguarding controversies. COVID-19 would add another layer of complexity and vulnerability for these protégés.

All these youngsters should be pursuing the twin ambitions of acquiring scholarly and sporting skills. With COVID-19, not only were sporting ambitions thwarted but with schools and colleges closed and public examinations cancelled there was a risk of double disappointment. This particularly affected those about to 'graduate' from an academy to senior ranks, trying to chase first professional contracts.

Elite sport has a fast-moving conveyor belt of young talent that is constantly being assessed, promoted or rejected. Gifted youngsters are coming up in the years behind. It is a ruthless business. It was clear from early pandemic days that there would be a financial fallout. Economic cuts and restricted competition would affect some youngsters who might be denied their final opportunity to pass muster.

Academies had to try and be inventive. Dundee United football club launched their Academy at Home initiative. However, trying to teach young teenagers tactics and skills on Zoom could never replicate time on the paddock. Andy Goldie, director of Dundee United's academy, remarked, 'We probably won't see the impact either way for a few months, or even years, in the decision-making, game intelligence and tactical awareness.' Added to that could be the period lost in acquiring physical competencies. During critical periods of youngsters' physical development, there would be retarded attainment of muscle memory skills so vital to performance.

Stories began to surface of youngsters and their coaches being released by football clubs as finances became tauter. When some form of training returned, reduced opportunities for matches and restrictions on travel raised further barriers. Earlier sections have recorded how rugby league academies ceased to function normally for two years. The 18 first-class cricket counties extended senior academy contracts by a year.

The truth is that nobody will ever know how many future stars were lost from the senior ranks following the pandemic. They simply disappeared from the elite radar screen.

The long game

Earlier sections chronicled the struggles community sports like football, cricket and the two rugby codes underwent to stay afloat during 2020–21. Some sports, like golf, boomed. Other activities, like netball, proved its resilience and bounced back once restrictions were lifted.

Walking for leisure, taken up enthusiastically during lockdown, remained popular once restrictions were lifted. Sport England estimated an extra 2.6 million people continued to follow the footpaths. Conversely, after a rush to run in 2020, numbers declined to 700,000 less than pre-pandemic. 'Fitness activity' participation fell by 1.4 million in 2022 compared to 2019. Swimming numbers had not fully recovered.

Team sports fared better in 2022. An extra half a million amateur footballers took to the public parks. There were reassuring rises in netball, basketball and cricket. Overall, participation in team sports at 3.1 million was equivalent to 2019.

Was the 2020 enthusiasm for cycling maintained? Were government initiatives and monies spent successful? The early figures were not encouraging.

The average number of cycle trips taken in 2021 dropped by a quarter compared to 2020. Similarly, miles cycled per person fell by 37 per cent in 2021 compared to one year earlier and reverted to pre-pandemic averages. Cycling trips and miles as a proportion of total transport modes reverted back to pre-pandemic levels of two per cent and one per cent respectively.

The boom in bike sales during the pandemic did not last. By 2022, new purchases had slumped by a quarter. It was estimated that less than half of people who invested in 'lockdown bikes' were still using them three years later. It rendered the national strategy of achieving half of all urban journeys by cycle or shanks's pony by 2030 a distant ambition.

The state and safety of British roads, the inflated prices of new bikes, the cost-of-living-crisis and laziness were all blamed. Government and local councils had spent a king's ransom on creating new cycling infrastructure since 2020. By 2023, the white flag seemed to have been run up. The Department for Transport would cut the infrastructure budget for walking and cycling by over £200m.

The indoor fitness lockdown success Peloton doubled their revenues in 2020 and repeated the trick in 2021. However, their share value nosedived 80 per cent over 2021. The company were left over-stocked in the belief that the boom would continue inexorably. It didn't. People had bought their $2,000 fitness machine once. They didn't want another one soon and embraced the gyms again once they reopened. PR disasters and product recalls tarnished their brand. Wiggle, the UK online supplier of cycling products, boomed during the height of the pandemic. It did not last. It posted pre-tax losses of £97m in 2023. In October 2023, it announced its intention to file for insolvency.

It appeared that you could put bicycle clips on the person, but not get them to mount their steeds. It would take more than a deadly virus to positively change some of the nation's exercise habits.

Looking back to look forward

Recreational sport, like its elite cousin, showed remarkable resilience in many ways. However, beneath the surface, the effects were more nuanced. The pandemic caused large swathes of the UK population to overindulge and lose focus on whatever exercise regime they had been pursuing. Like other pandemic outcomes, it would be poorer sections of society and ethnic minorities who struggled most to regain a degree of normality in their physical activity.

The real tragedy was with the young. Their education was parked. Their physical activities benched. The pandemic was the catalyst for ballooning weight and psychological fragility for many. Adolescents lost time developing skills, fitness and mental resilience – all key ingredients for success in competitive sport.

Various governments have made political capital on the 'levelling-up agenda'. Boris Johnson wanted to address chronic economic and opportunity inequalities but, also, tackle issues like differing levels of mental illness, obesity and life expectancies. The pandemic taught us the value in raising the overall population's fitness and reducing its BMI – some of the best tools we can have to fight future health crises. It is where education and resources need to be targeted.

Is it too much to hope that the lessons learned will inform future public policy on health priorities and enabling sport for all?

Chapter 34

For Richer, for Poorer, in Sickness and in Health

THREE WEEKS. Disappointing but manageable.

That was the hope offered by football authorities when games were suspended on Friday 13th. Commentators were less optimistic. The pandemic was not expected to peak until mid-summer. Within days, the full financial and health disaster was laid bare. Governments do not volunteer a £350bn rescue package to the nation's businesses for a short hiccough.

'We're doomed'

Words spoken by Private Frazer in *Dad's Army*. 1968–77

Sport began wrestling with the financial implications: TV contracts, sponsorship monies, merchandising sales and spectators' season tickets. The prescient amongst them (tennis and golf) dusted off their insurance policies.

The Premier League contemplated the £1.6bn in transfer fees due for settlement that summer; the £762m repayment to TV if the season did not restart. Financial experts predicted a 'watershed moment' for huge transfer deals.

The Premier League's CEO, Richard Masters, told the DCMS of a £1bn loss if the season was not completed. The EFL faced a £200m deficit by the autumn. Its chairman,

389

Rick Parry, told the DCMS that, in 2018, the Premier League earned £3bn from TV and paid £2.9bn in wages. The EFL paid £1bn in wages, but only took £100m from TV. Parry admitted that it was a crazy model requiring a reset.

Cricket calculated a £380m loss if no play was possible in 2020. The RFU would lose £106m if the final Six Nations games and autumn internationals were cancelled. Six Olympic and Paralympic sports faced insolvency by the summer. The delay of the Tokyo Olympics by one year was causing a funding gap for many sports.

'We've Gotta Get Out of This Place'

Song by the Animals. 1965

Psychologists describe the stages of grief – shock, denial, anger, bargaining, guilt, depression, acceptance and hope. Millions of families around the world went through this process during the pandemic. Sport did the same.

What were the financial means out of this crisis? Essentially, it was to beg, borrow or 'cut your cloth' accordingly. Once the Treasury, banks and sports' finance officers had crunched the numbers, various rescue packages appeared.

As in other sectors of the economy, the government rode to sport's rescue. The cavalry coming over the hill. Three days before lockdown, the Coronavirus Job Retention Scheme (CJRS) committed the government to pay 80 per cent of employees' salaries. Furlough had arrived. Both the lifeline and PR problems this created for professional sport were outlined earlier. The scheme ran for 18 months.

The government were generous with grants and loans at all levels of the sporting landscape. Within weeks, Sport England, using lottery and government funding, announced £195m for grassroots sport and physical activity. It would top up with £16.5m in October. The same month, the government announced £100m for public gyms, leisure centres and swimming pools to keep them afloat.

In November, the government produced a £300m winter survival package of loans and grants for 11 major participation and spectator sports; £135m in loans were allocated to rugby union and £40m to horse racing. Sports Minister Tom Huddleston had to defend himself against accusations of supporting 'posh sports'. The politician defended the decision not to support men's elite football, noting that 'the Premier League has just spent £1.2 billion on transfers' in the autumn transfer window. He said football had 'enough money to go around'.

Rugby league was the first British sport to be bailed out by the government. A £16m emergency loan arrived on 1 May with further injections of £12m in November and £16.7m in March 2021. The sport was devastated by the pandemic in 2020. Half of BSL fixtures were lost, the cup needed reorganising, its Canadian franchise was virtually 'stillborn', and the first Australian tour for 17 years was cancelled. No women's or junior games took place in 2020 and, at the end of the year, its Sky TV deal would expire.

Governments abroad were performing similar good Samaritan acts. Across the Channel, French TV refused to pay the next instalment of its £637m deal to broadcast Ligue 1. Its government lent monies to the top two football leagues to cover losses from television after their 2019/20 season was abandoned.

Financial houses chimed in. The Bank of England lent Tottenham Hotspur £175m (at a very favourable interest rate of 0.5 per cent) in June 2020 to offset income loss from matchdays and other planned events at their new stadium. NatWest lent the WRU £18m in November 2020 as part of the Coronavirus Large Business Interruption Loan Scheme (CLBILS). It borrowed a further £2m from World Rugby and passed the entire £20m on to its four regional sides to save them from bankruptcy. The monies were scheduled to be repaid over three years.

Major national and international organisations came to the rescue of struggling clubs and individuals. British Darts provided an emergency hardship fund for members experiencing oche exile. The Lawn Tennis Association gave £20m to tennis venues, coaches, officials and players. Globally, the WTA and ATP announced a $6m hardship war chest. Athletics' bodies offered funds to individuals.

World Rugby tendered £80m to struggling national unions. UEFA announced £61m worth of relief to football clubs across its 55 countries. FIFA provided £121m to its 211 nations. By mid-June, the ECB had pumped nearly £100m into first-class and recreational cricket, of which £30m to the FCCs was monies promised from the abandoned Hundred competition.

Within football, teams further up the food chain helped those less well off. In early April, the Premier League advanced £125m to the EFL and National Leagues. In June, the league offered £1m to women's football to allow the WSL to implement testing protocols for 2020/21. Later, in December 2020, the Premier League reached an agreement to give a further £50m to Leagues One and Two and an interest-free loan of £200m to the Championship.

By the end of March, professional sport was in full 'money-belt tightening mode'. Many of sport's senior administrators, coaches and leading athletes announced pay cuts or deferrals. Abroad, USA Rugby filed for bankruptcy and Rugby Australia laid off 75 per cent of its staff – 'the toughest decision in the game's history'.

Hard assessments had to be made to concentrate on the most profitable sources of income. International men's cricket was prioritised. The women's equivalent went into hibernation.

To make further savings, various sports looked at cuts in financial caps, limiting expenditure by teams. In June, English rugby union's Premiership agreed to reduce each club's salary cap from £6.4m to £5m for 2021. Players and clubs had already agreed in March to introduce a 25 per cent voluntary salary reduction throughout the crisis. Previously, clubs had lost a combined £89m in the two pre-pandemic seasons. It made them less competitive compared to the French Top 14 whose cap was £8.5m.

Formula 1 had decided pre-pandemic to introduce a budget cap for 2021 to limit teams' spending on car performance. The original limit was $175m but lowered to $145m within months of the pandemic. It would be further reduced to $140m for 2022 and $135m in 2023. Although it excluded other items, like driver salaries, it was a considerable restriction for some of the wealthier teams, whose pre-pandemic overall budgets topped $500m.

Football's EFL looked to reduce players' salaries. In May 2020, it was proposed to limit League One clubs to a salary cap of £2.5m per year and League Two clubs to £1.25m from the beginning of the 2020/21 season. Some clubs would need to adjust. When Sunderland were relegated into League One in 2018, their wage bill was £40m. When it was ratified in August, many clubs and the PFA were unhappy. The latter called it 'unlawful and unenforceable'. Its appeal was upheld by an independent arbitration panel in February 2021. The EFL was forced to withdraw its plans. Not for English football an American-style sporting cap – more like a Stetson. Carry on with the Wild West show and bank with Wells Fargo in the hope of a Gold Rush.

'Can we have the bill now, please?'

By the summer of 2021, the true cost of the pandemic became clear as sports announced their annual accounts.

Empty grounds cost Premier League clubs a combined £1.1 billion with some clubs losing £5m per game. Deloitte's annual review of football finance estimated that the loss of fans, commercial partners and TV rebates had cost the top 20 wealthiest European clubs £1.7bn across 2019/20 and 2020/21. In Europe, overall, the 2019/20 season saw revenues fall by £3.4bn.

The pandemic costs to individual clubs were announced. Tottenham Hotspur claimed COVID-19 cost them over £150m in two years, Liverpool £70m, Juventus £43.5m, West Ham £40m, Derby County £20m and Glasgow Rangers £10m. In Spain, La Liga president Javier Tebas estimated his clubs would still lose £265m despite temporary pay cuts. Scottish football was reported to be facing a 'doomsday scenario' with most professional clubs showing signs of 'financial distress' and some insolvency was expected.

The ECB lost £16.1m in 2020/21. Its reserves had dwindled from £70m in 2016 to £2.2m by 2021; 2020 cost the 18 FCCs £100m, with most losses accrued by the richer counties with significant commercial revenue streams. Lancashire's revenue fell from £34m to £16m.

The RFU derives 85 per cent of its income from Twickenham-based activities. In late 2021, it announced a £23m loss and £70m drop in revenues. Apart from redundancies, it reduced spending in the professional game by £21m and there was an £11m cut in investment projects. Astonishingly, the Rugby Football League announced a £25k profit over the same period.

The damage to the horse-racing industry became apparent. The 13 courses owned by the Jockey Club lost £100m in revenues during 2020. By August 2022, the total loss to British racecourses was estimated to be £400m with a significant fall in prize monies offered.

'Please, Sir, I want some more'

Quote from *Oliver Twist* by Charles Dickens. 1838

With the crisis continuing into 2021 and beyond, it was clear that many within sport would require extra financial support. Sport England announced a further £50m for grassroots sport in new year 2021. It would be particularly targeted at indoor sports and outdoor sports, such as rugby, that had seen no action for nearly a year.

In March 2021, a summer sports recovery package was announced by the government; £300m would be available, principally for cricket, tennis and horse racing. The FA announced a £180m four-year investment in grassroots football. The EFL negotiated a £177m loan from an institutional investor for the Championship. As late as January 2021, Arsenal would take a £120m government loan to cover the income lost from its closed ground.

In the midst of the recovery programmes in April 2021, 12 European football clubs, including six from the Premier League, announced the formation of a breakaway European Super League. The condemnation was swift. 'Pure greed' was a common sentiment. It even united the leaders of Britain's two major parties – Boris Johnson and Keir Starmer – in opposition. Three days later all six English clubs withdrew.

A year later, some Premier League clubs were squabbling. Everton were claiming to have lost £170m from COVID-19 – which was reported to dwarf other similar clubs' losses. Leeds and Burnley wanted the 'Toffees' investigated over potential irregularities as COVID-19 losses could be deducted to remain compliant with Financial Fair Play rules. The investigation lasted through until late 2023 and Everton were deducted ten Premier League points.

Tripping over hurdles

UK Athletics (UKA) fell into difficult financial currents. Its flagship events were responsible for a high proportion of its income. Losing the July 2020 Goodwill Games in London created a £2m hole in its revenues. Its annual BBC TV deal worth £3m expired at the end of 2020. No new deal was signed until 2022. Domestic athletics' coverage on terrestrial screens suffered accordingly.

In 2016, the organisation had £4.6m in reserve. This more than halved one year after the first lockdown and dwindled to £400,000 in March 2022. Over 90 per cent of its cushion had gone during the pandemic. By May 2023, the organisation announced the closure of its Birmingham base, admitted not being able to pay coaches for months and was making redundancies. Its CEO, Jack Buckner, had to reassure athletes and the public that UKA was not about to go bust and that the team's preparation, for Paris 2024 would be unaffected. For a sport that has delivered its nation more than double the number of Olympic medals of any other, it represented a sad state of affairs. In the circumstances, the delivery of a record-equalling medal haul at the Budapest World Championships in August 2023 was nothing short of miraculous.

A collapsing scrum

The English Premiership lost three of its 13 teams in the 2022/23 season: Worcester Warriors, Wasps and London Irish. Welsh rugby faced a mutiny from its players in the middle of the 2023 Six Nations. How did these crises arise?

It all looked so different in 2015. The RFU had hosted a successful World Cup contributing to a total annual profit of £102m. The next year, the RFU signed a new eight-year deal with the Premiership clubs, paying them £220m over that period. The teams hiked their salary cap accordingly. However, the sting was in the 'small print'. Payments for the last half of the contract could be varied according to the RFU's financial performance. Enter COVID-19 stage left. With projected revenue losses of £150m from 2020–24, central monies to clubs fell. In 2018, the latter had sold a 27 per cent share in the league to the private equity firm CVC. The monies pumped into the clubs had been swallowed by the virus. The 'magical money tree' had developed Dutch elm disease. The 2021 accounts revealed that 12 of the clubs held a combined £470m in debt – Worcester were bankrupt and did not file accounts. Calls for greater financial transparency amongst the clubs were becoming deafening. In September 2023, it was reported that the RFU was expecting to make a loss for eight of the next nine years, totalling £161m.

Over in Wales, the £20m bailout fund was hanging over its four provinces. In early 2022, the repayment period was extended from three to 20 years. It would still cause distress. In March 2023, the WRU and provinces signed a new six-year agreement on funding. Delays in its implementation, which required buy-in from the Welsh government, caused the provinces cash-flow problems. Salary caps were to be reduced for 2023/24 and further shrunk for the season after. In the middle of the Six Nations, the players threatened not to play against England. The dispute was resolved but it did not stop an exodus of players abroad at the end of the season.

'It's a rich man's world'

Lyrics from 'Money, Money, Money' by ABBA. 1976

Despite many predictions, none of the 92 clubs in the Premier League or EFL disappeared in the three years after the pandemic struck. Admittedly, some clubs, such as Derby County, teetered on the brink but managed a Houdini escape. Southend United were relegated out of the EFL and staggered from crisis to crisis and Macclesfield quickly folded after relegation from League Two.

But was the game more resilient than previously believed? Premier League revenue reached an all-time high in 2018/19 of £5.1 billion. The pandemic reduced 2019/20 revenues – but only by 13 per cent to £4.5bn.

The 2020/21 season's accounts saw a variance across the major European leagues. Most differences can be credited to television revenues. Despite continuing national restrictions and the absence of fans, Premier League income returned to pre-pandemic levels. Comparatively, in Spain and Germany, revenues fell by eight per cent and in France increased by one per cent. The success story was Italy's Serie A, which was the first major league to exceed pre-pandemic income with a record £2.1bn – an increase of 23 per cent on the year before.

The pandemic had put a minor blip into the steep upward slope of revenue generation of Europe's elite clubs. By

2022/23, Premier League income was expected to hit £6bn. Its income sources had proved impervious to the pandemic. A veritable cash cow.

An indicator of confidence and cash within football is the size of spending in summer and winter transfer windows. Deloitte analyse these transactions within the English game. Premier League clubs splashed out £1.4bn in summer 2019 and £230 million in January 2020 – just two months before the virus struck.

The summer 2020 window was extended to October to reflect Project Restart. Spending decreased by nine per cent. However, clubs still shelled out £1.3bn. Hardly the actions of a group of businesses fearful for their survival. English spending represented 43 per cent of total global outlay on football transfers. Many hoped the worst of the pandemic was behind them.

As the country suffered its third lockdown, the realisation hit that this might be more than a six-month glitch. January 2021 spending fell by more than two-thirds to £70m. The readjustment continued into the summer. Gross transfer fees fell by 11 per cent to £1.1bn – the lowest total for six years.

Perhaps this was the readjustment some experts had predicted? Not a chance.

The 2022 winter transfer window indicated 'normality' was returning: £295m spent, quadrupling expenditure from one year earlier. Summer 2022 smashed all records: £1.9bn, One third higher than the previous record summer madness of 2017. The Premier League spent more than the Bundesliga, La Liga and Serie A put together. It did not stop there. Winter 2023 saw further records: £815m. It obliterated the previous record of £430m in 2018. Chelsea spent more in the window than the four other main European leagues combined. By summer 2023, the Premiership recorded another record: a gross spend of £1.92bn.

Gross spend is one thing. What about net spend? In summer 2022, the Premier League exceeded the £1bn barrier for the first time. Net spending on transfers, as a percentage of total revenue, averaged 15 per cent in the five pre-pandemic seasons. Summer 2020 saw it rise to 16 per cent and, for the three seasons after, an average of 17 per cent.

The English Championship was a little more circumspect in the transfer market. Its business model suggests it should be. The 2017–19 gross transfer summer expenditures averaged £169m. In the three summers after the pandemic's onset, the clubs spent £55m (2020), £35m (2021) and £86m (2022). Indeed, many Championship clubs made a net profit in the summer transfer markets; £110m in 2022 between the 20 clubs.

As ever, it was broadcast rights that oiled the Premiership wheels. In early 2022, it was announced that the new 2022–2025 deals would exceed £10bn for the first time. In the face of a global rights recession occasioned by COVID-19, the enduring appeal of domestic English football was remarkable. However, the gloss from such riches hid another story underneath.

In 2023, the London finance firm LCP reported on English football's finances. It was bleak. Over two-thirds of the 92 clubs made combined losses of £1.2bn in 2021/22. Only one third were profitable – a combined £300m. The Premier League accounted for 85 per cent of revenue in the top four tiers. Total net debt across the 92 was £5.6bn. Half that debt was due to owners – who could call on it at any time. LCP likened the financial risks within the game as akin to 'a pack of cards'.

Reliance on wealthy benefactors placed the sport at significant risk.

The gamblers within the football pyramid remained the Championship clubs. In trying to reach the Premier League's promised land, they were prepared to stake the family silver. No lessons had been learned from the pandemic. In 2020/21, net debt for the 20 clubs increased by one third to £1.8bn and the wages/revenue ratio at 125 per cent. Even with some correction the year after, wages still outstripped revenue.

In EFL Leagues One and Two, revenues and wages are dwarfed by the leagues above. In 2021/22, League One revenues fell by 22 per cent to £129m and for the first time ever their wages/revenue ratio peaked above 100 per cent. League Two income fell by four per cent to £94m but wages remained better contained with an 80 per cent ratio.

The economic picture of the sport remained one of 'fantasy football'. The scenario of the 'Emperor's new clothes' remained a risk for many clubs.

However, while we rail against unstable English economic models, it is worth reflecting upon the struggles of Spanish giant Barcelona. In 2021/22, Barcelona's income was £174m below 2018/19 levels. In early 2021, Spanish media were reporting that the club was on the edge of bankruptcy.

Barcelona's woes came to a head in August 2021. They announced that after 778 games and 35 trophies, Lionel Messi was leaving and joining Paris Saint Germain. Barça's net worth was reported to be a negative £387m with £1.2bn of gross debt. Their 2020/21 wage bill was £529m – 103 per cent of its total revenue. The club had resorted to 'payday loans' at high interest rates to keep afloat. Messi earned a reputed £125m annually. La Liga had limited Barça's maximum spending on transfers and wages for 2021/22 to one quarter of the £562m it paid out in 2019/20. Barça simply could not afford Messi anymore. Unsurprisingly, Barça finished the 2021/22 season trophyless.

With concerns over English football's finances, its attraction for unscrupulous 'chancers', and the risk of damaging the cultural heritage of its clubs, the government announced its intention to introduce an independent regulator for the sport in April 2022. It met with a lukewarm response from the major clubs.

For richer or poorer?

What was the long-term economic cost to sport of the COVID-19 years? It can be difficult to distil the viral effects from other financial pressures leaning on the industry in recent years. Similarly, it is difficult to discount some of the questionable business models in sport that existed pre-pandemic. However, the health crisis posed major monetary stresses on many sports and, in some cases, pushed them to the brink of collapse, and, for a few, beyond.

The top echelon of English football sailed serenely on. The virus caused little more trouble than a piece of flotsam would to a passing battleship. Beneath it, all was not well. The crisis heightened awareness of the need for greater independent regulation and transparency of institutions which form such an important part of our social fabric. It took an enormous effort from government and other institutions to keep sport afloat. Hopefully, their efforts will be rewarded. Without accessible grassroots sporting opportunities, the detrimental effect on our future nation's health is too painful to contemplate.

Chapter 35

Conflict, Climate and Contagion

Lessons from history

Sport in 2020 had become a major part of society's fabric: personal crusades to remain fit, our fascination with elite sport, the media industry surrounding it, sport's economic importance, and the boost to national prestige from international sporting success. There is no denying its central role in our day-to-day lives.

It is why sport's collapse in early 2020 had such a profound effect. Lost opportunities for personal and collective sporting escapism intensified society's perception of personal restrictions, economic meltdown and the horror of the unfolding health tragedy.

However, in the previous century, organised sport has been stopped in its tracks. Often. Cumulatively, more than a decade was lost to the ravages of war, climatic conditions and previous pandemics. However, sport recovered. These 'roadblocks' changed sport – sometimes for the better. Residents of the 21st century were not the first to suffer sporting deprivations.

World War I

When war broke out in July 1914, the military required fit, healthy men. Physical unpreparedness was not confined to Britain. In America, up to a half of recruits were unfit for service. Athletes were role models – moral leaders with inherent fitness ready to fight.

Prominent people appealed to sportsmen. Posters from the FA secretary appeared: 'Good sportsmen enlist now and help the other good sportsmen who are so bravely Fighting Britain's Battle against the world's enemies'. Sherlock Holmes's creator, Sir Arthur Conan Doyle, entreated people to enlist during half-time at soccer matches. Recruiting officers scoured games looking for volunteers.

Cricket shut up shop quicker than football. It stopped five weeks after hostilities commenced following many players' enlistment. Jack Hobbs moved his benefit match from the Oval to Lord's after the army requisitioned the venue. W.G. Grace wrote, 'I should like to see all first-class cricketers of suitable age set a good example and come to the help of their country without delay in its hour of need.' He took to waving his fist in defiance at Zeppelins flying over his house.

The Lord's outfield became home to a flock of geese. The Old Trafford pavilion converted to a Red Cross hospital. Military matches continued to be played at home and abroad. In 1915, at Gallipoli, the Aussies played a game in view of the Turkish troops as a ruse while ANZAC forces were evacuated from the beach. First-class cricket would not return in England until May 1919. At least 210 first-class cricketers fought and 34 were killed. Hundreds more amateurs and officials perished.

Rugby union was an amateur sport in 1914. Many players were already members of the Territorial Army and team ranks dwindled rapidly in the late 1914 summer. By early September, British club rugby was abandoned. The RFU called upon all players between 19 and 35 years old to enlist and called for the formation of a rugby players' battalion. One hundred and sixty England internationals fought in the war and 28 died. Scotland lost 30 internationals and Wales 11 players. The Bristol rugby club alone lost 300 members.

Like cricket, military rugby sides continued with large crowds – 20,000 at Leicester on New Year's Day 1915. The question of rugby league players involved in union games arose. League players had been banned for life since 1895. However, a pragmatic truce was reached, allowing league players back into the fold for the war's duration.

English football continued throughout the 1914/15 season but not without controversy. *Punch* magazine depicted a cartoon of Mr Punch talking to a footballer, with the caption, 'No doubt you can make money in this field, my friend, but there's only one field today where you can get honour'. With public approval wavering and players unavailable, league football was suspended until August 1919. Games contested by amateurs continued and raised funds for the war effort. Matches entertained returning and wounded troops. Sides varied from week to week. Many 'ex-professionals' played when they were stationed close to grounds. Amongst the 887,000 British military deaths, thousands of sportsmen perished including at least 337 professional English and Scottish footballers.

Nine hundred thousand women joined the war effort by working in munitions factories and numerous ladies' football teams emerged. The female game's popularity continued briefly after the war. The Preston-based Dick, Kerr Ladies took on St Helen's at Everton's Goodison Park on Boxing Day 1920; 53,000 people attended with an estimated 14,000 locked outside. In 1921, the FA banned ladies from Football League stadiums on the grounds that the spectacle was 'distasteful' and the 'game was quite unsuitable for females'.

Sport was encouraged in order to maintain fitness and morale and offset boredom amongst the troops. Football was more popular in the conflict zones. The famous Christmas 1914 match in no-man's land between British and German troops has become the stuff of legend. Rugby was difficult to play on uneven terrain and more injury-prone. Football was described as 'a practical exercise in class collaboration'.

However, football, which had been dominant pre-war in public and grammar schools, became supplanted by rugby union in the 1920s. Rugby had rapidly called its players to arms and positioned itself during the war as 'unequalled by any other game as a school of true manhood and leadership'.

In 1914, Pals' battalions were recruited, comprising young men from local communities. Tragically, they often died together, devastating families and neighbourhoods. It was a natural corollary that military companies of sports people should band together. The first sportsman's unit came from Scotland. The Hearts team signed up *en bloc* and, joined by four other clubs, formed 'McCrae's Battalion'. In their wake followed 650 football supporters. Two hundred and fifty sportsmen joined the Northamptonshire Regiment under the command of England rugby player Edgar Mobbs. The latter died in 1917 but his name was commemorated in the annual East Midlands Mobbs Memorial Match and the Ella-Mobbs Cup played between Australia and England.

America entered the war in April 1917. To stay 'in step' with public opinion, some MLB teams 'drilled' pre-game using bats as substitute guns. It would not be enough. The public questioned why baseball players remained exempt from the national effort. In 1918, the government issued a 'work or fight' mandate. Non-essential jobs, including sport, could not continue. Athletic men were needed on the battlefield. Baseball negotiated an extension for ten weeks. Thirty games were shaved off the regular season, but the World Series was completed. Boston Red Sox won the title – their last until 2004.

Spanish flu pandemic

The 1918 Spanish flu pandemic was one of the deadliest in history. Estimates hover between 20 million and 50 million deaths worldwide claiming more victims than the Great War; 228,000 people in the UK succumbed. At home, the war effort took precedence. However, in November 1918, the *News of the World* advised, 'Wash inside nose with soap and water ... force yourself to sneeze ... breathe deeply. Do not wear a muffler ... walk home from work; eat plenty of porridge.'

The source of Spanish flu is uncertain but unlikely to have been Spain. Cases were present in Kansas in March 1918 and Europe one month later. Like in 2020, the virus would attack in waves.

The 1918 world was different. Global population was a third of its size in 2020. The war had exacerbated pre-existing poverty, malnourishment and poor health. Overcrowded hospitals were struggling to cope with injured soldiers and vaccinations were unavailable. Repatriated soldiers helped spread the virus to their own communities.

The first wave was relatively mild, but it did not stop three-quarters of French troops, half of the British military and more than 900,000 German soldiers becoming sick. In autumn 1918, American troop ships were returning stateside with weary soldiers and the virus on board. From August 1918, disembarking platoons in Boston spread the disease to every military site within 30 miles. By October, it had spread across America and established the second wave. It was particularly serious for young adults.

Approximately 4,800 Bostonians died from flu in 1918, fuelled by the World Series games at Fenway Park. It is ironic that the 2020 owners of Liverpool Football Club should be the Fenway Sports Group. Anfield was seen as a super-spreader event after the decision to play the Atlético Madrid game.

The 1919 MLB season was 14 games shorter because of the continuing impact of the war. The 'work or fight' order continued to regard sport as 'unnecessary labor'. Babe Ruth contracted, but survived, the virus. A few other baseball luminaries were not so lucky. Many professional baseball players sported masks on the diamond. Many colleges' baseball and football games were cancelled.

The 1919 ice hockey Stanley Cup Final play-offs were abandoned following an outbreak of flu at the Montreal Canadiens. The sixth and final game with the Seattle Metropolitans was abandoned hours before the start. The Canadiens had only three fit players. One died four days later, and the manager never recovered health and died two years afterwards. It was the only time in the competition's history, dating back to 1893, that no winner has been declared.

The third wave started in the Australian summer of January 1919 and spread globally. It lasted until mid-1919. Although not as virulent as the second wave, the third coming killed more people than the first 1918 wave.

In Britain, league football remained suspended until August 1919. Wartime regional matches continued as did the women's games. There was no attempt to restrict crowds. English cricket resumed in May 1919. Yorkshire were awarded the title on a 'win percentage to matches played' formula. They played more than twice as many matches as some other counties. Games were played over two rather than three days. There was a concern that county cricket may have lost its allure after the conflict – which proved erroneous. The epidemic attracted little attention in the contemporary annual *Wisden Cricketers' Almanack* – the population was just relieved to welcome back sport after the war. However, the 1919 and 1920 editions listed 20 cricketing obituaries with influenza listed as the cause of death.

World War II

Britain declared war on Germany in September 1939. The football season was three games old. Contracts were declared null and void. Players returned home, enlisted or volunteered for essential work. To maintain morale and appease angry fans, the FA created seven regional leagues, as non-essential travel was limited to 50 miles. The season restarted after a six-week hiatus. One year later, two league tables were created – North and South.

Initially, crowds were limited to 8,000 for fear of Luftwaffe bombing. Preston North End and England star Tom Finney recalled the team bus being caught in an air raid returning from Anfield. Teams changed weekly according to player availability. Northampton Town put out nine different 'number 9s' in the 1941/42 season. The 'guest' system allowed players billeted locally to turn out. Players could appear for and against the same team on successive Saturdays. Military movement meant internationals turning out for some unfashionable clubs. Northampton fielded numerous internationals including the later, great Liverpool manager Bill Shankly, and 1966 World Cup-winning trainer Harold Shepherdson. Crowds were called upon to supply players and officials in emergencies. One game was abandoned mid-match as the referee had to return to barracks and another match terminated when a German bomber appeared. The referee began shooting at the invader using a nearby anti-aircraft gun.

In 1940, a bomb landed in the unoccupied Chelsea stands and their manager, Billy Birrell, defused it. Many grounds were damaged by enemy bombing including Wembley, Highbury and Old Trafford. Manchester United shared with Manchester City and Arsenal with Tottenham Hotspur. White Hart Lane became a temporary mortuary during the Blitz. Aston Villa did not play until 1942 after the army requisitioned their ground for varying functions including an ammunition store. English league football would not return until August 1946. Seven seasons had been lost to the war.

English cricket ceased upon declaration of war. The visiting West Indies had been sent home for their own protection. The rest of the season was cancelled and remained in abeyance until 1946. The Oval and Lord's prepared to receive prisoners of war but were never called upon. County clubs ceased to function. Contracts were ripped up, but supporters requested to continue with their annual subscriptions. The RAF occupied Lord's practice grounds, but the venue became the game's surviving spiritual home. Numerous games were played there involving mostly the military. Sir Pelham Warner felt it enabled 'cricket to provide a healthy and restful antidote to war strain'. Most matches were one-day affairs because of military commitments – several decades before it gained popularity again in the professional ranks.

Lord's was attacked twice. It was bombed in 1941 without casualties. In 1944, a V-1 doodlebug landed adjacent during a match. The players hit the square and then resumed play. The batsman dispatched the next ball for six. A year later, the Victory five-match series took place between an Australian Services XI and an England team. A total of 367,000 spectators attended.

America joined the war after the Japanese bombed Pearl Harbor in December 1941. At that time, the major spectator sports were baseball, boxing, horse racing and college football. The NFL started in 1920 and was gaining in popularity while professional basketball had yet to achieve prominence.

President Roosevelt declared that all sports, professional and amateur, should continue during wartime given their inherent 'morale benefits'. However, 350 colleges stopped football for the war's duration. By May 1942, one third of NFL players had signed up. Eventually over 1,000 NFL personnel enlisted, creating powerful teams for each military wing. In the summer of 1942, all car and motorcycle racing stopped because of petrol and rubber rationing. Baseball continued – although many of its stars were in uniform. Ex-players came out of retirement and less-talented players filled the team rosters.

To plug the gap, an All-American Girls Professional Baseball League was established in 1943. It combined elements of baseball and softball. Its rules could be fierce. Players were obliged to attend 'charm school' classes, have long hair, not smoke or drink in public, and always wear lipstick. There were 15 teams at varying times and it attracted

900,000 spectators in 1948. It folded in 1954 but its memory was rekindled by the 1992 film *A League of Their Own*.

Winter wonderland

The 1946/47 English football season would witness the first full programme for seven years. A return to 'normal sport' seemed just the tonic the country needed after the long war and continuing food rationing. Instead, they got rained and snowed on from above. The Football League published the fixture list that had been intended for the cancelled 1939/40 season.

The winter of 1947 was believed to be the snowiest since records began. From late January, the cold and blizzards started. Power cuts were required and transport ground to a halt. In early March, snow drifts piled up over 23ft (7m) deep in Scotland. March was the wettest for over 300 years and the melt caused widespread flooding. Australian and Canadian charities provided support and food parcels.

As in 2020, the government summoned sports' representatives, on 12 March. Prime Minister Attlee wanted 'all hands to the pump' to minimise economic disruption. Midweek sport would distract the workforce from their labours. The government wanted it banned. Protests from sports' administrators and fans (including a greyhound supporters' demonstration outside the Home Office) failed to change minds. There would be no 1947 equivalent of a 'cold, rainy midweek fixture at Stoke' to test the players' mettle.

The Epsom Derby had been run on a weekday since 1780. In 1942–45, it was held on Saturdays before reverting to Wednesday in 1946; 1947 saw it back in its weekend spot. The Aintree Grand National had recommenced in 1946. The course had been requisitioned by the military during the war. It raced traditionally on a Friday. To placate Home Secretary James Chuter Ede, the 1947 episode moved to a Saturday and has stayed there ever since.

Football faced a huge backlog of fixtures. *The Guardian* reported that 'many grounds are flooded, some are still frozen, and others are covered with varying amounts of ice, water and snow'. Like in 2020, authorities were left with a dilemma. *The Guardian* summarised, 'The league are asked ... to choose between abandoning this season's championship ... or playing on halfway through the summer, or ... playing behind closed doors the games needed to conclude the league programme.' They played on. With only Saturdays and Bank Holidays available, the season was extended to 14 June. Northampton Town in Division Three (South) played only once between 25 January and 8 March. They played seven games in April including four games over the Easter weekend. On Easter Monday, they beat Brighton at home 6-1 before losing 0-8 away to Walsall the next day.

On the final weekend, several clubs remained poised to win the First Division title – Stoke, Liverpool, Wolves and Manchester United. If Stoke City could win their final game against Sheffield United, they would claim their first-ever league championship. Confident, the Potters took the team to Buxton to celebrate the century-old Well Dressing Festival 48 hours before they met the Blades. After lunching well, they repaired to the sports fields to indulge in bowls, tennis and putting. They lost the game 2-1, finished fourth, and have still never won the title. The longest season in English football history ended with the title going to Anfield, a feat repeated in 2020. At the other end of the table, Brentford were relegated in June 1947. It would be another 74 years, at the end of the COVID-19 season in May 2021, before they would return to the top echelon.

The Big Freeze

The Big Freeze of 1963 trumped 1947. It was one of the coldest winters on record and, certainly, the worst of the 20th century. Snow blizzards started after Christmas. Scottish temperatures in Januuary reached -19.4°C and seas froze for a mile off the Kent coast. From New Year's Day 1963, Britain woke up to 64 consecutive frosts until 6 March. As the snow melted, the release of water was reported to be of biblical proportions.

The English FA Cup third round took 66 days to complete. Lincoln City versus Coventry City was postponed 15 times while, in Scotland, Stranraer against Airdrie was postponed 33 times. Games were played under extreme conditions. On Boxing Day 1962, 42,000 fans attended Roker Park to see Sunderland play Bury in atrocious weather. The referee allowed the game to be played. Sunderland's centre-forward, Brian Clough, sustained a severe knee injury. He took two years to return and retired after only three games back. He went on to manage Derby and Nottingham Forest to the Division One titles and the latter to back-to-back European titles.

Brighton used a local builder's tarmac-laying equipment to thaw the turf and destroyed the pitch. They were relegated at the end of the season. Chelsea tried a tar burner. Norwich employed a flamethrower, but the ice refroze as fast as it melted. Subsequently an ice breaker was tried at Carrow Road. Blackpool asked players to clear the ice and snow. Halifax turned their pitch into a skating rink and charged fans to use it. Blackpool's international duo, Jimmy Armfield and Tony Waiters, ice skated on the Bloomfield Road pitch.

Some clubs sought warmer climes. Jimmy Hill took Coventry west to Ireland where they played friendlies against Manchester United and Wolves. Tommy Docherty took Chelsea south to Malta.

Upon resumption, games came thick and fast. Games could be played on neutral grounds if home pitches were unfit. Coventry played five FA Cup ties (including two replays) and two league matches in just over two weeks. Northampton Town played only twice between Boxing Day and 2 March, and then completed nine matches in April.

The season was extended by four weeks and finished the day before the delayed FA Cup Final on 25 May. Some leagues below the professional ranks never completed. The Pools Panel was created to predict the results of postponed matches and keep afloat Pools companies and millions of weekly punters' dreams. The panel comprised ex-international footballers and referees. Its first chairman was John Theodore Cuthbert Moore-Brabazon, 1st Baron Brabazon of Tara. The ex-Conservative MP's idea of sport was, in 1909, to tie a piglet in a wastepaper basket to the wing of his aeroplane to prove that 'pigs could fly'. He was replaced by a Second World War flying ace, Group Captain Douglas Bader, who had lost both his legs in action and, subsequently, two MPs.

Both rugby codes were severely affected. There was no horse racing in England between 23 December and 7 March with 94 meetings lost because of the Big Freeze.

However, sports survived and later flourished. This was despite support and leadership from government and sporting organisations that was less than fulsome.

Conservative Prime Minister Harold Macmillan recognised the need for a senior politician to keep a watching brief on sport. Sir John Wolfenden, an educationalist and author of the 1957 eponymous report on 'Homosexual Offences and Prostitution', chaired the 'Sport in the Community' committee of 1960. It made far-reaching recommendations for sport's governance and advised the creation of a Sports Development Council. Instead 'Super Mac' turned to an Old Etonian for leadership. The ex-Viscount Hailsham, Quentin Hogg, was assigned special responsibility for sport from 1962 to 1964. He was also simultaneously responsible for unemployment in the North East between 1963 and 1964 and for higher education between 1963 and 1964. Hogg had little interest in sports and later wrote that '[t]he idea of a Minister for Sport has always appalled me. It savours of dictatorship and the nastiest kind of populist or Fascist dictatorship at that.' He spent most of his spare time shooting and fishing. To cover his absences, an assistant was appointed. The ex-governor of Honduras, Guyana and Kenya took the role. Admitting that he had no knowledge of sport, he remarked that 'I'll be starting from scratch'.

To these two men fell the government's responsibility of supporting sport during the Big Freeze. It would not be until 1964 that Labour's Harold Wilson appointed Denis Howell as Britain's first minister for sport.

So, we have been here before

COVID-19 was not the first nor will be the last calamity to close sport. Threats from war, weather and microbes will never leave us. Increasing globalisation and ease of international travel means that other pandemics inevitably will visit us.

Since the 1918 Spanish flu, the world has experienced seven further pandemics of which COVID-19 has been the deadliest. Looking back to historical pandemic patterns, coupled with modern virology knowledge, it was fanciful to expect the world could escape COVID-19 with one 'wave' – especially in the initial absence of effective immunisation. Future salvation will be in measures such as improved surveillance, enhanced testing capabilities, rapid isolation, better tracing, sufficient PPE, access to adequate hospital beds and improved pharmacological capabilities.

COVID-19 was a terrifying and deadly experience for many. However, Spanish flu killed many more than the First World War or COVID-19. Sport's responses to previous catastrophes can teach us a lot. In the 20th century, sport was more in tune with national priorities.

In history, sport has proven resourceful and flexible and rolled with the punches. It was prepared to rip up existing fixtures and formats to find acceptable alternatives. Professional cricket and football lost many seasons without income, survived, and came back strongly. In 1914, as in 2020, professional football wanted to go at a different pace to other sports. Twenty-first-century athletes have not been asked to shovel snow, dodge bombs, or parade with oxygen cylinders in support of the NHS. Wars showcased female sport and one-day cricket. Even if these experiments failed initially, the experiences were not forgotten. Previous inclement weather forced footballers to endure periods of intolerable fixture congestion. Despite modern sports medicine and science knowledge, financial imperatives caused the same mistakes in 2020.

Governments and sport must learn both the lessons from history and recent experiences to protect the public and athletes of the future.

Chapter 36

A Game Changer?

THE PANDEMIC supplied sport with its greatest convulsion since the Second World War. The repercussions were probably even greater than 80 years beforehand. By 2020, sport had grown global tentacles, its timetables interlocked, and homage duly paid to sponsors and broadcasting media.

Increasing professionalism led to ever-improving standards on the field of play and burgeoning financial burdens off it. It had spawned numerous supporting industries. Businesses spend fortunes investing in sport to enhance their brands by association. Fans devour sports news, follow individuals' and teams' fortunes, and are encouraged to mimic their heroes by taking up exercise themselves.

Once sport had recovered its voice following the initial lockdown anaesthetic, fears were expressed for the survival of sport in its present form and reflections on how its excesses and sense of entitlement should not be repeated. The Liverpool manager, Jürgen Klopp, tried to reposition football early in the piece by declaring that his sport 'is the most important of the least important things'.

'Lessons need to be learned' was a recurring theme. But were they? Despite best endeavours, once the starter's flag was waved, were good intentions replaced by the need to pursue glory and replenish depleted coffers?

'Suffer little children and forbid them not'
Matthew 19; verse 14. The Bible

Children suffered a double whammy. Education and exercise. The positive effect of sport on learning was blunted. The pandemic gave rocket fuel to the growing obesity crisis. The failure to acquire a love of exercise and sport-specific skills during a vital two years of maturation threatens future participation in exercise at all levels for this generation.

The lessons for schools need to be learned in planning responses to similar future threats.

At grassroots level, the prohibition of most exercise had wide-ranging consequences. It supercharged the industry developing around remote exercise classes and home fitness equipment but did not offset the loss of access to our local gyms and sports clubs. Esports (electronic sports) experienced considerable growth. Health concerns were expressed regarding altered diet, alcohol intake and homeworking. The knowledge gleaned during lockdowns demonstrated that sensible outside exercise did not carry the transmission risks originally feared. By autumn 2020, SAGE admitted that indoor gyms' closures were marginal in combatting the disease.

With the post-pandemic crisis within our health services, our government has majored on illness prevention. Exercise should play a pivotal role. Greater investment in school and grassroots sport should be a central plank in any planning.

Safety-first measures in spring 2020 were understandable. Subsequent wisdom suggests that future decision-making in similar circumstances should be more balanced in recognising the detrimental effects of lockdowns for the majority, while protecting the elderly and infirm.

'Oh Doctor, I'm in trouble!'
Lyrics from 'Goodness Gracious Me' by Peter Sellers and Sophia Loren. 1960

Sports medicine was recognised as a UK clinical speciality only 15 years before the pandemic. COVID-19 would be its biggest test. Senior sports doctors affiliated to clubs and associations were thrust centre stage. Their knowledge, experience and contacts within the wider medical community would be critical in shaping responses. The government convened medical leaders in many major sports to advise on 'return protocols'. Some, like Bill, were co-opted on to club boards to advise its members.

The crisis created a need for accurate but rapid research to underpin global decision-making. Later, more considered work would appear to document the virus's longer-term effects upon athletic bodies and minds. This has added hugely to our knowledge on the risks within sport for the spread of illnesses. It will be important in countering any future such catastrophe.

Keeping body and mind together

Elite sport had to pivot rapidly from performance orientation to welfare considerations. Many organisations were ill-equipped, but most responded positively by providing support for staff, their families, fans and the wider community.

But has the momentum been maintained? A case can be made for a division between individual clubs and the overarching sporting federations. The latter are charged with strategic and financial decision-making to grow 'their brands'. It is the clubs who had to be the protectors of their employees.

Young, fit athletes were not immune from the acute and longer-term effects of the virus whereas acquired immunity, via vaccination, reduced risks without impeding physical performance. Going forward, time should be spent on greater education within sport of these balances.

Coaches and clinicians understood intuitively the response to inadequate preparation time, compressed fixture lists and compromised recovery intervals. Some sports reacted positively while others chose to avert their gaze. Subsequent evidence has reinforced prior predictions. Viral disease, and enforced detraining during isolation, increases injury risk on return. Even the best-prepared athletic machines have their limits.

Many sports' administrators seem reluctant to listen. Athlete burnout had been a topic for many years. Football knows one way of reducing injury. Use mid-season breaks. The Premier League jettisoned it in early 2021. Playing back-to-back games repeatedly will exceed the breaking point for many. In football, various new and expanded international competitions threaten to bring players to their knees. In 2023, rugby union announced a new biennial competition, the Nations Championship. Its only obvious motivation was money. The clear downside was shortening some players' careers. Conrad Smith, the International Rugby Players' Association welfare lead, commented, 'As soon as we don't put players first, don't say player welfare is the priority any longer, say commerciality is. Players are getting tired of it. The players have had enough.'

It will be years before we know how many athletes' careers were shortened by the indecent haste to complete competitions, minimise revenue losses and plan extra future commitments.

However, the pandemic has increased awareness around mental health. Elite athletes have access to various professionals to discuss matters outside of the performance arena – psychologists, doctors, 'trade union' representatives and club chaplains. Since COVID-19, sport has increasingly appreciated the need to invest in welfare as well as the performance sector of its operation with increased co-ordination of this support structure. Organisations are increasingly introducing mental health 'first aid kit' courses to equip all staff to recognise and signpost fellow colleagues for professional support. The crisis accelerated the drive to de-stigmatise declarations of mental health struggles. Many activities embrace sports psychologists to enhance athletic performance. COVID-19 increased the realisation that clinical psychologists were equally important in addressing wider 'life issues' beyond the playing field.

Bio-secure bubbles ensured sporting organisations' health but came at a price for individuals' health. The short tolerance of goldfish bowl existences was predicted in advance. By the end of 2020, bio-bubble ceilings were estimated to be three to four weeks before 'parole' was appropriate in cricket. Rest rotations were instituted. Clinical psychologists were added to support those held behind bio-secure shields. The lessons of intolerance for lengthy separation and the requirement for early professional support should be heeded by all sports for the future.

Sport would benefit from an independent ombudsman to adjudicate in the powerplay between economics and individual athlete well-being.

Stress-testing sports' savings

COVID-19 shook the world's financial markets and economies. In sport, it caused everybody from the volunteer local tennis club treasurer to the finance directors of global sporting organisations to bury their heads in their hands.

The doom and gloom merchants predicted financial meltdown across sport. UK governmental largesse, in terms of furlough provision, grants and loans, staved off initial collapse for most sporting enterprises. However, there would be a sting in the tail for many with a time for reckoning.

Teasing out the exact impact of COVID-19 on sports' economies is not easy. Within the UK, the effect of Brexit, the Ukraine–Russian war, and the energy and cost-of-living crises blew balance sheets off course.

The banana republic-style financial model of many British football clubs is a matter of record. However, all 92 clubs in the Premier and Football League survived – against many forecasts. Similarly, the 18 professional cricket counties, who benefitted from central funding and the ECB's ability to stage international cricket in 2020. It was sports like rugby union and athletics where the financial pain was most apparent in terms of loss of teams, contracting of budgets and redundancies.

COVID-19 certainly delineated between the sporting 'haves, think they haves, and have nots'. The Plimsoll line level appeared lower on the side of the hull of HMS *Sport*. For some, who believed that their heads were above water financially pre-pandemic, it would be difficult to surface again. Expenditure and income loss during the crisis added to the cargo tonnage. Everybody was deeper in the water. Some were beyond the reach of a lifebelt.

Pre-pandemic, over 4.3 million people were employed in the UK sports industry. Sport and physical activity provided £39bn to the economy. If the health and mental well-being argument was not persuasive enough for government and sporting bodies, the central and considerable contribution sport makes to the financial health of the country should be. It is imperative that the necessary checks and balances are in place to ensure that the sector is run within its means and with sufficient headroom to provide some protection against future calamities.

'All change, please!'

Sport had to re-learn flexibility. Elite sport is timetabled years in advance. Olympic and FIFA World Cup hosts are nominated seven years beforehand. Individual sports and the whole sporting edifice have schedules synchronised to avoid clashes and maximise media coverage.

The pandemic demonstrated that plans can be unpicked and repackaged at surprisingly short notice. Major Games had to be moved wholesale and individual fixtures slid. Not ideal. But the crisis proved that sport could function at short notice. Sponsors still wanted to be associated with high-profile events. Television remained hungry to fill its rosters. The sporting spectacle survived not being planned in the minutest detail ages in advance.

The crisis demonstrated that where there is a will there is a way. It was something to put in the 'back pocket' and hang on to for when the next 'rainy day' arrives.

UK versus the world

What were the differences in the way sports handled the pandemic around the world?

English football wanted a 'perfect' Project Restart. As little deviation as possible from the original fixtures, please. Suggestions for limited grounds, neutral venues, player and staff isolation from families were swatted away. The Premier League is used to mostly getting its way. Cricket provided the blueprint for bio-secure bubbles – but required significant understanding and co-operation from visiting teams and its own players.

In America, basketball and ice hockey employed neutral venues with strict hotel lockdowns. Some players were away from home for months. Baseball reverted to restricted locations at the end of its truncated season. Cities and states employed their own rules and regulations. It resulted in a few players being forced out of chunks of seasons due to their anti-vax stance. American sport came down heavily on miscreants. Huge fines and even contract terminations were employed. The Canadian government stood firm on its pandemic principles. Some franchises were forced to locate 'south of the border'. It employed draconian security and penalties for sporting rule-breakers. The censure of wayward individuals and institutions in UK sport was anaemic in comparison.

North American players' representatives had more clout at the 'top table' when formulating COVID-19 countermeasures. It reflected the historical power built during strikes, managing lockouts and collecting bargaining. Our own PFA, PCA and RPA looked like 'innocents abroad' in comparison.

Football looked for a privileged position compared to other sports from early in the pandemic. The government appeared to treat all sports equitably, but politicians realised that sport (i.e., Premier League football) would provide a distraction from the horrors unfolding in our hospitals and parry worries over alcoholism and domestic abuse.

The UK government was proactive in centrally convening experts from across sport, science and medicine. The DCMS established groups like that tasked with returning elite sport safely, the Entertainment and Events and Broadcasting groups, and the Science Board for the ERP. They were all pivotal in helping sport recover.

European decision-making varied. French, Dutch and Belgian football shut up shop for the summer of 2020. Their governments were firm on saying *'Non'* or *'Nee'*. French regulations affected all three cycling grand tours' timings and itineraries. In contrast, football in the four richest European leagues resumed – Germany, Italy, Spain and England. Once the Bundesliga had kicked off, wild horses would not have stopped the Premier League's insistence on returning despite the more precarious British general situation at the time.

Further afield, the fortress constructed around Australian and New Zealand borders had a major impact on Antipodean sport. Athletes were afforded privileges not granted to thousands of residents stranded abroad but none could escape the strict quarantine regulations that extended much longer than in the UK.

Society and sport

What did the pandemic teach us about our relationship with sport and vice versa?

The multiple anxieties created within society by COVID-19 frequently coloured people's opinions about elite sport. There were strong feelings that fairness and priorities should reign. Especially when PPE and testing kits were scarce and hospital saturation points were uppermost in our thoughts. Many societies were polarised when it came to elite sport. Witness the strong support in Japan for abandoning the Olympics.

There seemed to be three notable pinch points during the crisis. The first comes when the media reported multiple acts of lockdown-breaking by athletes in spring 2020. Probably no more than others of their generation but it threatened public health messaging and smothering news of the multiple acts of kindness performed by sportsmen and women to others.

Secondly, when the nation was plunged into further misery and even greater death tolls over Christmas and New Year 2020–21. Patience for parties, trips abroad and the flouting of guidelines that allowed sport to continue reached a nadir.

Finally came late 2021. Restrictions remained and new variants were on the rise. Sports people's low vaccination rates could influence others. Requests to crisscross the world while softening quarantine requirements on return added insult to injury for the suffering general populace.

Despite vast amounts spent on PR, elite sport did not always cover itself in glory. It proved itself ill-equipped at times to 'read the room'.

For years pre-COVID-19, there had been a view that some elite sports' huge wealth was threatening to dislocate it from its core support. The costs of following 'your team' soared. Despite this, many within society take succour from strongly identifying with their clubs. Its abrupt attenuation added to the sense of disorientation from normal life as the virus struck.

It was loss of TV revenues that drove on the Premier League, international cricket and the IOC. However, the sterile atmospheres created by behind-closed-doors games were clear on our television screens. A major sporting contest is an 'event' to which attending fans contribute hugely to the common experience.

Sport realised the need to reach out to its core support. Burgeoning social media outlets proved invaluable. It was appreciated that televised sport could have positive well-being effects upon its fans. Sport upped its game in terms of improved presentation of its product. It came in the form of novel technologies and wider platforms to access. County cricket provided digital coverage of all games. Increasingly, sophisticated analysis and opinion combined with state-of-the-art, no-angle-excluded viewing of the action were all designed to improve spectator engagement.

'No man is an island'

17th-century poet John Donne

History has taught us that further crises will affect mankind and, by implication, sport. What legacy will COVID-19 leave? What lessons will future generations take from this dark chapter?

Sport survived and proved its resilience. Its contribution to our country's culture and wealth could not be denied. Accordingly, elite sport was granted special privileges because of its position within society. At times, it struggled to acknowledge the fact. Commentators hoped that the pandemic would teach elite sport greater social responsibility. Many sports and individuals within it rose to the challenge. Others failed miserably. Greater emphasis had to be placed on health and safety although some cynics would argue it was driven on only by financial necessity. Reappearing blinking in the sunlight at the other side, elite sport has jettisoned many of its ethical and welfare reflections in the quest to replenish its coffers. However, the way sport engages with its core support may have changed irrevocably.

Inevitably, it was those at the other end of sport's ecosystem who suffered most. Children and grassroots sport. Female and disabled sport. Lacking power and financial clout, these groups seemed at times to be regarded as 'having less skin in the game'. However, the health fallout may cascade down the decades. Exercise is one of the most important elements in maintaining fit bodies and minds. Improving access and quality of facilities to all should have been one of the central lessons from the pandemic.

COVID-19 taught us that within society no man is an island. Everything, and everybody, is interconnected and co-dependent. Elite sport and its participants walked on a very narrow tightrope at times. Some tottered and fell, most clung on, and a few walked tall.

Acknowledgements

MUCH HAS been written about the COVID-19 pandemic. More will appear in time to come. Rightly so. This health crisis has been the worst shared global disaster of our generation. This book should be dedicated to two groups. Firstly, health clinicians and scientists who have worked tirelessly to tend the sick and find solutions to protecting us all. Secondly, the victims and their families who suffered and succumbed at the hands of this virus.

The authors are two individuals whose friendship has been anchored by our mutual love and work within sport. Mark from a journalist's perspective, and Bill from a surgeon's viewpoint. Both witnessed first-hand the effect on sport of the pandemic and we have blended our experiences and opinions to produce this book.

We are indebted to the many people within sport and medicine who have been generous with their time and knowledge in providing insights into the management of this pandemic for the benefit of athletes. Often their contributions are hidden from sight but remain vital in allowing us to participate or follow sport in all its many wondrous guises.

The research for this book is a fusion of the contributions of our colleagues from within the media and experts from the scientific literature. Their unstinting hard work to observe, report and analyse has been inspiring and crucial to the delivery of this book.

All book projects need advocates. Jane Camillin and all the team at Pitch Publishing provided that support for the authors and the subject matter. Their professionalism combined with the skills of our editor, Andrea Dunn, proofreader Dean Rockett and creative colleagues Duncan Olner and Graham Hales enhanced the quality of the final product.

Finally, we must acknowledge our families for their encouragement, patience and enthusiasm throughout a three-year-long project. To Siân and Jane. Thank you.

Index

Index